Do you know that the Sanford Guide is available in two larger sized print editions and electronic editions for hand-held devices?

This pocket-sized edition (4 x 6 in) is handy to keep in your labcoat, but if the print is becoming a challenge, consider the bigger books:

Spiral-bound edition (5 x 8 in) and Desk/Library edition (7.250 x 11 in)

The spiral book still fits in a pocket and the desk book is great eye relief!

The electronic edition is available for Windows Mobile® devices, Palm® devices and for Blackberry®

For more information, go to www.sanfordguide.com

S0-DSN-432

SANFORD GUIDE®

Thirty-Seventh Edition

THE SANFORD GUIDE TO ANTIMICROBIAL THERAPY 2007

David N. Gilbert, M.D.
Chief of Infectious Diseases
Director, Earl A. Chiles Research Institute
Providence Portland Medical Center
Professor of Medicine
Oregon Health Sciences University
Portland, Oregon

Robert C. Moellering, Jr., M.D.
Shields Warren-Mallinckrodt Professor of Medical Research
Harvard Medical School
Boston, Massachusetts

George M. Eliopoulos, M.D.
Chief, James L. Tullis Firm, Beth Israel Deaconess Hospital
Professor of Medicine
Harvard Medical School
Boston, Massachusetts

Merle A. Sande, M.D.
Professor of Medicine
University of Washington School of Medicine
Seattle, Washington

THE SANFORD GUIDE TO ANTIMICROBIAL THERAPY 2007
37TH EDITION

Jay P. Sanford, M.D.
1928–1996

Editors

David N. Gilbert, M.D.
George M. Eliopoulos, M.D.

Robert C. Moellering, Jr., M.D.
Merle A. Sande, M.D.

The Sanford Guides are published annually by

ANTIMICROBIAL THERAPY, INC.
P.O. Box 276, 11771 Lee Hwy, Sperryville, VA 22740-0276 USA
Tel 540-987-9480   Fax 540-987-9486
Email: info@sanfordguide.com   www.sanfordguide.com

Printed in the United States of America
ISBN 978-1-930808-38-6
Pocket Edition (English)

PUBLISHER'S PREFACE

This edition marks the 37th revision of the SANFORD GUIDE TO ANTIMICROBIAL THERAPY. The manuscript has been significantly redesigned to improve the readability of the pocket-sized edition. For those who remain challenged by the small sized book, two larger editions are available as well as electronic editions for PDAs and smartphones. Our thanks to Lingua Solutions, Inc., for its redesign of the manuscript and to Gerette Braunsdorf for assistance in updating the manuscript for this edition.

Though many readers of the SANFORD GUIDE receive their copy from a pharmaceutical company representative, please be assured that the SANFORD GUIDE has been, and continues to be, independently prepared and published since its inception in 1969. Decisions regarding the content of the SANFORD GUIDE are solely those of the editors and the publisher. We welcome your questions, comments and feedback concerning the SANFORD GUIDE. All of your feedback is reviewed and taken into account in preparing the next edition.

NOTE TO READER

Every effort is made to ensure the accuracy of the content of this guide. However, current full prescribing information available in the package insert of each drug should be consulted before prescribing any product. The editors and publisher are not responsible for errors or omissions or for any consequences from application of the information in this book and make no warranty, express or implied, with respect to the currency, accuracy, or completeness of the contents of the publication. Application of this information in a particular situation remains the professional responsibility of the practitioner.

—TABLE OF CONTENTS—

2

SUMMARY OF ABBREVIATIONS

DRUG NAME ABBREVIATIONS

Antibacterial & Antimycobacterial Drugs

AG = aminoglycoside
AMK = amikacin
AM-CL = amoxicillin-clavulanate
AM-CL-ER = amoxicillin-clavulanate extended release
Amox = amoxicillin
AMP = ampicillin
AM-SB = ampicillin-sulbactam
AP Pen = antipseudomonal penicillins
APAG = antipseudomonal aminoglycoside (tobra, gent, amikacin)
Azithro = azithromycin
BL/BLI = beta-lactam/beta-lactamase inhibitor
CARB = carbapenems (ERTA, IMP, MER)
Cefpodox = cefpodoxime proxetil
Ceftaz = ceftazidime
CFP = cefepime
Chloro = chloramphenicol
CIP = ciprofloxacin; CIP-ER = CIP extended release
Clarithro = clarithromycin; ER = extended release
Clav = clavulanate
Clinda = clindamycin
Clot = clotrimazole
Dalba = dalbavancin
Dapto = daptomycin
Dirithro = dirithromycin
Doxy = doxycycline
EES = erythromycin ethyl succinate
ERTA = ertapenem
Erythro = erythromycin
ETB = ethambutol
FQ = fluoroquinolone (CIP, Oflox, Lome, Peflox, Levo, Gati, Moxi, Gemi)
Gati = gatifloxacin
Gemi = gemifloxacin
Gent = gentamicin
GNB = gram-negative bacilli
IMP = imipenem-cilastatin
INH = isoniazid
IVIG = intravenous immune globulin
Levo = levofloxacin
Lome = lomefloxacin
Macrolides = azithro, clarithro, dirithro, erythro, roxithro
MER = meropenem
Metro = metronidazole
Mino = minocycline
Moxi = moxifloxacin
NF = nitrofurantoin
O Ceph 1,2,3 = oral cephalosporins—see Table 10B
Oflox = ofloxacin

P Ceph 1,2,3,4 = parenteral cephalosporins—see Table 10B
P Ceph 3 AP = parenteral cephalosporins with antipseudomonal activity—see Table 10B
Peflox = pefloxacin
PIP-TZ = piperacillin-tazobactam
PZA = pyrazinamide
Quinu-dalfo = Q-D = quinupristin-dalfopristin
RFB = rifabutin
RFP = rifampin
RIF = rifampin
Roxi = roxithromycin
SM = streptomycin
Sub = sulbactam
Tazo = tazobactam
TC-CL = ticarcillin-clavulanate
Teico = teicoplanin
Telithro = telithromycin
Tetra = tetracycline
Ticar = ticarcillin
TMP-SMX = trimethoprim-sulfamethoxazole
Tobra = tobramycin
Vanco = vancomycin

Antifungal Drugs

Ampho B = amphotericin B
ABCC = ampho B cholesteryl complex
ABLC = ampho B lipid complex
LAB = liposomal ampho B
Clot = clotrimazole
Flu = fluconazole
Flucyt = flucytosine
Griseo = griseofulvin
Itra = itraconazole
Keto = ketoconazole
Vori = voriconazole

Antiparasitic Drugs

Atov = atovaquone
At/Pro = atovaquone/proguanil
CQ = chloroquine phosphate
MQ = mefloquine

PQ = primaquine
Pyri = pyrimethamine
QS = quinine sulfate

Antivirals; Anti-HIV Drugs

3TC = lamivudine
d4T = stavudine
ddC = zalcitabine
ddl = didanosine
FTC = emtricitabine
TDF = tenofovir
DLV = delavirdine
ADF = adefovir

ZDV = zidovudine
EFZ = efavirenz
NVP = nevirapine
ATV = atazanavir
FOS-APV = fos-amprenavir
IDV = indinavir
IFN = interferon

LP/R = lopinavir/ritonavir
NFR = nelfinavir
RTV = ritonavir
SQV = saquinavir
TPV = Tipranavir
ENT = entecavir

DRUG DOSAGE DRUG ADMINISTRATION

mcg = microgram
mg = milligram
gm = gram
DS = double strength

AD = after dialysis
div = divided
IP = intraperitoneal
IT = intrathecal

---

bid = twice a day
tid = 3 times a day
qid = 4 times a day
BW = body weight
DOT = directly observed therapy

po = per os (by mouth)
subcut = subcutaneous
dc = discontinue
rx = treatment

DRUG-RELATED

G = generic
I = investigational
IA = injectable agent
NB = name brand
NFDA-I = not FDA-approved indication
NUS = not available in the U.S.

ASA = aspirin
NSAIDs = non-steroidal anti-inflammatory drugs

DISEASE-ASSOCIATED

ARDS = acute respiratory distress syndrome
ARF = acute rheumatic fever
CAPD = continuous ambulatory peritoneal dialysis
CAVH = continuous arteriovenous hemodialysis
CSD = cat-scratch disease
DIC = disseminated intravascular coagulation
ESRD = endstage renal disease
HEMO = hemodialysis
PEP = post-exposure prophylaxis
PTLD = post-transplant lymphoproliferative disease
RTI = respiratory tract infection
STD = sexually transmitted disease
TBc = tuberculosis
UTI = urinary tract infection

ORGANISMS

CMV = cytomegalovirus
DGI = disseminated gonococcal infection
DRSP = drug-resistant S. pneumoniae
EBV = Epstein-Barr virus
GC = gonorrhea
HHV = human herpesvirus
HSV = herpes simplex virus
LCM = lymphocytic choriomeningitis virus
M. Tbc = Mycobacterium tuberculosis
MSSA/MRSA = methicillin-sensitive/resistant S. aureus
Rick = Rickettsia
RSV = respiratory syncytial virus
VISA = vancomycin intermediately resistant S. aureus
VZV = varicella-zoster virus

B. frag group = B. fragilis, B. distasonis, B. ovatus, B. thetaiotaomicron

ABBREVIATIONS (2)

MISCELLANEOUS

Diagnosis
C&S = culture & sensitivity
CXR = chest x-ray
ESBLs = extended spectrum β-lactamases
ESR = erythrocyte sedimentation rate
HLR = high-level resistance
LCR = ligase chain reaction
PCR = polymerase chain reaction
TEE = transesophageal echocardiography
VL = viral load

Organizations
ATS = American Thoracic Society
CDC = Centers for Disease Control
ICAAC = International Conference on Antimicrobial Agents & Chemotherapy
IDSA = Infectious Diseases Society of America
WHO = World Health Organization

Other
AUC = area under the curve
DBPCT = double-blind placebo-controlled trial
EDC = expected date of confinement
PRCT = Prospective randomized controlled trials
Pts = patients
S = resistant
S = potential synergy in combination with penicillin, AMP, vanco, telco

Sens = sensitive (susceptible)
VR = very rare

ABBREVIATIONS OF JOURNAL TITLES

AAC: Antimicrobial Agents & Chemotherapy
Adv PID: Advances in Pediatric Infectious Diseases
AIDS Res Hum Retrovir: AIDS Research & Human Retroviruses
AJM: American Journal of Medicine
AJRCCM: American Journal of Respiratory Critical Care Medicine
AJTMH: American Journal of Tropical Medicine & Hygiene
Aliment Pharmacol Ther: Experimental Pharmacology & Therapeutics
Am J Hlth Pharm: American Journal of Health-System Pharmacy
AnEM: Annals of Emergency Medicine
AnIM: Annals of Internal Medicine
AnPharmacother: Annals of Pharmacotherapy
AnSurg: Annals of Surgery
ArDerm: Archives of Dermatology
Antivir Ther: Antiviral Therapy
ARIM: Archives of Internal Medicine
ARRD: American Review of Respiratory Disease
BMJ: British Medical Journal
Brit J Derm: British Journal of Dermatology
Can JID: Canadian Journal of Infectious Diseases
CCM: Critical Care Medicine
CCTID: Current Clinical Topics in Infectious Disease
Clin Infect Dis: Clinical Infectious Diseases
Clin Micro & Infect: Clinical Microbiology and Infection
Clin Micro Rev: Clinical Microbiology Reviews
COID: Current Opinion in Infectious Disease
Curr Med Res Opin: Current Medical Research and Opinion
Derm Ther: Dermatologic Therapy

Dig Dis Sci: Digestive Diseases and Sciences
DMID: Diagnostic Microbiology and Infectious Disease
EID: Emerging Infectious Diseases
EJCMID: European Journal of Clin. Micro & Infectious Diseases
Eur J Neurol: European Journal of Neurology
Exp Mol Path: Experimental & Molecular Pathology
Gastro: Gastroenterology
Hpt: Hepatology
ICHE: Infection Control and Hospital Epidemiology
IDC No. Amer: Infectious Disease Clinics of North America
IDCP: Infectious Diseases in Clinical Practice
IJAA: International Journal of Antimicrobial Agents
Inf Med: Infections in Medicine
JAIDS: JAIDS Journal of Acquired Immune Deficiency Syndromes
J AIDS & HR: Journal of AIDS and Human Retrovirology
J All Clin Immun: Journal of Allergy and Clinical Immunology
J Am Ger Soc: Journal of the American Geriatrics Society
J Chemother: Journal of Chemotherapy
JCI: Journal of Clinical Investigation
J Clin Micro: Journal of Clinical Microbiology
J Clin Virol: Journal of Clinical Virology
J Derm Treat: Journal of Dermatological Treatment
J Hpt: Journal of Hepatology
J Inf: Journal of Infection
J Med Micro: Journal of Medical Microbiology
J Micro Immunol Inf: Journal of Microbiology, Immunology, & Infection
J Ped: Journal of Pediatrics

JAC: Journal of Antimicrobial Chemotherapy
JAMA: Journal of the American Medical Association
JAVMA: Journal of the Veterinary Medicine Association
JID: Journal of Infectious Diseases
JNS: Journal of Neurosurgery
JTMH: Journal of Tropical Medicine and Hygiene
J Viral Hep: Journal of Viral Hepatitis
Ln: Lancet
LnID: Lancet Infectious Disease
Mayo Clin Proc: Mayo Clinic Proceedings
Med Lett: Medical Letter
Med Mycol: Medical Mycology
MMWR: Morbidity & Mortality Weekly Report
NEJM: New England Journal of Medicine
Neph Dial Transpl: Nephrology, Dialysis Transplantation
Ped Ann: Pediatric Annals
Peds: Pediatrics
Pharmacother: Pharmacotherapy
PIDJ: Pediatric Infectious Disease Journal
QJM: Quarterly Journal of Medicine
Scand J Inf Dis: Scandinavian Journal of Infectious Diseases
Sem Resp Inf: Seminars in Respiratory Infections
SMJ: Southern Medical Journal
Surg Neurol: Surgical Neurology
Transpl: Transplantation
Transpl Inf Dis: Transplant Infectious Diseases
TRSM: Transactions of the Royal Society of Medicine
West J Med: Western Journal of Medicine

TABLE 1 – CLINICAL APPROACH TO INITIAL CHOICE OF ANTIMICROBIAL THERAPY*

Treatment based on presumed site or type of infection. In selected instances, treatment and prophylaxis based on identification of pathogens (Abbreviations on page 2)

ANATOMIC SITE/DIAGNOSIS/ MODIFYING CIRCUMSTANCES	ETIOLOGIES (usual)	SUGGESTED REGIMENS*		ADJUNCT DIAGNOSTIC OR THERAPEUTIC MEASURES AND COMMENTS
		PRIMARY	ALTERNATIVE†	
ABDOMEN: See PERITONEUM, page 42, Gallbladder, page 15, and Pelvic Inflammatory Disease, page 22				
BONE: Osteomyelitis. Microbiologic diagnosis is essential. If blood culture negative, need culture of bone. Culture of sinus tract drainage not predictive of bone culture. Review: Ln 364:369, 2004				
Hematogenous Osteomyelitis				
Empiric therapy—Collect bone and blood cultures before empiric therapy				
Newborn (<4 mos.) See Table 16 for dose	S. aureus, Gm-neg. bacilli, Group B strep	**MRSA possible: (Nafcillin or oxacillin) + P Ceph 3**	**MRSA unlikely: (Nafcillin or oxacillin) + P Ceph 3**	Table 16 for dose. Severe allergy or toxicity (**Linezolid**[HMA+]10mg/kg IV/po q8h + **aztreonam**). Could substitute **clindamycin** for nafcillin
Children (>4 mos.)—Adult: Osteo of extremity	S. aureus, Group A strep, Gm-neg. bacilli rare	**MRSA possible: Vanco** Add:**P Ceph 3** if Gm-neg. bacilli on Gram stain. Doses: Table 16	**MRSA unlikely: Nafcillin or oxacillin**	Severe allergy or toxicity: **Clinda** or **TMP-SMX** or **linezolid**[HMA]. Dosages in Table 16. See Table 16 for adverse reactions to drugs.
Adult (>21 yrs) **Vertebral osteo ± epidural abscess,** other sites (NEJM 355:2012, 2006)	S. aureus most common but variety other organisms. **Blood & bone cultures essential.**	**MRSA possible: Vanco 1 gm IV q12h**	**MRSA unlikely: Nafcillin or oxacillin 2gm IV q4h**	**Dx: MRI early to look for epidural abscess.** Allergy or toxicity: **TMP-SMX** 8-10mg/kg/d div q8h or **linezolid** 600mg IV/po q12h (AJM 138:135, 2003)[HMA]. See MRSA specific therapy comment. Epidural abscess ref.: JVIM 164:2409, 2004.
Specific therapy—Culture and in vitro susceptibility results known				
MSSA		**Nafcillin or oxacillin** 2gm IV q4h or **cefazolin** 2gm IV q8h	**Vanco** 1gm q12h IV	**Other options if susceptible in vitro and allergy/toxicity issues:** 1) **TMP-SMX** 8-10mg/kg/d IV div q8h – Minimal data on treatment of osteomyelitis. 2) **Clinda** 600-900mg IV q8h – have lab check for inducible resistance esp if erythro. Resistant (CID 40:280,2005). 3) **Clp** 750mg po bid or **levo** 750mg po q24h) + **rif** 300mg po q8h or bid 4) **Daptomycin** 6mg/kg IV q24h – based on eval of pts in bacteremia trial (ISDA Abst. 2006) clinical failure secondary to resistance reported (J Clin Micro 44:595, 2006). 5) **Linezolid** 600mg po/IV bid – anecdotal reports of efficacy (J Chemother 17:643,2005), optic & peripheral neuropathy with long-term use (Neurology 64:926, 2005). 6) **Fusidic acid**[NUS] 500mg IV q8h + **rif** 300mg po bid (CID 42:394, 2006)
MRSA—See Table 6, page 73		**Vanco** 1 gm IV q12h	**Linezolid** 600mg q12h IV/po ±**RIF** 300mg po/IV bid	
Contiguous Osteomyelitis Without Vascular Insufficiency				
Empiric therapy: Get cultures!				
Foot bone osteo due to nail through tennis shoe	P. aeruginosa	**CIP** 750mg po bid or **Levo** 750mg IV q12h	**Ceftaz** 2gm IV q8h or **CFP** 2gm IV q12h	See Skin—Nail puncture, page 50. Need debridement to remove foreign body.
Long bone, post-internal fixation of fracture	S. aureus, Gm-neg. bacilli, P. aeruginosa	**Vanco** 1gm IV q12h + (**ceftaz** or **CFP** [see footnote†]). See Comment	**Linezolid** 600mg IV/po bid[NUS] + (**ceftaz** or **CFP**). See Comment	Often necessitates removal hardware to allow bone union. May need revascularization. Regimens listed are empiric. Adjust after culture data available: If susceptible Gm(+), can use **Levo** 750mg po bid or **CIP** 750mg po bid. Gm(-) bacilli: **CIP** 750mg po bid or **Levo** 1 gm IV q12h. For other S. aureus options: See Hem. Osteo. Specific Therapy, Table 1(1).
Hemoglobinopathy: Sickle cell/thalassemia	Salmonella, other Gm-neg. bacilli	**CIP** 400mg IV q12h	**Levo** 750mg IV q24h	Thalassemia: transfusion and iron chelation risk factors.

* **DOSAGES SUGGESTED** are for adults (unless otherwise indicated) with clinically severe (often life-threatening infections, and not severe hepatic dysfunction. † **ALTERNATIVE THERAPY INCLUDES** these considerations: **allergy, pharmacology/pharmacokinetics, compliance, costs, local resistance profiles.** Dosages also assume **normal renal function, and not severe hepatic dysfunction.**

† Drug dosage: **ceftazidime** 2 gm IV q8h; **CFP** 2 gm IV q12h; **metro** 1 gm IV q12h; **vanco** 1 gm loading dose and then 0.5 gm IV/po q8h or 1 gm IV q12h; **aztreonam** 2 gm IV q8h; **vanco** 1 gm IV q12h

TABLE 1 (2)

ANATOMIC SITE/DIAGNOSIS/ MODIFYING CIRCUMSTANCES	ETIOLOGIES (usual)	SUGGESTED REGIMENS*		ADJUNCT DIAGNOSTIC OR THERAPEUTIC MEASURES AND COMMENTS
		PRIMARY	ALTERNATIVE†	
BONE/Contiguous Osteomyelitis Without Vascular Insufficiency/Empiric therapy (continued)				
Prosthetic joint	See prosthetic joint, page 29			
Sternum, post-op	S. aureus, S. epidermidis	**Vanco** 1gm IV q12h	**Linezolid** 600mg po/IV[MRSA] bid	Sternal debridement for cultures & removal of necrotic bone. For S. aureus options: Hem/Osteo, Specific Therapy, Table 1(1).
Contiguous Osteomyelitis With Vascular Insufficiency				
Most pts are **diabetics** with peripheral neuropathy & infected skin ulcers (see *Diabetic foot, page 14*)	Polymicrobic: (Gm+ cocci (to include MRSA) (aerobic & anaerobic) and Gm-rods/bacilli (aerobic & anaerobic))	Debride overlying ulcer & submit bone for histology & culture. Select antibiotic on culture results & treat for 6 weeks. **No empiric therapy unless acutely ill.** If acutely ill, see suggestions, Diabetic foot, page 14. Revascularize if possible. Full contact cast.		**Diagnosis of osteo:** Culture of biopsied bone gold standard. Marrow edema on MRI best imaging. Probe to bone has high predictive value. Poor concordance of culture results between swab of ulcer and bone -- need bone. (CID 25:1257, 63:2006). **Treatment:** (1) Revascularize if possible. (2) Culture bone. (3) Specific antimicrobial(s). (4) Full contact cast.
Chronic Osteomyelitis: Specific therapy By definition, implies presence of dead bone. **Need valid cultures**	S. aureus, Enterobacteria-ceae, P. aeruginosa	**Empiric rx not indicated.** Base systemic rx on results of culture, sensitivity testing. If acute exacerbation of chronic osteo, rx as acute hematogenous osteo		Important adjuncts: removal of orthopedic hardware, surgical debridement, vascularized muscle flaps, distraction osteogenesis (Ilizarov) techniques. Antibiotic-impregnated cement & hyperbaric oxygen adjunctive. **NOTE: RIF + (vanco or β-lactam)** effective in animal model and in a clinical trial of S. aureus chronic osteo (SMJ 79:947, 1986).
BREAST: Mastitis—Obtain culture; need to know if MRSA present. Review with definitions. Ob.& Gyn Clin No Amer 29:89, 2002				
Postpartum mastitis				
Mastitis without abscess Ref. JAMA 289:1609, 2003	S. aureus; less often (S. pyogenes (Gp A or B), E. coli, bacteroides species, maybe Corynebacterium sp. & selected coagulase-neg staphylococci (e.g. .S lugdunensis)	**NO MRSA: Outpatient: Dicloxacil-lin** 500mg po qid or **cephalexin** 500mg po qid **Inpatient: Nafcillin/oxa-cillin** 2gm IV q4h	**MRSA Possible: Outpatient:** TMP-SMX-DS po bid **Inpatient: Vanco** 1gm IV q12h	If no abscess, ↑ freq. of nursing may hasten response; no risk to infant. Coryne-bacterium sp. assoc. with chronic granulomatous mastitis (CID 35:1434, 2002). Bartonella henselae infection reported (Ob.& Gyn 85:1027, 2000). With abscesses, d/c nursing, I&D standard; needle aspiration reported successful (Am J Surg 182:117, 2001). Resume breast feeding from affected breast as soon as pain allows.
Mastitis with abscess				
Non-puerperal mastitis with abscess	S. aureus; less often Bacter-oides sp., peptostreptococ-cus, & selected coagulase-neg. staphylococci			If subareolar & odoriferous, most likely anaerobes; need to **add metro** 500 mg IV/po tid. If not subareolar, staph. Need pretreatment aerobic/anaerobic cultures. Surgical drainage for abscess
Breast implant infection	Acute: S., pyogenes ,S TSS reported Chronic: Look for rapidly growing Mycobacteria	Acute: **Vanco** 1gm IV q12h pending culture results	Chronic: Await culture results. See Table 12 for mycobacteria treatment	Lancet Infect Dis 5:94, 462, 2005

NOTE: All dosage recommendations are for adults (unless otherwise indicated) and assume normal renal function.

TABLE 1 (3)

ANATOMIC SITE/DIAGNOSIS/ MODIFYING CIRCUMSTANCES	ETIOLOGIES (usual)	SUGGESTED REGIMENS*		ADJUNCT DIAGNOSTIC OR THERAPEUTIC MEASURES AND COMMENTS
		PRIMARY	ALTERNATIVE‡	
CENTRAL NERVOUS SYSTEM				
Brain abscess				
Primary or contiguous source Ref.: CID 25:763, 1997	Streptococci (60–70%), bacteroides (20–40%), Enterobacteriaceae (25–33%), S. aureus (10–15%). Rare: Nocardia (Table 11A, page 100) Listeria (CID 40:907, 2005)	P Ceph 3 (cefotaxime 2gm IV q4h or ceftriaxone 2gm IV q12h) + metro 7.5mg/kg q6h or 15mg/kg IV q12h	Pen G 3–4 million units IV q4h + metro 7.5mg/kg q6h or 15mg/kg IV q12h	If CT scan suggests cerebritis (JNS 59:972, 1983), abscesses <2.5 cm and pt neurologically stable and conscious, start antibiotics and observe. Otherwise, surgical drainage necessary. Neurologic deterioration usually mandates surgery. Experience with Pen G (HD) + metro without P Ceph 3 or nafcillin/oxacillin has been good. We use P Ceph 3 because of frequency of isolation of Enterobacteriaceae. **S. aureus rare without positive blood culture; if S. aureus, include vanco until susceptibility known.** Strep. milleri group esp. prone to produce abscess.
		Duration rx unclear; rx until response by neuroimaging (CT/MRI)		
Post-surgical, post-traumatic	S. aureus, Enterobacteriaceae	(Nafcillin or oxacillin) 2gm IV q4h + P Ceph 3	Vanco 1gm IV q12h + P Ceph 3	**If MRSA a consideration, substitute vanco for nafcillin or oxacillin.** P Ceph 3 dose as for brain abscess, primary.
HIV-1 infected (AIDS)	Toxoplasma gondii	See Table 13A, page 126		
Subdural empyema: In adult 60–90% are extension of sinusitis or otitis media. Rx same as primary brain abscess. Surgical emergency; must drain (CID 20:372, 1995).				
Encephalitis/encephalopathy Ref.: Ln 359:507, 2002 (See Table 14A, page 139, and for rabies, Table 20, page 182)	Herpes simplex, arboviruses, rabies, West Nile virus. Rarely: listeria, cat-scratch disease	Start IV acyclovir while awaiting results of CSF PCR for H. simplex.		Newly recognized strain of bat rabies. May not require a break in the skin. Eastern equine encephalitis causes focal MRI changes in basal ganglia and thalamus (NEJM 336:1867, 1997). Cat-scratch ref.: PIDJ 23:1161, 2004). Ref. on West Nile & related viruses: NEJM 351:370, 2004.
Meningitis, "Aseptic": Pleocytosis of 100s of cells, CSF glucose normal, neg. culture for bacteria (see Table 14A, page 134)	Enteroviruses, HSV-2, LCM, HIV, other viruses, drugs (NSAIDs, metronidazole, carbamazepine, TMP-SMX, IVIG), rarely leptospirosis	For all but leptospirosis, IV fluids and analgesics. D/C drugs that may be etiologic. For lepto (doxy 100mg IV/po q12h) or (Pen G 5 million units IV q6h or (AMP 0.5–1gm IV q6h). Repeat LP if suspect partially-treated bacterial meningitis.		If available, PCR of CSF for enterovirus. HSV-2 unusual without concomitant genital lesion. Drug-induced aseptic meningitis: AnIM 159:1185, 1999. For lepto, positive epidemiologic history and concomitant hepatitis, conjunctivitis, dermatitis, nephritis.
Meningitis, Bacterial, Acute: Goal is empiric therapy, then specific therapy. Do CSF exam within 30min. If focal neurologic deficit, give empiric rx, then head CT, then LP. (CID 39:1267,2004; NEJM 354:44,2006) NOTE: In children, treatment caused CSF cultures to turn neg. in 2 hrs with meningococci & partial response with pneumococci in 4 hrs (Peds 108:1169, 2001)				
Empiric Therapy—CSF Gram stain is negative—Immunocompetent				
Age: Preterm to <1 mo Ln 361:2139, 2003	Group B strep 49%, E. coli 18%, listeria 7%, misc. Gm-neg. 10%, misc. Gm-pos. 10%.	AMP + cefotaxime Intraventricular rx not recommended. Repeat CSF exam/culture 24–36hr after start of rx For dosage, see Table 16	AMP + gentamicin	Primary & alternative reg active vs Group B strep, most coliforms, & listeria. If premature infant with long nursery stay, S. aureus, enterococci, and resistant coliforms potential pathogens. Optional empiric regimens: [nafcillin + (cefotaxime or cefotaxime)]. If high risk of MRSA, use vanco + cefotaxime. Alter regimen after culture/sensitivity data available.

NOTE: All dosage recommendations are for adults (unless otherwise indicated) and assume normal renal function.

TABLE 1 (1)

ANATOMIC SITE/DIAGNOSIS/ MODIFYING CIRCUMSTANCES	ETIOLOGIES (usual)	SUGGESTED REGIMENS* PRIMARY	ALTERNATIVE[1]	ADJUNCT DIAGNOSTIC OR THERAPEUTIC MEASURES AND COMMENTS
CENTRAL NERVOUS SYSTEM/Meningitis, Bacterial, Acute/Empiric Therapy *(continued)*				
Age: 1mo.–50yrs See footnote[1] for empiric treatment rationale	S. pneumo, meningococci, H. influenzae now very rare, **listeria unlikely if young & immuno-competent** (add ampicillin if suspect listeria 2gm IV q4h)	Adult dosage: ((**Cefotax-ime** 2gm IV q4–6h **OR ceftriaxone** 2gm IV q12h) + (**dexametha-sone**) + **vanco** (see footnote)[3] Peds: see footnote[3] **Dexamethasone**[4] 0.15mg/kg IV q6h x 2–4 days. **Give with or just before 1st dose of antibiotic (see Comment).** See footnote[4] for ped. dosage	((MER 2gm IV q8h) (Peds: 40mg/kg IV q8h)] + IV **dexamethasone + vanco** (see footnote)[3] Peds: see footnote[3]	For pts with severe pen. allergy: Chloro 12.5mg/kg IV q6h (max. 4gm/day) (for meningococcal) + **TMP-SMX** 5mg/kg q6-8h for listeria (if immunocom-promised) + **vanco**. Rare meningococcal isolates chloro-resistant (NEJM 339:868, 1998). The standard alternative for pts with severe pen. allergy was chloro. However, high failure rate in pts with DRSP (JID 39:405, 1992; Ln 339:405, 1992). **So far, no vanco-resistant S. pneumo.** Value of dexamethasone documented in children with H. influenzae & now confirmed in adults with S. pneumo & N. meningitidis (NEJM 347:1549 & 1613, 2002; LnID 4:139, 2004). **Give 1st dose 15–20min. prior to or con-comitant with 1st dose of antibiotic. Dose: 0.15mg/kg IV q6h x 2–4 days. For meningococcal immunization, see Table 20B, page 178.**
Age: >50yrs or alcoholism or other **debilitating assoc diseases** or **impaired cellular immunity**	S. pneumo, listeria, Gm-neg. bacilli. Note absence of meningo-coccus	**AMP** 2gm IV q4h) + (**ceftriaxone** 2gm IV q12h or **cefotaxime** 2gm IV q6h) + **vanco** + IV **dexamethasone** For vanco dose, see footnote[3] **Dexamethasone** 0.15mg/kg IV q6h x 2–4 days, 1st dose before or concomitant with 1st dose of antibiotic.	MER 2gm IV q8h + **vanco** + IV **dexamethasone** **For severe pen. Allergy, see Comment**	**Severe penicillin allergy:** Vanco 500-750mg IV q6h + **TMP-SMX** 5mg/kg q6-8h pending culture results. Chloro has failed vs DRSP (Ln 342:240, 1993).
Post-neurosurgery, post-head trauma, or post-cochlear implant (NEJM 349:435, 2003)	S. pneumoniae most common, esp. if CSF leak. Other: S. aureus, coliforms, P. aeruginosa	**Vanco** (until known for MRSA) 500–750mg IV q6h[3] + (**cefepime** or **ceftazidime** 2gm IV q8h)(see footnote)	MER 2gm IV q8h + **vanco** 1gm IV q6-12h	Vanco alone not optimal for S. pneumo. If/when suscept. S. pneumo identified, quickly switch to **ceftriaxone** or **cefotaxime**. If coliform or pseudomonas meningitis, some add intrathecal gentamicin (4 mg q12h into lateral ventricles). Cure of acinetobacter meningitis with intrathecal colistin (JAC 53:290, 2004)
Ventriculitis/meningitis due to infected ventriculo-peritoneal (atrial) shunt	S. epidermidis, S. aureus, coliforms, diphtheroids (rare), P. acnes	**Vanco** 500–750mg IV q6h[3] + (**cefepime** or **cef-tazidime** 2gm IV q8h) If unable to remove shunt, consider intraventricular	**Vanco** 500-750mg IV q6h[3] + **ceftriaxone** 2gm IV q12h + timed **dexa-methasone** If unable to remove shunt, see footnote[3]	Usual care: 1st, remove infected shunt & culture, external ventricular catheter for drainage/pressure control, antimicrobics x14 days. For timing of new shunt, see CID 39:1267, 2004.
Empiric Therapy—Positive CSF Gram stain				
Gram-positive diplococci	S. pneumoniae	Either (**ceftriaxone** 2gm IV q12h or **cefotaxime** 2gm IV q4–6h) + **vanco** 500–750mg IV q6h + timed **dexa-methasone** 0.15mg/kg IV q6h x 2–4 days		Alternatives: **MER** 2gm IV q8h or **Moxi** 400mg IV + **dexamethasone**
Gram-negative diplococci	N. meningitidis	(**Cefotaxime** 2gm IV q4-6h or **ceftriaxone** 2gm IV q12h) + timed **dexamethasone** (dose above)		Alternatives: **Pen G** 4 mill. units IV q4h or **AMP** 2gm q4h or **Moxl** 400mg IV q24h or **chloro** 1gm IV q6h

---

[1] **Rationale**—Hard to get adequate CSF concentrations of anti-infectives, hence MIC criteria for susceptibility are lower for CSF isolates (ArM 161:2538, 2001).

[2] Low & erratic penetration of **vanco** into the CSF (PIDJ 17:895, 1997). Rec **children's dosage** 15mg/kg IV q6h (2x standard adult dose) is suggested: **500–750mg IV q6h**.

[3] **Dosage of drugs used to rx children ≥1mo or age:** Cefotaxime 200mg/kg per day IV div q6–8h; ceftriaxone 100mg/kg per day IV div q12h; vanco 15mg/kg IV q6h.

[4] Dosages for intraventricular therapy. The following are daily adult doses in mg: amikacin 30, gentamicin 4–8, polymyxin 8 (Colistin) 10, tobramycin 5–20, vanco 10–20. Ref. CID 39:1267, 2004.

Abbreviations on page 2. NOTE: All dosage recommendations are for adults (unless otherwise indicated) and assume normal renal function.

TABLE 1 (5)

ANATOMIC SITE/DIAGNOSIS/ MODIFYING CIRCUMSTANCES	ETIOLOGIES (usual)	SUGGESTED REGIMENS*		ADJUNCT DIAGNOSTIC OR THERAPEUTIC MEASURES AND COMMENTS
		PRIMARY	**ALTERNATIVE†**	
CENTRAL NERVOUS SYSTEM/Meningitis, Bacterial, Acute (continued)				
Gram-positive bacilli or cocco-bacilli	Listeria monocytogenes	**AMP** 2 gm IV q4h ± **gentamicin** 2mg/kg loading dose then 1.7mg/kg q8h		If pen-allergic, use **TMP-SMX** 5mg/kg q6–8h or **MER** 2gm IV q8h
Gram-negative bacilli	H. influenzae, coliforms, P. aeruginosa	**(Ceftazidime** or **cefepime** 2gm IV q8h) + **gentamicin** 2mg/kg 1st dose then 1.7mg/kg q8h		Alternatives: **CIP** 400mg IV q8–12h; **MER** 2gm IV q8h
Specific Therapy—Positive culture of CSF with in vitro susceptibility results available. Interest in monitoring/reducing intracranial pressure: CID 38:384, 2004				
H. influenzae	β-lactamase +	**Ceftriaxone** (peds) 50mg/kg IV q12h		Pen.-allergic: **Chloro** 12.5mg/kg IV q6h (max. 4gm/day)
Listeria monocytogenes (CID 43:1233, 2006)		**AMP** 2gm IV q4h ± **gentamicin** 2mg/kg loading dose, then 1.7mg/kg q8h		Pen. allergic: **TMP-SMX** 20mg/kg per day div. q6–12h. One report of greater efficacy of AMP + TMP-SMX as compared to AMP + gentamicin (JID 33:79, 1996). **Altern: MER** 2gm IV q8h. Success reported with **linezolid + RIF** (CID 40:1060, 2005).
N. meningitidis	MIC 0.1–1 mcg per mL	**Ceftriaxone** 2gm IV q12h x 7 days (see Comment); if pen. allergic, **chloro** 12.5mg/kg (up to 1gm) IV q6h		Rare isolates chloro-resistant (NEJM 339:368 & 917, 1998). Alternatives: **MER** 2gm IV q8h or **Moxi** 400mg q24h.
S. pneumoniae	Pen G MIC			
NOTES:	<0.1mcg/mL	**Pen** G 4 million units IV q4h or **AMP** 2gm IV q4h		Alternatives: **Ceftriaxone** 2gm IV q12h, **chloro** 1gm IV q6h
1. Assumes dexamethasone just prior to 1st dose & x4 days.	0.1–1mcg/mL	**Ceftriaxone** 2gm IV q12h or **cefotaxime** 2gm IV q4–6h		Alternatives: **Cefepime** 2gm IV q8h or **MER** 2 gm IV q8h
2. If MIC >1: repeat CSF exam after 24–48h.	>2mcg/mL	**Vanco** 500–750mg IV q6h + **(ceftriaxone** or **cefotaxime** as above)		Alternatives: **Moxi** 400mg IV q24h
3. Treat for 10–14 days	Ceftriaxone MIC ≥1mcg/mL	**Vanco** 500–750mg IV q6h + **(ceftriaxone** or **cefotaxime** as above)		Alternatives: **Moxi** 400mg IV q24h; If MIC to ceftriaxone >2mcg/mL, add **RIF** 600mg 1x/day.
E. coli, other coliforms, or P. aeruginosa	Consultation advised—need susceptibility results	**(Ceftazidime** or **cefepime** 2gm IV q8h) ± **gentamicin**		Alternatives: **CIP** 400mg IV q8–12h; **MER** 2 gm IV q8h. For discussion of intraventricular therapy: CID 39:1267, 2004
Prophylaxis for H. influenzae and N. meningitides				
Haemophilus influenzae (type b (Neisseria on page 9) Household and/or day care contact: reading with index case or 24hrs. Day care contact: same day care as index case for 5–7 days before onset		**RIF** 20mg/kg po (not to exceed 600mg) x 4 doses. **Adults: RIF** 600mg q24h x 4 days		**Household:** If there is one unvaccinated contact ≤4yr in the household, RIF rec for all household contacts (except all pregnant women). **Child Care Facilities:** With 1 case, if attended by unvaccinated children <2yr, consider prophylaxis. With vaccinate susceptibles. If all contacts >2yr; no prophylaxis. If ≥2 cases in 60 days & unvaccinated children attend, prophylaxis recommended for children & personnel (Am Acad Ped Red Book 2006, page 313).

Abbreviations on page 2.   *NOTE: All dosage recommendations are for adults (unless otherwise indicated) and assume normal renal function.*

TABLE 1 (6)

ANATOMIC SITE/DIAGNOSIS/ MODIFYING CIRCUMSTANCES	ETIOLOGIES (usual)	SUGGESTED REGIMENS*		ADJUNCT DIAGNOSTIC OR THERAPEUTIC MEASURES AND COMMENTS
		PRIMARY	ALTERNATIVE⁵	
CENTRAL NERVOUS SYSTEM/Meningitis, Bacterial, Acute/Prophylaxis for H. influenzae and N. meningitidis *(continued)*				
Neisseria meningitidis exposure (close contact) *MMWR 46(RR-5):1, 1997.* CDC recommends informing college freshmen living in dormitories & residence halls of available vaccine *(MMWR 46(7):1, 2000 & 50/23:487, 2001)*		**[CIP** (adults) 500mg po (single dose)] **OR [Ceftriaxone** 250mg IM x 1 dose (child <15yr 125mg IM x 1)] **OR [RIF** 600mg po q12h x 4 doses. (Children >1mo 10mg/kg po q12h x 4 doses, <1mo 5mg/kg q12h x 4 doses)]* **OR Spiramycin**⁽ᴺᴬ⁾ 500mg po q6h x 5 days. Children 10mg/kg po q6h x 5 days.		Spread by respiratory droplets, not aerosols, hence dose contact req. ↑risk if: close contact for at least 4hrs during wk before illness onset (e.g., housemates, day care contacts, cellmates) or exposure to pt's nasopharyngeal secretions (e.g., kissing, mouth-to-mouth resuscitation, intubation, nasotracheal suctioning). Since RIF-resistant N. meningitidis documented post-prophylaxis(*EID 11/977, 2005*), prefer Cip or ceftriaxone (*Cochrane, CD 004785, 2005*). Primary prophylactic regimen in many European countries.
Meningitis, chronic. Defined as symptoms + CSF pleocytosis for ≥4 wks	M. tbc 40%, cryptococcus 7%, Lyme, syphilis, Whipple's disease	Treatment depends on etiology. No urgent need for empiric therapy.		Long list of etiologies: bacteria, parasites, fungi, viruses, neoplasms, vasculitis, and other miscellaneous etiologies—see chapter on chronic meningitis in latest edition of Harrison's Textbook of Internal Medicine. Whipple's: *JID 188:797 & 801, 2003.*
Meningitis, eosinophilic *AJM 114:217, 2003.* (See Table 13A, page 127)	Angiostrongyliasis, gnathostomiasis, rarely others	Corticosteroids	Not sure antihelminthic rx works.	1/3 lack peripheral eosinophilia. Need serology to confirm dx. Steroid ref.: *NEJM 346:668, 2002.*
Meningitis, HIV-1 infected (AIDS) (See Table 11, Sanford Guide to HIV/AIDS Therapy)	As in adults, >50yr, also consider cryptococci, M. tuberculosis, syphilis, HIV aseptic meningitis, Listeria monocytogenes	If etiology not identified: rx as adult, >50yr + obtain CSF/serum crypto-coccal antigen (see Comments)	For crypto rx, see Table 11A, page 94	C. neoformans most common etiology in AIDS. H. influenzae, pneumococci, Tbc, syphilis, viral, histoplasma & coccidioides also need to be considered. Obtain blood cultures. L. monocytogenes risk >60x if 1% present as meningitis (*CID 17:224, 1993*).
EAR				
External otitis				
"Swimmer's ear" *PIDJ 22:299, 2003.*	Pseudomonas sp., Enterobacteriaceae, Proteus sp. (Fungi rare.) Acute infection usually 2° S. aureus	Eardrops: **Ofloxa 0.3% soln bid** or **(polymyxin B + neomycin + hydrocortisone)** qid or **(CIP** + **hydrocortisone)** qid. For acute disease: **dicloxacillin** 500mg po qid-qid.		Rx should include gentle cleaning. Recurrences prevented (or decreased) by drying with alcohol drops (1/3 white vinegar, 2/3 rubbing alcohol) after swimming, then antibiotic drops or 2% acetic acid solution. Ointments should not be used in ear. Do not use neomycin if tympanic membrane punctured.
Chronic	Usually 2° to seborrhea.	Eardrops: **[(polymyxin B + neomycin + hydrocortisone)** qid] **+ selenium sulfide**		Control seborrhea with dandruff shampoo containing selenium sulfide (Selsun) or [(ketoconazole shampoo) + (medium potency steroid solution, triamcinolone 0.1%)].
"Malignant otitis externa" Risk groups: Diabetes mellitus, AIDS, chemotherapy.	Pseudomonas aeruginosa in >90%.	**IMP** 0.5gm IV q6h) or **(MER** 1gm IV q8h) or **(CIP** 400mg IV q12h (or 750mg po q12h)) or **(ceftaz 2gm** IV q8h) or **(PIP 2gm** q12h) or **(PIP** 4-6gm IV q4-6h + **tobra** dose Table 10D) or **TC 3gm** IV q4h + **tobra** dose Table 10D)		CIP especially useful for outpatient rx with early disease. Surgical debridement usually required, but not radical excision. R/O osteomyelitis, CT or MRI scan more sensitive than x-ray. If bone involved, rx for 4–6wks. Ref.: *LnID 4:34, 2004*

TABLE 1 (7)

ANATOMIC SITE/DIAGNOSIS; MODIFYING CIRCUMSTANCES	ETIOLOGIES (usual)	SUGGESTED REGIMENS*		ADJUNCT DIAGNOSTIC OR THERAPEUTIC MEASURES AND COMMENTS
		PRIMARY	ALTERNATIVE[1]	

EAR *(continued)*

Otitis media—infants, children, adults

Acute *(NEJM 347:1169, 2002; Peds 113:1451, 2004).* For correlation of bacterial eradication from middle ear & clinical outcome, see LnID 2:593, 2002.

Initial empiric therapy of acute otitis media (AOM) in **children <2yr old**. If > 2yr old, no treatment may be an option, see Comment. **NOTE:** Pending new data, rx children <2yr old. **NOTE:** In children with non-severe disease & uncertain diagnosis, consider analgesic treatment without antimicrobials. Favorable results in mostly afebrile pts with waiting 48hrs before deciding on antibiotic use (*JAMA 296:1235, 1290, 2006*)	Overall detection in middle ear fluid: No pathogen ... 25% Virus ... 5–48% Bac + virus ... 55% Bacteria only ... 55% Role of viruses: *Clin Micro Rev 16:230, 2003* Pathogens from middle ear, 2000–2003: S. pneumo 31%, H. influenzae, & M. catarrhalis 11% (*PIDJ 23:829, 2004*)	**If NO antibiotics in prior month:** Amox po HD[1] **Duration of rx:** <2yr old x 10 days; ≥2yr x 5–7 days. Approp. duration unclear. 5 days may be inadequate for severe disease (*NEJM 347:1169, 2002*). **For adult dosages, see Sinusitis, pages 44–45, and Table 10**	**If allergic to β-lactam drugs?** If history unclear or rash, effective oral ceph OK; avoid ceph if IgE-mediated allergy; e.g., anaphylaxis. High failure rate with TMP-SMX if etiology is DRSP or H. influenzae (*PIDJ 20:260, 2001*); **azithro x 5 days or clarithro x 10 days** (both have↓ activity vs DRSP). **Up to 50% S. pneumo resistant to macrolides.** AM-CL superior to azithro in recent bacterial clinical trial (*JAMA 290:1633, 2003, 2004*). Rationale & data to single dose azithro, 30 mg per kg, *PIDJ 23:S102 & S108, 2004.* **Spontaneous resolution:** 90% pts infected with M. catarrhalis, 50% with H. influenzae, 10% with S. pneumoniae; overall 80% resolve within 2–14 days (*Ln 363:465, 2004*). **Risk of DRSP** if age <2yr, antibiotics last 3mo, &/or daycare attendance. Source/cause of drug (1) effectiveness against β-lactamase producing H. influenzae & M. catarrhalis & (2) effectiveness against S. pneumo, inc. DRSP. Cefaclor, loracarbef, & ceftibuten less active vs DRSP than other agents listed. Variable acceptance of drug taste/smell by children 4–8 y.o. (*PIDJ 19 (Suppl 2):S174, 2000*).
Treatment for clinical failure after 3 days rx	Drug-resistant S. pneumoniae main concern	**NO antibiotics in prior month:** AM-CL extra-strength[1] or cefdinir or cefpodoxime or cefprozil or cefuroxime. **For dosage, see footnotes[1] and[2]. All doses are pediatric**	**Received antibiotics in prior month:** Amox HD[1] or AM-CL extra-strength[1] or cefdinir or cefpodoxime or cefprozil or cefuroxime axetil For dosage, see footnotes[1] and[2] **All doses are pediatric**	**Clindamycin** not active vs H. influenzae or M. catarrhalis. S. pneumo resistant to macrolides are usually also resistant to clinda. Definition of failure: no change in ear pain, fever, bulging TM or otorrhea after 3 days of rx. Tympanocentesis will allow culture. **Newer FQs active vs DRSP, but not approved for use in children** (*PIDJ 23:390, 2004*). **Vanco is active vs DRSP.** Ceftriaxone IM x 3 days superior to 1-day treatment vs DRSP (*PIDJ 19:1040, 2000*). AM-CL HD reported successful for pen-resistant S. pneumo AOM (*PIDJ 20:829, 2001*).
After >48hrs of nasotracheal intubation	Pseudomonas sp., Klebsiella, enterobacter	**Antibiotics in mo prior to last 3 days:** [(IV) ceftriaxone] or (clinda-mycin) (after tympanocen-tesis) See clinda/pen Comments		With nasotracheal intubation >48 hrs, about ½ pts will have otitis media with effusion.
		Ceftazidime or CFP or IMP or MER or (Pip-Tz) or TC-CL or CIP For dosages, see Ear, Malignant otitis externa, page 9		

---

[1] **Amoxicillin UD or HD** = amoxicillin usual dose or high dose. **AM-CL HD** = amoxicillin-clavulanate high dose. Data supporting amoxicillin HD: *PIDJ 22:405, 2003*.

[2] **Drugs & peds dosage (all po unless specified) for acute otitis media: Amoxicillin UD** = 40mg/kg per day div q12h or q8h. **Amoxicillin HD** = 90mg/kg per day div q12h or q8h; **AM-CL HD** = 90mg/kg per day of amox component. **Extra-strength AM-CL oral suspension** (Augmentin 20–30mg/kg per day with 600mg AM & 42.9mg CL / 5mL—dose: 90/6.4mg/kg per day div bid. **Cefuroxime axetil** 30mg/kg per day div q12h. **Ceftriaxone** 50mg/kg IM x 3 days. **Clindamycin** 20–30mg/kg per day (may be effective vs DRSP but no activity vs H. influenzae). **Other drugs suitable for clinical use (e.g., penicillin)-sensitive S. pneumo: TMP-SMX** 8mg/kg of TMP q12h; **Erythro-sulfisoxazole** 50mg/kg per day of erythro div q6–8h; **Clarithro** 15mg/kg per day div q12h; **Azithro** 10mg/kg per day x 1 day then 5mg/kg per day on days 2–5; **Cefdinir** 14mg/kg per day div q12–24h x 3 days & 30mg/kg q24h x 1; **Cefpodoxime proxetil** 10mg/kg per day as single dose; **cefaclor** 40mg/kg per day div q8h; **loracarbef** 15mg/kg per day div q12h; **cefprozil** 15mg/kg q12h; **cefpodoxime proxetil** 10mg/kg per day. *NOTE: All dosage recommendations are for adults (unless otherwise indicated) and assume normal renal function.*

Abbreviations on page 2.

TABLE 1 (8)

ANATOMIC SITE/DIAGNOSIS/ MODIFYING CIRCUMSTANCES	ETIOLOGIES (usual)	SUGGESTED REGIMENS*		ADJUNCT DIAGNOSTIC OR THERAPEUTIC MEASURES AND COMMENTS
		PRIMARY	ALTERNATIVE†	
EAR/Otitis media *(continued)*				
Prophylaxis: acute otitis media *PIDJ 22:10, 2003*	Pneumococci, H. influenzae, M. catarrhalis, Staph. aureus, Group A strep **(see Comments)**	**Sulfisoxazole** 50mg/kg po at bedtime or **amoxicillin** 20mg/kg po q24h	**Use of antibiotics to prevent otitis media is a major contributor to emergence of antibiotic-resistant S. pneumo!** Pneumococcal protein conjugate vaccine decreases freq. AOM in general & due to vaccine serotypes. Adenoidectomy at time of tympanostomy tubes + need for future hospitalization for AOM (*NEJM 344:1188, 2001*).
Mastoiditis				
Acute				
Outpatient	Strep. pneumoniae 22%, S. pyogenes 16%, Staph. aureus 7%, H. influenzae 4%, P. aeruginosa 4%, others < 1%	Empirically, same as Acute otitis media, above, need **vanco** or **nafcillin/oxacillin** if culture + for S. aureus. **Ceftriaxone** 1–2gm IV q24–8h (depends on severity) or **(ceftriaxone** 2gm IV q24h <age 60, 1gm IV q24h > age 60)		Has become a rare entity, presumably as result of the aggressive rx of acute otitis media. Small ↑ in incidence in Netherlands where use of antibiotics limited to children with complicated course or high risk (*PIDJ 20:140, 2001*).
Chronic	Often polymicrobic: anaerobes, S. aureus, Enterobacteriaceae, P. aeruginosa	Treatment for acute exacerbations or perioperatively. Ideally, no treatment until surgical cultures obtained. Examples of empiric regimens: **IMP** 0.5 gm IV q6h, **TC-CL** 3.1gm IV q6h, **PIP-TZ** 3.375gm IV q4–6h or 4.5gm q8h, **MER** 1gm IV q8h.		May or may not be associated with chronic otitis media with drainage via culture+ tympanic membrane. Antimicrobials given in association with surgery. Mastoidectomy indications: chronic drainage and evidence of osteomyelitis by MRI or CT, evidence of spread to CNS (epidural abscess, supurative phlebitis, brain abscess).
EYE—General Reviews: *CID 21:479, 1995; IDCP 7:447, 1998*				
Eyelid: Little reported experience with CA-MRSA *(Ophtha 111:455, 2006)*				
Blepharitis	Etiol. unclear. Factors include Staph. aureus & Staph. epidermidis, seborrhea, rosacea, & dry eye	Lid margin care with baby shampoo & warm compresses q24h. Artificial tears if assoc. dry eye (see Comment).		Usually topical ointments of no benefit. If associated rosacea, add doxy 100mg bid for 2wk and then q24h.
Hordeolum (Stye)				
External (eyelash follicle) or Internal (Meibomian gland): Can be acute, subacute or chronic.	Staph. aureus Staph. aureus, MSSA Staph. aureus, MRSA-CA Staph. aureus, MRSA-HA	Hot packs only. Will drain spontaneously Oral **nafcillin/oxacillin** — hot packs TMP/SMX-DS, tabs ii po bid Unizolid 600mg po bid possible therapy if multi-drug resistant.		Infection of superficial sebaceous gland. Also called acute meibomianitis. Rarely drain spontaneously; may need I&D and culture. Role of fluoroquinolone eye drops is unclear. MRSA often resistant to lower conc.; may be susceptible to higher concentration of FQ in ophthalmologic solutions of gati, levo or moxi.
Conjunctiva: *NEJM 343:345, 2000*				
Conjunctivitis of the newborn (**ophthalmia neonatorum**): by day of onset post-delivery—all doses pediatric				
Chemical (due to AgNO₃ prophylaxis)		None		Usual prophylaxis is erythro ointment; hence, AgNO₃ irritation rare.
Onset 1st day				
Onset 2–4 days	N. gonorrhoeae	**Ceftriaxone** 25–50mg/kg IV x 1 dose (see Comment), not to exceed 125mg		Treat mother & her sexual partners. Hyperpurulent. Topical rx inadequate. **Treat neonate for both gonococcal & chlamydia**
Onset 3–10 days	Chlamydia trachomatis	**Erythro base or ethylsuccinate syrup** 12.5mg/kg q6h x 14 days). No topical rx needed		Diagnosis by antigen detection. Azithro susp 20mg/kg po q24h x 3 days reported efficacious (*PIDJ 17:1049, 1998*). Treat mother & sexual partner
Onset 2–16 days	Herpes simplex types 1,2	See keratitis on page 12		Consider IV acyclovir if concomitant systemic disease.
Ophthalmia neonatorum prophylaxis.	**Silver nitrate** 1% x 1 or **erythro** 0.5% ointment x 1 or **tetra** 1% ointment x 1 application		

Abbreviations on page 2.   NOTE: All dosage recommendations are for adults (unless otherwise indicated) and assume normal renal function.

TABLE 1 (9)

ANATOMIC SITE/DIAGNOSIS/ MODIFYING CIRCUMSTANCES	ETIOLOGIES (usual)	SUGGESTED REGIMENS*		ADJUNCT DIAGNOSTIC OR THERAPEUTIC MEASURES AND COMMENTS
		PRIMARY	ALTERNATIVE§	
EYE (continued)				
Pink eye (viral conjunctivitis). Usually unilateral	Adenovirus (types 3 & 7 in children, B, 11 & 19 in adults)	No treatment. If symptomatic, cold artificial tears may help.		Highly contagious: Onset of ocular pain and photophobia in an adult suggests associated keratitis—rare.
Inclusion conjunctivitis (adult). Usually unilateral	Chlamydia trachomatis	Doxy 100mg bid po x 1–3wk	Erythro 250mg po qid x 1–3wk	Oculogenital disease. Diagnosis by culture or antigen detection or PCR—availability varies by region and institution. Treat sexual partner.
Trachoma	Chlamydia trachomatis	Azithro 20mg/kg po single-dose—78% effective in children	Doxy 100mg po bid x days or tetracycline 250mg po qd tx 1-6 days.	Starts in childhood and can persist for years with subsequent damage to cornea. Topical therapy of marginal benefit. Avoid doxy/tetracycline in young children. Mass treatment works (JAMA 292:721, 2004)
Suppurative conjunctivitis:				
Non-gonococcal; non-chlamydial *Med Lett 46:25, 2004*	Staph. aureus, S. pneumoniae, H. influenzae, et al. Outbreak due to atypical S. pneumo. *NEJM 348:1112, 2003*	Ophthalmic solution: Gati 0.3%, Levo 0.5%, or Moxi 0.5%. All 1–2 gtts q2h while awake 1° 2 days, then q4–8h up to 7 days.	Polymyxin B + trimethoprim solution 1-2 gtts q3–6h x 7-10 days.	FQs best spectrum for empiric therapy but expensive: $40–50 for 5mL. High concentrations 1° likelihood of activity vs S. aureus—even MRSA. TMP spectrum may include MRSA. Polymyxin B spectrum only Gm-neg. bacilli but not ophthal. prep of only TMP. Most S. pneumo resistant to gent & tobra.
Gonococcal (peds/adults)	N. gonorrhoeae	Ceftriaxone 25-50mg/kg IV/IM (not to exceed 125mg) as one dose in children; 1gm IV/IM as one dose in adults		
Cornea (keratitis): Usually serious and often sight-threatening. Prompt ophthalmologic consultation essential! Herpes simplex most common etiology in developed countries; bacterial and fungal infections more common in underdeveloped countries.				
Viral:				
H. simplex	H. simplex, types 1 & 2	Trifluridine, one drop q2h, 9x/day for up to 21 days.	Vidarabine ointment— useful in children. Use 5x/day for up to 21 days.	Fluorescein staining shows topical figures. 30-50% rate of recurrence within 2 years. 400mg acyclovir po bid ↓ recurrences, p 0.005 (NEJM 339:300, 1999). If child fails vidarabine, try trifluridine.
Varicella-zoster ophthalmicus	Varicella-zoster virus	Famciclovir 500mg po tid or valacyclovir 1gm po tid x 10 days	Acyclovir 800mg po 5x/day x 10 days	Clinical diagnosis most common: dendritic figures with fluorescein staining in patient with varicella-zoster staining of ophthalmic branch of trigeminal nerve.
Bacterial (Med Lett 46:25, 2004)		**All rx listed for bacterial, fungal, & protozoan is topical**		
Acute: No comorbidity	S. aureus, S. pneumo, S. pyogenes, Haemophilus sp.	Moxi: eye gtts. 1 gtt tid x 7 d.	Gati: eye gtts. 1-2 gtts q2h while awake x 2 d. then q4h x MRSA.	Prefer Moxi due to enhanced lipophilicity & penetration into aqueous humor. Survey of Ophthal 50 (suppl 1) 1, 2005. despite high conc. may fail vs MRSA.
Contact lens users	P. aeruginosa	Tobra or gentamicin (14mg/mL) + piperacillin or ticarcillin eye drops (6-12mg/ml) q15-60 min around clock x 24-72 hrs, then slow reduction	Cip 6.6% or Levo 0.5% drops q15-60min around clock x 24-72 hrs	Pain, photophobia, impaired vision. Recommend alginate swab for culture and sensitivity testing.

Abbreviations on page 2.   NOTE: All dosage recommendations are for adults (unless otherwise indicated) and assume normal renal function.

TABLE 1 (10)

ANATOMIC SITE/DIAGNOSIS/ MODIFYING CIRCUMSTANCES	ETIOLOGIES (usual)	SUGGESTED REGIMENS* PRIMARY	ALTERNATIVE†	ADJUNCT DIAGNOSTIC OR THERAPEUTIC MEASURES AND COMMENTS
EYE/Cornea (Keratitis)/Bacterial *(continued)*				
Dry/cornea, diabetes, immunosuppression	Staph. aureus, S. epidermidis, S. pneumoniae, S. pyogenes, Enterobacteriaceae, listeria	**Cefazolin** (50mg/mL) + **gentamicin or tobra** (14mg/mL) q15-60 min around clock x 24-72 hrs, then slow reduction	**Vanco** (50mg/mL) + **ceftaz-idime** (50mg/mL), q15-60 min around clock x 24-72 hrs, then slow reduction. See *Comment*	Specific therapy guided by results of alginate swab culture and sensitivity. CIP 0.3% found clinically equivalent to cefazolin + tobra; only concern was efficacy of CIP vs. S. pneumoniae (*Ophthalmology* 163:1854, 1996).
Fungal	Aspergillus, fusarium, candida. No empiric therapy—see *Comment*	**Natamycin** (5%) drops q3-4 hrs with subsequent slow reduction	**Ampho B** (0.05-0.15%) q3-4 hrs with subsequent slow reduction	No empiric therapy. Wait for results of Gram stain or culture in Sabouraud's medium.
Mycobacteria: Post-Lasik	Mycobacterium chelonae	**Moxi** eye gtts. 1 gtt qid	**Gati** eye gtts. 1 gtt qid	Ref. *Ophthalmology* 113:950, 2006
Protozoan Soft contact lens users (overnight † risk 10-15 fold)	Acanthamoeba, hartmannella	**Propamidine** 0.1% + **neomycin/gramicidin/ polymyxin** Eyedrops q waking hour for 1wk, then slow taper	**Polyhexamethylene biguanide (PHMB)** 0.02% or **chlorhexidine** 0.02%	Uncommon. Trauma and soft contact lenses are risk factors. Corneal scrapings stained with calcofluor white show characteristic cysts with fluorescent microscopy. PHMB source: Leiter's Park Ave. Pharm.; 800-292-6773. Ref. *CID* 35:434, 2002
Lacrimal apparatus				
Canaliculitis	Actinomyces most common. Rarely, Arachnia, fusobacterium, nocardia, candida	Remove granules & irrigate with **pen G** (100,000mcg/mL)	If fungi, irrigate with **nystatin** approx. 5mcg/mL + 1 gtt t/d	Digital pressure produces exudate at punctum; Gram stain confirms diagnosis. Hot packs to punctal area qid.
		Child: AM-CL or O Ceph 2		
Dacryocystitis (lacrimal sac)	S. pneumo, S. aureus, H. influenzae, S. pyogenes, P. aeruginosa	Often consequence of obstruction of lacrimal duct. Empiric rx based on Gram stain of aspirate—see *Comment*		Need ophthalmologic consultation. Can be acute or chronic. Culture to detect MRSA.
Endophthalmitis. For post-op endophthalmitis, see *CID* 38:542, 2004				
Bacterial: Haziness of vitreous key to diagnosis: Needle aspirate of both vitreous and aqueous humor for culture prior to therapy. Intravitreal administration of antimicrobials essential				
Postocular surgery (cataracts) Early; acute onset (incidence 0.05%)	S. epidermidis 60%, Staph. aureus, streptococci, & enterococci each 5-10%, Gm-neg. bacilli 6%	**Immediate ophthal. consult.** If only light perception or worse, immediate vitrectomy + intravitreal vanco 1mg, & intravitreal ceftazidime 2.25mg. No clear data on intravitreal steroid. May need to repeat intravitreal antibiotics in 2-3 days. Can usually leave lens in.		
Low-grade, chronic	Propionibacterium acnes, S. epidermidis, S. aureus (rare), Staph. sp. & fungi	May require removal of lens material. Intraocular **vanco** ± vitrectomy.		
Post filtering blebs for glaucoma	Strep. species (viridans & others), H. influenzae	Intravitreal and topical agent as above + systemic **clinda or vanco**. Use topical antibiotics post-surgery (tobra & cefazolin drops).		
Post-penetrating trauma	Bacillus sp. & S. epidem			
None, suspect hematogenous	S. pneumoniae, N. meningitidis, Staph. aureus	Intravitreal agent + (systemic **clinda or vanco**) as with early post-operative.	**P Ceph 3** (**cefotaxime** 2gm IV q4h or **ceftriaxone** 2gm IV q24h) + **vanco** 1gm IV q12h pending cultures.	
IV heroin abuse	Bacillus cereus, Candida sp.	Intravitreal agent + (systemic **clinda or vanco**)		

NOTE: All dosage recommendations are for adults (unless otherwise indicated) and assume normal renal function.

Abbreviations on page 2

TABLE 1 (11)

ANATOMIC SITE/DIAGNOSIS/ MODIFYING CIRCUMSTANCES	ETIOLOGIES (usual)	SUGGESTED REGIMENS*		ADJUNCT DIAGNOSTIC OR THERAPEUTIC MEASURES AND COMMENTS
		PRIMARY	ALTERNATIVE¹	
EYE: Endophthalmitis (continued)				
Mycotic (fungal) Bacteremia, i.e. antibiotics, often corticosteroids, indwelling venous catheters	Candida sp., Aspergillus sp.	Intravitreal **ampho B** 0.005-0.01mg in 0.1mL. Also see Table 11A, page 97 for concomitant systemic therapy. See Comment.		With moderate/marked vitritis, options include systemic rx + vitrectomy ± intra-vitreal ampho B (CID 27:1130 & 1134, 1998). Report of failure of ampho B lipid complex (CID 28:1177, 1999).
Retinitis Acute retinal necrosis	Varicella zoster, Herpes simplex	IV **acyclovir** 10-12mg/kg IV q8h x 5-7 days, then 800mg po 5x/day x 6wk.		Strong association of VZ virus with atypical necrotizing herpelic retinopathy (CID 24:603, 1997).
HIV+ (AIDS) CD4 usually <100/mm³	Cytomegalovirus	See Table 14, page 137		Occurs in 5-10% of AIDS patients
Orbital cellulitis (see page 46 for erysipelas, facial)	S. pneumoniae, H. influenzae, M. catarrhalis, S. aureus, anaerobes, group A strep, occ. Gm-neg. bacilli post-trauma	**Nafcillin** 2gm IV q4h (or if MRSA-**vanco** 1gm IV q12h) + **ceftriaxone** 2gm IV q24h + **metro** 1gm IV q12h		**If penicillin/ceph allergy: Vanco + levo** 750mg IV once daily + **metro** IV. Risk of cavernous sinus thrombosis. Image orbit (CT or MRI). If vanco intolerant, another option for s. aureus is dapto 6mg/kg IV q24h.
FOOT				
"**Diabetic**"—Empiric therapy. Refs.: CID 39:885, 2004; NEJM 351-48, 2004; Ln 366:1725, 2005				**General:**
Ulcer without inflammation	Colonizing skin flora.	No antibacterial therapy		1. Glucose control, no weight-bearing 2. Assess for peripheral vascular disease—very common (CID 39-437, 2004)
Ulcer with <2cm of superficial inflammation	S. aureus (assume MRSA), S. agalactiae (Gp B), Enterobacteriaceae	**Oral therapy: TMP-SMX-DS** ² or **minocycline** plus (**Pen VK** IV or selected **Dosages in footnote**		**Principles of empiric antibacterial therapy:** 1. Include drug predictably active vs MRSA. 2. Community-acquired MRSA (CA-MRSA) can outpatient, can assume
Ulcer with ≥2cm of inflammation with extension to fascia	As above, plus coliforms possible	**Oral therapy: (AM-CL-ER** plus **TMP-SMX-DS)** (CIP or **Levo** or **Moxi**) plus **linezolid** **Dosages in footnote**		active until culture results available. 2. As culture results dominated by S. aureus & Streptococcus species, empiric drug regimens should include strep & staph. Role of enterococci uncertain.
Extensive local inflammation plus systemic toxicity. Other treatment modalities, lmtd efficacy & expensive: Neg pressure (wound vac) (Ln 366:1704, 2005), and hyperbaric oxygen (CID 43:188, 193; 2006)	As above plus anaerobic bacteria. Role of enterococci unclear.	**Parenteral therapy: (Vanco** plus β-lactam/β-lactamase inhibitor) or (**vanco** plus **carbapenem**). Other alternatives: 1. **Dapto** or **linezolid** for vanco 2. **CIP** or **Levo** or **Moxi** or **aztreonam** plus **metronidazole** **Dosages in footnote**		3. Severe limb threatening infections require initial parenteral therapy with predictable activity vs Gm-positive cocci, coliforms & other aerobic Gm-neg. rods, & anaerobic Gm-negative bacilli. **NOTE:** The regimens listed are suggestions consistent with above principles. Other alternatives exist & may be appropriate for individual patients.
Onychomycosis See Table 11, page 100, fungal infections				
Puncture wound: Nail/Toothpick	P. aeruginosa	Cleanse. Tetanus booster. Observe.		See page 4 , 1–2% evolve to osteomyelitis. After toothpick injury (PIDJ 23-80, 2004): S. aureus, Strep sp. and mixed flora.

¹ **TMP-SMX-DS** 2 tabs po bid, **minocycline** 100mg po bid, **Pen VK** 500mg po bid, **cefprozil** 500mg po qid, **cefpodoxime** axetil 500mg po q12h, **cefuroxime** axetil 500mg po q12h, **cefdinir** 300mg po q12h or 600mg po q24h, **cefpodoxime** 200mg po q12h, **CIP** 750mg po bid, **Levo** 750mg po bid, **TMP-SMX-DS** 2 tabs po bid, **CIP** 750 mg po bid, **Levo** 750 mg po bid, **Moxi** 400mg po q24h, **linezolid** 600 mg po bid
² **AM-CL-ER** 2000/125 po bid. **TMP-SMX-DS** 2 tabs po bid. **CIP** 750 mg po bid, **Levo** 750 mg po bid, **Moxi** 400mg po q24h, **Moxi** 400mg po q24h, **AM-SB** 3gm IV q6h, **PIP-TZ** 3.375gm IV q6h or 4.5gm IV q8h, **PIP-TZ** 3.375gm IV q6h or 4.5gm IV q8h, **carbapenems**: **ERTA** 1gm IV q24h; **IMP** 0.5gm IV q6h; **MER** 1gm IV q8h; **parenteral β-lactam/β-lactamase inhibitors**: **AM-SB** 3gm IV q6h, **daptomycin** 6mg per kg IV q24h, **linezolid** 600mg IV q12h, **aztreonam** 2gm IV q8h, **CIP** 400mg IV q12h, **Levo** 750mg IV q12h, **Moxi** 400mg IV q24h, **metro** 1gm IV q12h
³ **Vanco** 1gm IV q12h; loading dose & then 0.5gm IV q6h or 1gm IV q12h

NOTE: All dosage recommendations are for adults (unless otherwise indicated) and assume normal renal function.

Abbreviations on page 2

TABLE 1 (12)

ANATOMIC SITE/DIAGNOSIS/ MODIFYING CIRCUMSTANCES	ETIOLOGIES (usual)	SUGGESTED REGIMENS*		ADJUNCT DIAGNOSTIC OR THERAPEUTIC MEASURES AND COMMENTS
		PRIMARY	ALTERNATIVE[1]	
GALLBLADDER				
Cholecystitis, cholangitis, biliary sepsis, or common duct obstruction (partial, 2° to tumor, stones, stricture)	Enterobacteriaceae 68%, enterococci 14%, bacteroides 10%, Clostridium sp. 7%, rarely candida	**PIP-TZ** or **AM-SB** or **TC-CL** or **ERTA** or **MER** If life-threatening: **IMP**	OR **IP Ceph 3 + metro** OR **Aztreonam + metro** OR **CIP + metro OR Moxi** Dosages in footnote 3 previous page	For severely ill pts, antibiotic rx is complementary to adequate biliary drainage. 15–30% pts will require percutaneous, surgical, percutaneous or ERCP-placed stent. Whether empirical rx should always cover pseudomonas & anaerobes is uncertain. Ceftriaxone associated with biliary sludge of drug(by ultrasound 50%, symptomatic 9%, *NEJM 322:1821, 1990*); clinical relevance still unclear but has led to surgery (*MMWR 42-39, 1993*).
GASTROINTESTINAL				

Gastroenteritis—Empiric Therapy (laboratory studies not performed or culture, microscopy, toxin results NOT AVAILABLE) (Ref.: *NEJM 350:38, 2004*)

Premature Infant with necrotizing enterocolitis	Associated with intestinal flora	Treatment and rationale as for diverticulitis/peritonitis, page 19. See Table 16, page 168 for pediatric dosages		Pneumatosis intestinalis on x-ray confirms dx. Bacteremia-peritonitis in 30–50%. If *Staph. epidermidis* isolated, add vanco.
Mild diarrhea (<3 unformed stools/day, minimal symptomatology)	Bacterial (see below), viral, parasitic. Viral usually causes mild to moderate disease. For traveler's diarrhea, see page 17	Fluids only + lactose-free diet, avoid caffeine		**Rehydration: For po fluid replacement, see Cholera, page 17.** **Antimotility:** Loperamide (Imodium) 4 mg po, then 2 mg after each loose stool to max. of 16 mg per day. Bismuth subsalicylate (Pepto-Bismol) 2 tablets (262 mg) q.i.d. Do not use if suspect hemolytic uremic syndrome
Moderate diarrhea (≥4 unformed stools/day &/or systemic symptoms)		Antimotility agents (see Comments) + fluids		**Hemolytic uremic syndrome (HUS):** Risk in **children** infected with E. coli 0157:H7 is 6–10%. Early treatment with TMP-SMX or FQs ↑ risk of HUS (*NEJM 342:1930 & 1990, 2000*). Controversial meta-analysis: *JAMA 288:996 & 3111, 2002*.
Severe diarrhea (≥6 unformed stools/day, &/or temp ≥101°F, tenesmus, blood, or fecal leukocytes) NOTE: Severe afebrile bloody diarrhea should ↑ suspicion of E. coli 0157:H7 infection—causes only ↓↓<3% all cases diarrhea in US but can cause up to 38% cases of bloody diarrhea (*CID 32:573, 2001*)	Shigella, salmonella, C. jejuni, E. coli 0157:H7, toxin-positive C. difficile, Ent. histolytica. For typhoid fever, see page 54	**FQ** (**CIP** 500 mg po q12h or **Levo** 500 mg q24h) 3–5 days. Campylobacter resistance to FQ common in tropics. *If recent antibiotic therapy:* C. difficile toxin possible) **add** **Metro** 500 mg po tid times 10–14 days	**TMP-SMX-DS** po bid times 3-5 days. **C. difficile toxin colitis** **Vanco** 125 mg q.i.d. times 10–14 days	**Norovirus:** Etiology of over 90% of non-bacterial diarrhea (± nausea/vomiting). Lasts 12-60 hrs. Hydrate. No effective antiviral. **Other potential etiologies:** Cryptosporidium—no treatment in immunocompetent host (see Table 13A & JID 170:272, 1994). Cyclospora—usually responds to TMP-SMX (see Table 12A & AIM 123:409, 1996). **Cases** of severe diarrhea treated with CIP 500 mg po tid decreases duration of diarrhea and other symptoms without changing duration of fecal carriage. Increasing resistance of campylobacter to FQs.

Gastroenteritis—Specific Therapy (results of culture, microscopy, toxin assay AVAILABLE) (Ref.: *NEJM 350:38, 2004*)

If culture negative, probably Norovirus (Norwalk) or rarely (in adults) Rotavirus—see Norovirus, page 144 NOTE: In 60 hospital pts w unexplained WBCs ≥ 15,000, 35% had C. difficile toxin present (*AJM 115:543, 2003; CID 34:1585, 2002*)	**Aeromonas/Plesiomonas**	**CIP** 500 mg po bid times 3 days	**TMP-SMX-DS** po bid times 3 days	Although no absolute proof, increasing evidence as cause of diarrheal illness.
	Amebiasis (Entamoeba histolytica), Cyclospora, Cryptosporidia (and Giardia), see Table 13A			
	Campylobacter jejuni See Comment on FQ resistance Fever in 53-83%, H/O bloody stools 37%	**Azithro** 500mg po q24h x 3 days or **CIP** 500mg po bid (See Comment)	**Erythro stearate** 500mg po q.i.d x 5 days	↑ **worldwide resistance to FQs** varies by region from 10% (USA) to 84% (Thailand) (*AAC 47:2358, 2003*). Erythro resistance rarely reported (*CID 37:131, 2003*). **Post-Campylobacter Guillain-Barré:** assoc. 15% of cases (*Ln 366:1653, 2005*) Assoc. with small bowel lymphoproliferative disease, may respond to antimicrobials (*NEJM 350:239, 2003*). **Reactive arthritis** another potential sequelae.

[1] **H/O** = history of
Abbreviations on page 2.

NOTE: All dosage recommendations are for adults (unless otherwise indicated) and assume normal/renal function.

TABLE 1 (13)

ANATOMIC SITE/DIAGNOSIS/ MODIFYING CIRCUMSTANCES	ETIOLOGIES (usual)	SUGGESTED REGIMENS*		ADJUNCT DIAGNOSTIC OR THERAPEUTIC MEASURES AND COMMENTS
		PRIMARY	ALTERNATIVE[1]	
GASTROINTESTINAL/Gastroenteritis—Empiric Therapy (continued)				
(Continued from above)	**C. difficile toxin positive antibiotic-associated colitis** (CID 43:428, 2006)			
	C. difficile: Mild: WBC po mildly okay. WBC <20,000	Metro 500mg po bid or 250mg po qid x 10-14 days	Vanco 125mg po qid x 10-14 days Teicoplanin 400mg po bid x 10 days	**D/C antibiotic if possible; avoid antimotility agents, hydration, enteric isolation.** Relapse in 10-20% Nitazoxanide 500mg po bid for 7-10 days equivalent to Metro po in phase 3 study (CID 43:428, 2006)
	No meds okay. Sicker: WBC >20,000	Vanco 125 mg po q.i.d. x 10-14 days	Metro 500mg po tid x 10 days	Hints that metro not as effective in more severely ill pts (CID 40:1586, 1591,& 1598, 2005). Relapse in 10-20% not due to resistance (JAC 56:988, 2005)
	Post-treatment relapse	**1st relapse** Metro 500 mg p.o.t.i.d. x 10 days	**2nd relapse** Vanco as above + riff 300mg po bid **3rd relapse**	**3rd relapse** Vanco taper (all doses 125mg po): week 1 – qid; week 2 – bid; week 3 – q24h; week 4 – qod; wks 5&6 – q 3 d. Last resort: stool transplant (CID 36:580, 2003).
	Post-op ileus, severe disease with toxic megacolon			For vanco installation into bowel, add 500mg vanco to 1 liter of saline and perfuse at 1-3ml/min to maximum of 2gm in 24 hrs (CID 690,2002). **Note: IV vanco not effective.** Anecdotal reports of use of IVIG 400mg/kg for 1-3 doses (AAC 53:882, 2004).
	E. coli O157:H7? H/O bloody stools 63%	**NO TREATMENT** with antimicrobials or anti-motility drugs, may precipitate toxin release and ↑ risk of hemolytic uremic syndrome (HUS) (NEJM 342:1930 & 1990, 2000). Hydration important (Ln 365:1073, 2005).		**NOTE:** 5-10% of pts develop HUS (approx. 10% with HUS die or have permanent renal failure; 50% HUS pts have some degree of renal impairment (CID 38:1298, 2004).
	Listeria monocytogenes	AMP 50mg/kg IV q6h	**TMP-SMX** 20mg/kg per day IV div. q6-8h	Recently recognized cause of food poisoning, manifest as febrile gastroenteritis. Percentage with complicating bacteremia/meningitis unknown. Not detected in standard stool culture (NEJM 336:100 & 130, 1997).
	Salmonella, non-typhi For typhoid (enteric) fever, see page 54 Fever in 71–91%, H/O bloody stools in 34%	If pt asymptomatic or illness mild, antimicrobial therapy not indicated. Treat if <1yr old or >50yr old, if immunocompromised, CIP 500mg po bid x 5-7 days. Resistance ↑ (Ln 353:1590, 1999)	if vascular graft or prosthetic joints (see typhoid fever, page 54) **Azithro** 1gm po once, then 500mg q24h x 6 days (AAC 43:1441, 1999)	resistance to TMP-SMX and chloro. Ceftriaxone usually active (see footnote, page 22, for dosage). FQ resistance in SE Asia (CID 40:1315, 2005; Ln 363:1285, 2004). Primary treatment of children is ceftriaxone: electrolyte replacement. No adverse effects from FQs in children (Ln 348:547, 1996). If immunocompromised, rx 14 days.
	Shigella Fever in 58%, H/O bloody stools 51%	FQs p.o.: [CIP 500mg bid] or (Levo 500mg q24h) 3 days	**TMP-SMX-DS,** po bid x 3 days) or (azithro 500mg po x1, then 250 mg q24h x4 days)	**Peds doses:** TMP-SMX 5/25mg/kg po x 3 days. For severe disease, ceftriaxone 50-75mg/kg per day x 2-5 days. CIP suspension 10mg/kg bid x 5 days. (Ln 352:522, 1998) CIP superior to ceftriaxone in children (LnID 3:537, 2003). **Immunocompromised children & adults: Treat for 7-10 days.** Azithro superior to cefixime in trial in children (PIDJ 22:374, 2003).
	Staphylococcus aureus See Comment	See Comment for peds x per dose		Case reports of toxin-mediated pseudomembranous enteritis/colitis (pseudo-membranes in small bowel) (CID 39:747, 2004). **Clinda** to stop toxin production possibly, not validated in specific situations.
	Spirochetosis (Brachyspira pilosicoli)	Vanco 1gm IV q12h + 125mg po q6h	Benefit of treatment unclear. Susceptible to **metro.** ceftriaxone, and **Moxi** (AAC 47:2354, 2003)	Anaerobic intestinal spirochete native to colon of domestic & wild animals plus humans. Case reports of diarrhea with large numbers of the organism (AAC 39:347, 2001; Am J Clin Path 120:828, 2003)

[1] H/O = history of
Abbreviations on page 2.

NOTE: All dosage recommendations are for adults (unless otherwise indicated) and assume normal renal/renal function.

TABLE 1 (14)

ANATOMIC SITE/DIAGNOSIS/ MODIFYING CIRCUMSTANCES	ETIOLOGIES (usual)	SUGGESTED REGIMENS*		ADJUNCT DIAGNOSTIC OR THERAPEUTIC MEASURES AND COMMENTS
		PRIMARY	ALTERNATIVE†	
Gastrointestinal/Gastroenteritis—Specific Therapy (continued)				
(continued from above) **Vibrio cholerae**	Treatment decreases duration of disease, vol. losses, & duration of excretion CID 37:272, 2003; Ln 363:223, 2004	**Primary: Rx is hydration** (see Comment). **Azithromycin** 1gm po once. (NEJM 354:2452, 2500, 2006) Increasing number of failures (11/06).	**Primary: Rx is hydration**. **CIP** 1gm po once but high failure rate. Peds dosage in Comments	Primary: Rx is fluid. **IV** use (per liter): 4gm NaCl, 1gm KCl, 5.4gm Na lactate, 8gm glucose. **PO** use (per liter: potable water): 1 level teaspoon table salt + 4 heaping teaspoons sugar (JTMH 84:73, 1981). Add orange juice or 2 bananas for K+. Volume given — fluid loss. Mild dehydration: give 5% body weight, for moderate, 7% body weight. (Refs. CID 20:1485, 1995; TRSM 89:103, 1995) Peds azithro: 20mg/kg (to 1gm max.) x 1 (Ln 360:1722, 2002); CIP 20mg/kg (Ln 366:1085, 2005).
Vibrio parahaemolyticus		**Antimicrobial rx does not shorten course**. Hydration.		Shellfish exposure common. Treat severe disease: **FQ**, **doxy**, **P. Ceph 3**.
Vibrio vulnificus		(Usual presentation is skin lesions & bacteremia: life-threatening; treat early: **ceftaz** + **doxy**—see page 49.		
Yersinia enterocolitica Fever in 68%, bloody stools in 26%		No treatment unless severe. If severe, combine **doxy** 100mg IV bid + (**tobra** or **genta** 5mg/kg per day once q24h). **TMP-SMX** or **FQs** are alternatives.		Mesenteric adenitis pain can mimic acute appendicitis. Lab diagnosis difficult: requires "cold enrichment" and/or yersinia selective agar. Desferoxamine rx ↑ severity, discontinue if on it. Iron overload states predispose to yersinia (CID 21:1362 & 1367, 1998).
Gastroenteritis—Specific Risk Groups–Empiric Therapy				
Anoreceptive intercourse Proctitis (distal 15 cm only)	Herpes viruses, gonococci, chlamydia, syphilis. See Genital Tract, page 19			
Colitis	Shigella, salmonella, campylobacter, E. histolytica (see Table 13A)			
HIV-1 infected (AIDS): >10 days diarrhea	Cryptosporidium parvum, Cyclospora cayetanensis, Isospora belli, microsporidia (Enterocytozoon bieneusi, Septata intestinalis)			**FQ** (e.g., **CIP** 500mg po) q12h x 3 days. See Table 13A
Acid-fast organisms:				See Table 13A
Other:	As for perirectal abscess, diverticulitis, pg 19. Ensure empiric regimen includes **Clo-** species: e.g., **pen G**, **AMP** or **clinda** (see Comment re: resistance) and activity vs P. aeruginosa also.			See Table 13A Tender right lower quadrant. Surgical resection controversial but may be necessary (see Comment). **NOTE:** Resistance of clostridia to clindamycin reported.
Neutropenic enterocolitis or "typhlitis" (CID 27:695 & 700, 1998)	Usually bacteremia: Occasionally caused by C. sordellii or P. aeruginosa			
Traveler's diarrhea self-medication. Patient usually afebrile	Acute 60% due to toxigenic E. coli, shigella, salmonella, C. jejuni, vibrio, aeromonas, & rarely cyclospora, C. difficile, amebiasis (see Table 13). If chronic: cyclospora, giardia, isospora	**Levo** 500mg po x 1 dose. Alternative: **CIP** or **other FQ** bid x 3 days (see footnote¹). **Imodium** optional: 4mg x 1, then 2mg after each loose stool to max.16mg/day.	**Azithro** 1gm po x 1 dose or 500mg once daily x 3 days or 400mg po bid x 3 days (does not treat Shigella). Alternative during ‡ 3wk & only if activities similar to placebo.	Treatment based on randomized trial (CID 37:1165, 2003). Peds & pregnancy: Avoid FQs. Azithro peds dose: 5–10mg/kg x 1 dose. Rifaximin approved for age 12 or older. Adverse effects similar to placebo. No loperamide if fever or blood in stool. **CIP and rifaximin**-equivalent efficacy vs non-invasive pathogens (AJTMH 74:1060, 2006)
Prevention		Not routinely indicated. Current recommendation is to take **FQ** + **Imodium** with 1st loose stool.	Alternative during ‡ 3wk & only if activities indicated are essential. **Rifaximin** 200mg po bid (AJTMH 74:1060, 2006)	No lopermaide; if fever or blood in stool, the ‡ 3wk & only if activities are essential. **Rifaximin** 200mg po bid (AIM 142:805 & 861, 2005)

¹ **FQ** dosage po for self-rx for traveler's diarrhea—mild disease: **CIP** 750mg x 1; severe 500mg bid x 3 days. **Oflox** 300mg po bid x 3 days. **Levo** 500mg; **Moxi** 400mg probably would work, but not FDA-approved indication.
Abbreviations on page 2. *NOTE: All dosage recommendations are for adults (unless otherwise indicated) and assume normal renal function.*

TABLE 1 (15)

ANATOMIC SITE/DIAGNOSIS/ MODIFYING CIRCUMSTANCES	ETIOLOGIES (usual)	SUGGESTED REGIMENS*		ADJUNCT DIAGNOSTIC OR THERAPEUTIC MEASURES AND COMMENTS
		PRIMARY	ALTERNATIVE¹	
GASTROINTESTINAL (continued) **Gastrointestinal Infections by Anatomic Site: Esophagus to Rectum**				
Esophagitis		See SANFORD GUIDE TO HIV/AIDS THERAPY and Table 11A, page 98		
Duodenal/Gastric ulcer; gastric cancer, MALT lymphomas (not ²⁻⁹ NSAIDs) (NEJM 347:1175, 2002; Can J Gastro 19:399, 2005; Ann Intern Med 144:94, 140, 2006)	**Helicobacter pylori** See Comment Prevalence of pre-treatment resistance increasing	**Rx po for 14 days:** (Omeprazole 20mg¹ + rabeprazole 20mg¹ + amox (gm) + clarithro 500mg. Efficacy 85–95% OR (Rabeprazole 20mg + amox (gm) + clarithro 500mg bid x 5 d. then (rabeprazole 20mg + clarithro 500mg + tinidazole 500mg) bid for another 5 days.	**Rx po for 14 days: Bismuth** (see footnote²), **bismuth subsalicylate 2** tabs qid + **metronidazole** 500mg tid + **tetracycline** 500mg qid x14 + **omeprazole**¹ 20mg bid. Efficacy 90–99%	**Dx: Stool antigen**—Monoclonal EIA >90% sens. & specific. (Amer J Gastro. 101:921, 2006) Other tests: Urea breath test, if endoscoped, rapid urease &/or histology &/or culture. **Antimicrobial resistance: Predicts rx failure** (AnIM 139:463, 2003). Resistance to amox & tetra uncommon; clarithro resistance, up to 23%, metro 20–30% (Dig Liver Dis 35:541, 2003). **Treatment success:** Correlates with active drugs & pt compliance. Suggested **rx duration** varies between 7–14 days; we suggest (big regimen times 14 days to ↑ compliance & hopefully efficacy (7–9% ↑ cures with 14 days) (Aliment Pharmacol Ther 14:603, 2000). **Test of cure:** Repeat stool antigen and/or urea breath test >8 wks post-treatment.
Small intestine: Whipple's disease (CID 32:457, 2001; Ln 363:654, 2004) See Infective endocarditis, culture-negative, page 27	Tropheryma whipplei	**Initial 10–14 days** (Pen G 6–24 million units IV q24h + **streptomycin** 1gm IM/IV q24h) OR **ceftriaxone** 2gm IV q24h **Then, for approx. 1 year** TMP-SMX-DS 1 tab bid	TMP-SMX-DS 1 tab po bid **Doxy** 100mg po bid) or (cotrim 400mg po bid) or (Pen VK 500mg po qid)	Rx regimen based on empiricism and retrospective analyses. TMP-SMX: CNS relapses during TMP-SMX reported. Interesting in vitro susceptibility study: combination of doxy & hydroxychloroquine bactericidal (AAC 45:747, 2004). Cultivated from CSF in pts with intestinal disease and no neurologic findings (JID 188:797 & 801, 2003).
Inflammatory bowel disease: Ulcerative colitis, Crohn's disease Mild to moderate Ref. Ln 359:331, 2002	Unknown	Sulfasalazine 1gm po q6h or mesalamine (5ASA) 1gm po q6h	Coated mesalamine (Asacol) 800mg bid or qid equally effective. Corticosteroid enemas (Gastro 123:33, 2002).	Check stool for E. histolytica. Try aminosalicylates 1³ in mild/mod. disease. See review article for more aggressive therapy.
Severe Crohn's	Unknown	Etanercept	In randomized controlled trial, CIP + metro had no benefit (Gastro 114:A323, 1998). Infliximab/adalimumab¹	Screen for latent TBc before blocking TNF (MMWR 53:683, 2004). If possible, delay anti-TNF drugs until TBc prophylaxis complete. For other anti-TNF risks: NEJM 351:42, 2004

* Can substitute other **proton pump inhibitors** for omeprazole or rabeprazole—all bid: esomeprazole 20mg (FDA-approved), lansoprazole 30mg (FDA-approved), pantoprazole 40mg (not FDA-approved for this indication)

² **3 bismuth preparations:** (1) In U.S., **bismuth subsalicylate** (Pepto-Bismol) 262mg tabs: adult dose for helicobacter is 2 tabs (524 mg) qid. (2) Outside U.S., colloidal bismuth subcitrate (De-Nol) 120mg + metro (or tinidazole) is 1 tablet (120 mg) qid. (3) Another treatment option: Ranitidine bismuth citrate 400mg; give with metro 500mg and clarithro 500mg—all bid times 7 days. Worked despite metro/clarithro resistance (Gastro 114:A323, 1998).

NOTE: All dosage recommendations are for adults (unless otherwise indicated) and assume normal renal function.

Abbreviations on page 2.

TABLE 1 (16)

ANATOMIC SITE/DIAGNOSIS/ MODIFYING CIRCUMSTANCES	ETIOLOGIES (usual)	SUGGESTED REGIMENS* PRIMARY	ALTERNATIVE‡	ADJUNCT DIAGNOSTIC OR THERAPEUTIC MEASURES AND COMMENTS
GASTROINTESTINAL/Gastrointestinal Infections by Anatomic Site: Esophagus to Rectum (continued)				
Diverticulitis, perirectal abscess; occ. P. aeruginosa Also see Peritonitis, page 42 CID (in press)	Enterobacteriaceae, occ. P. aeruginosa, Bacteroides sp., enterococci	**Outpatient rx—mild diverticulitis, drained perirectal abscess:** [TMP-SMX-DS bid] or CIP 750mg bid or **Levo** 750mg bid + **metro** 500mg q6h. All po x 7-10 days **Inpatient rx—moderate disease** (e.g., focal peri-appendiceal phlegmon, peri-diverticular abscess, endomyometritis): **PIP-TZ** 3.375gm IV q6h or 4.5gm IV q8h or **AM-SB** 3gm IV q6h, **or TC-CL** 3.1gm IV q4-6h **or ERTA** 1gm IV q24h **or MOXI** 400mg IV q24h **Severe life-threatening disease, ICU patient:** **IMP** 500mg IV q6h or **MER** 1gm IV q8h	**AM-CL-ER** 1000/62.5mg (2 tabs po bid x 7-10 days) **OR Moxi** 400mg po q24h **—Inpatient—Parenteral Rx:** (**CIP** 400mg IV q12h) or **Levo** 750mg IV q24h) + **metro** 500mg IV q6h or 1gm IV q12h) **OR tigecycline** 100mg IV x1 dose & then 50mg IV q12h **OR APAG** (see Table 10D, page 93) **AMP + metro + (CIP** 400mg IV q12h or **Levo** 750mg IV q24h) **OR AMP** 2gm IV q6h + **metro** 500mg IV q6h + **APAG** (see Table 10D, page 93)	Must "cover" both Gm-neg, aerobic & Gm-neg, anaerobic bacteria. **Drugs active vs anaerobes:** clinda, cefotetan, cefoxitin, AP Pen, CIP, Levo. **Drugs active vs aerobic Gm-neg bacilli:** APAG, P-Ceph 2/3/4, aztreonam, AP Pen, CIP. **Drugs active vs both aerobic/anaerobic Gm-neg. bacteria:** cefotetan, cefoxitin, TC-CL, PIP-TZ, AM-SB, ERTA, IMP, MER, Moxi, & tigecycline. Increasing resistance of Bacteroides species: Cefoxitin Cefotetan Clindamycin % Resistant: 4-25 17-87 16-44 Resistance to metro, PIP-TZ rare (CID 35(Suppl 1):S126, 2002). Few case reports of metro resistance (CID 40:e67, 2005; J Clin Micro 42:4127, 2004). Resistance mechanisms reviewed: CID 39:92, 2004). **Ertapenem** less active vs P. aeruginosa/Acinetobacter sp., than IMP or MER. Concomitant surgical management important, esp. with moderate-severe disease. **Role of enterococci remains debatable.** Probably pathogenic in infections of biliary tract. Probably need drugs active vs enterococci in pts with valvular heart disease.
GENITAL TRACT: Mixture of empiric & specific treatment. Divided by sex of patient. For sexual assault (rape), see Table 15A, page 159. See Guidelines for Dx of Sexually Transmitted Diseases, MMWR 55 (RR-11), 2006.				
Both Women & Men:				
Chancroid	H. ducreyi	**Ceftriaxone** 250mg IM single dose OR **azithro** 1gm po single dose.	**CIP** 500mg bid po x 3 days OR **erythro base** 500mg po qid po x7 days	In HIV+ pts, failures reported with single-dose azithro & N gonorrhoeae. Evaluate after 7 days, ulcer should objectively improve.
Chlamydia, et al. non-gonococcal or post-gonococcal urethritis, cervicitis. **NOTE: Assume concomitant gonorrhea.** Chlamydia conjunctivitis, see page 11	Chlamydia 50%, Mycoplasma hominis. Other known etiologies (10-15%): trichomonas, herpes simplex virus, Mycoplasma genitalium. Ref: JID 193:333, 336, 2006.	(**Doxy** 100mg bid po x 7 days) or (**azithro** 1gm po as single dose). Evaluate & rx sex partner **In pregnancy: erythro base** 500mg po qid x 7 days OR **amox** 500mg po tid x 7 days	(**Erythro base** 500mg po q6h x 7 days) or (**Oflox** 300mg q12h po x 7 days) or (**Levo** 500mg q24h x 7 days) **In pregnancy: azithro** 1gm po x1 dose **Doxy & Oflox contra-indicated**	**Diagnosis:** Nucleic acid amplification tests for C. trachomatis & N. gonorrhoeae on urine samples equivalent to cervix or urethra specimens (AnIM 142:914, 2005). **For recurrent or persistent disease:** either metro 2gm po x1 + either erythro base 500mg po qid x 7 days or erythro ethylsuccinate 800mg po qid x 7 days Evaluate & treat sex partners. **For recurrent or persistent NGU** (metro or tinidazole 2gm po x 1 dose) plus azithro 1 gm po x1 dose.
Recurrent/persistent urethritis	Occult trichomonas, tetra-resistant U. urealyticum	**Metro** 2gm po x1 + **erythro base** 500mg po qid x 7 days	**Erythro ethylsuccinate** 800mg po qid x 7 days	In men with NGU, 20% infected with trichomonas (JID 188:465, 2003).

* APAG = antipseudomonal aminoglycosidic aminoglycoside, e.g., amikacin, gentamicin, tobramycin

‡ NOTE: All dosage recommendations are for adults (unless otherwise indicated) and assume normal renal function.

Abbreviations on page 2.

TABLE 1 (17)

ANATOMIC SITE/DIAGNOSIS/ MODIFYING CIRCUMSTANCES	ETIOLOGIES (usual)	SUGGESTED REGIMENS*		ADJUNCT DIAGNOSTIC OR THERAPEUTIC MEASURES AND COMMENTS
		PRIMARY	ALTERNATIVE[1]	
GENITAL TRACT: Both Women & Men (continued)				
Gonorrhea [MMWR 55 (RR-11), 2006]				
Conjunctivitis (adult)	N. gonorrhoeae	**Ceftriaxone** 1gm IM or IV times one dose		Consider saline lavage of eye times 1
Disseminated gonococcal infection (DGI, dermatitis-arthritis syndrome)	N. gonorrhoeae	[**Ceftriaxone** 1gm IV q24h) or **cefotaxime** 1gm q8h IV) or (**ceftizoxime** 1gm q8h IV)—see Comment	**Spectinomycin** 2gm IM q12h or **CIP** 400mg IV q12h or **Oflox** 400mg IV q12h or **Levo** 250mg IV q24h—see Comment	Continue IM or IV regimen for 24hr after symptoms ↓; reliable pts may be discharged 24hr after sx resolve to complete 7 days rx with **cefixime 400mg po bid or Oflox 400 mg po bid or Levo 500mg po q24h**. **Treat presumptively for concomitant C. trachomatis**. Avoid FQs in MSM.
Endocarditis	N. gonorrhoeae	**Ceftriaxone** 1–2gm IV q12h x 4wk		R/O meningitis/ endocarditis. Avoid FQs in MSM
Pharyngitis	N. gonorrhoeae	**Ceftriaxone** 125mg IM x 1	**CIP** 500mg po x 1 or **Levo** 250mg po x 1. Avoid FQs in MSM.	If chlamydia not ruled out: Azithro 1gm po x 1 or doxy 100mg po bid x 7 days. Some suggest test of cure culture after 1wk. Spectinomycin not effective
Urethritis, cervicitis, proctitis (uncomplicated) For prostatitis, see page 23 **Diagnosis**: Nucleic acid amplification test (NAAT) on urine or urethral swab—see MMWR 51 (RR-15), 2002	FQ-sensitive N. gonorrhoeae (50% of pts with urethritis, cervicitis have concomitant C. trachomatis —**treat for both unless NAAT indicates single pathogen**).	[(**Ceftriaxone** 125mg IM x 1) or (**cefpodoxime** 400mg po x 1) or (**Oflox** 400mg po x 1) or (**Azithro** 1gm po x 1)] **PLUS** — **if chlamydia infection not ruled out**: [(**doxy** 100mg po q12h x 7 days)]	[(**Ceftriaxone** 125mg IM x 1) or (**cefpodoxime** 400mg po x 1) or (**CIP** 500mg po x 1) or (**Levo** 250mg po x 1)] **PLUS** — **if chlamydia infection not ruled out**: [(**Azithro** 1gm po x 1) or (**doxy** 100mg po q12h x 7 days)]	**Treat for both GC and C. trachomatis unless single pathogen by NAAT.** Screen for syphilis. Other alternatives for **GC**: Spectinomycin[²] 2 gm IM x 1 Other single-dose cephalosporins: ceftizoxime 500mg IM, cefoxitin 2gm IM + probenecid 1gm po, cefotaxime 500mg IM. Azithro 1gm po x1 effective for chlamydia but need 2gm po for GC; not recommended for GC due to GI side-effects and expense. Should not use quinolones in MSM or if recent foreign travel or infection acquired in California or Hawaii or other areas with ↑ FQ resistance
	Risk of FQ-R gonorrhoeae	Treatment for (see comment): Ceftriaxone 125mg IM x 1 dose. **No FQ. PLUS**, if Chlamydia not ruled out: **azithro** 1gm po x 1 dose or **doxy** 100mg po q12h x 7 days.	Treatment for men-sex-with men or heterosexuals with recent travel (see comment): **Ceftriaxone** 125mg IM x 1 dose or **cefixime** 400mg po x 1 dose. **No FQ. PLUS**, if Chlamydia not ruled out: **azithro** 1gm po x 1 dose or **doxy** 100mg po q12h x 7 days.	
Granuloma inguinale (Donovanosis)	Klebsiella (formerly Calymmatobacterium) granulomatis	**Doxy** 100mg po bid x 3–4wks OR **TMP-SMX-DS** q12h x 3wk	**Erytho** 500mg po qid x 3wks OR **CIP** 750mg po qid x 3wks or **azithro** 1gm po wk x 3wks	Clinical response usually seen in 1wk. Rx until all lesions healed, may take 4wk. Treatment failures & recurrence seen with doxy & TMP-SMX. Report of efficacy with FQ and chloro. Ref: CID 25:24, 1997
Herpes simplex virus	See Table 14A, page 139			
Human papilloma virus (HPV)	See Table 14A, page 144			
Lymphogranuloma venereum	Chlamydia trachomatis, serovars L1, L2, L3	**Doxy** 100mg po bid x 21 days	**Erytho** 0.5gm po qid x 21 days	Dx based on serology; biopsy contraindicated because sinus tracts develop. Nucleic acid amplif tests for C. trachomatis will be positive. Specific LGV genotyping not widely available
Pthirus pubis (public lice, "crabs") & scabies	Phthirus pubis & Sarcoptes scabiei	See Table 13, page 130		

Abbreviations on page 2.   NOTE: All dosage recommendations are for adults (unless otherwise indicated) and assume normal renal/renal function.

TABLE 1 (18)

ANATOMIC SITE/DIAGNOSIS/ MODIFYING CIRCUMSTANCES	ETIOLOGIES (usual)	SUGGESTED REGIMENS*		ADJUNCT DIAGNOSTIC OR THERAPEUTIC MEASURES AND COMMENTS
		PRIMARY	ALTERNATIVE[1]	
GENITAL TRACT/Both Women & Men (continued)				
Syphilis (JAMA 290:1510, 2003), **Syphilis & HIV:** (JID LnID 4:456, 2004; MMWR 53:RR-15, 2004 and 55: RR-11, 2006				
Early: primary, secondary, or latent <1yr	T. pallidum NOTE: Test all pts with syphilis for HIV; test all HIV patients for latent syphilis.	**Benzathine pen G (Bicillin L-A)** 2.4 million units: IM x1 NOTE: **Azithro** 2gm po x1 dose efficacious. Worry about emerging azithro resistance. [See Comment]	**[Doxy** 100mg po bid x 14 days] or **[tetracycline** 500mg po qid x days] or **(ceftriaxone** 1gm IM/IV q24h x 8-10 days). Follow-up mandatory.	If early or congenital syphilis, **quantitate VDRL at 0**, 3, 6, 12 & 24 mo. after rx. If '1' or '2' syphilis, VDRL should ⤓ 4 titers by 6mo., 3 titers 12mo, & 4 titers 24mo. Early latent: 2 tubes→4 at 12mo. With '1', 50% will be RPR seronegative at 12mo.; 24% neg. FTA/ABS at 2-3yrs (AnIM 114:1005, 1991). If titers fail to fall: examine CSF; if CSF (+), treat as neurosyphilis; if CSF is negative, retreat with benzathine Pen G 2.4 m.u. IM x 3wks. **Azithro-resistant syphilis** documented in California, Ireland, & elsewhere (NEJM 351:122 & 154; 2004; SCID 28; 1291, 2005). NOTE: Use of **benzathine procaine penicillin G** is inappropriate!
More than 1 yr's duration (latent of indeterminate duration, cardiovascular, late benign gumma)		**Benzathine pen G (Bicillin L-A)** 2.4 million units: IM q.week x 3 = 7.2 million units total	**Doxy** 100mg po bid x 28 days or **tetracycline** 500mg po qid x 28 days	No published data on efficacy of alternatives. The value of routine lumbar puncture in asymptomatic late syphilis is being questioned in the U.S., i.e.: no LP, rx all patients except where neurologic symptoms, treatment failure, serum non-treponemal antibody titer ≥1:32, other evidence of active syphilis **Indications for LP (CDC): neurologic symptoms, treatment failure, serum non-treponemal antibody titer ≥1:32, other evidence of active syphilis (aortitis, gumma, iritis), and/or penicillin Tx, + HIV test.**
Neurosyphilis—Very difficult to treat. Includes ocular (retrobulbar neuritis) syphilis **All need CSF exam.**		**Pen G** 3-4 million units IV q4h x 10-14 days.	**(Procaine pen G** 2.4 million units: IM q24h + **probenecid** 0.5gm po qid) both x 10-14 days—See Comment	**Ceftriaxone** 2gm (IV or IM) q24h x 14 days. 23% failure rate reported (AJM 93:481, 1992). For penicillin allergy: either desensitize to penicillin or obtain infectious diseases consultation. **Serologic criteria for response to rx: 4-fold or greater ⤓ in VDRL titer over 6-12mo.** (CID 28 (Suppl. 1):S21, 1999).
HIV Infection (AIDS) (See SANFORD GUIDE TO HIV/AIDS THERAPY & refs. in Comments)		Treatment same as HIV uninfected in all stages of syphilis		HIV + plus RPR≥1:32 plus CD4 count ≤350/mcL increases risk of neurosyphilis (JID 189:369, 2004). Recommend CSF exam, of all HIV+ pts regardless of stage of syphilis. With treatment, VDRL/RPR titers slow to normalize (CID 38:1001, 2004). Reviews of syphilis & HIV: LnID 4:456, 2004; MMWR 53:RR-15, 2004.
Pregnancy and syphilis		Same as for non-pregnant, some recommend 2nd dose: (2.4 million units) **benzathine pen G** 1wk. after initial dose esp. in 3rd trimester or with 2° syphilis	Skin test for penicillin allergy. Desensitize if necessary, as parenteral pen G is only therapy with documented efficacy	Monthly quantitative VDRL or equivalent. If 4-fold ↑, re-treat. Doxy, tetracycline contraindicated. Erythro not recommended because of high risk of failure to cure fetus.
Congenital syphilis	T. pallidum	**Aqueous crystalline pen G** 50,000 units/kg/dose IV q12h x 7 days, then q8h for 10-day total	**Procaine pen G** 50,000 units/kg IM q24h for 10 days	Another alternative: Ceftriaxone ≥30 days old, 75mg/kg IV/IM q24h; or >30 days old 100mg/kg IV/IM q24h. Treat 10-14 days. If symptomatic, ophthalmologic exam indicated. If more than 1 day of rx missed, restart entire course. **Need serologic follow-up!**
Warts, anogenital		See Table 14, page 140		

Abbreviations on page 2.   *NOTE: All dosage recommendations are for adults (unless otherwise indicated) and assume normal renal function.*

TABLE 1 (19)

ANATOMIC SITE/DIAGNOSIS/ MODIFYING CIRCUMSTANCES	ETIOLOGIES (usual)	SUGGESTED REGIMENS*		ADJUNCT DIAGNOSTIC OR THERAPEUTIC MEASURES AND COMMENTS
		PRIMARY	ALTERNATIVE‡	
GENITAL TRACT (continued)				
Women:				
Amnionitis, septic abortion	Bacteroides, esp. Prevotella bivius; Group B, A strepto- cocci; Enterobacteriaceae; C. trachomatis	[(**Cefoxitin** or **TC-CL** or **IMP** or **MER** or **AM-SB** or **ERTA** or **PIP-TZ**) **+ doxy**] **OR** [**Clinda + (APAG** or **P Ceph 3**)] *Dosage: see footnote¹*		D&C of uterus. **In septic abortion,** Clostridium perfringens may cause fulminant intravascular hemolysis. **In postpartum patients** with enigmatic fever and/or pulmonary emboli, **consider septic pelvic vein thrombophlebitis** (see Vascular, septic pelvic vein thrombophlebitis, page 58). After discharge: doxy or continue clinda. **NOTE:** IV clinda effective for C. trachomatis, no data on po clinda (CID 19(720, 1994).
Cervicitis, mucopurulent Treatment based on results of nucleic acid amplification test	N. gonorrhoeae Chlamydia trachomatis	Treat for Gonorrhea, page 20 Treat for non-gonococcal urethritis, page 19		Criteria for dx: yellow or green pus on cervical swab, >10 WBC/oil field. Gram stain for GC, if negative rx for C. trachomatis. If in doubt, send swab or urine for culture, EIA or nucleic acid amplification test and rx for both.
Endomyometritis/septic pelvic phlebitis Early postpartum (1st–48 hrs) (usually after C-section)	Bacteroides, esp. Prevotella bivius; Group B, A strepto- cocci; Enterobacteriaceae; C. trachomatis	[(**Cefoxitin** or **TC-CL** or **ERTA** or **IMP** or **MER** or **AM-SB** or **PIP-TZ**) **+ doxy**] OR [**Clinda + (APAG** or **P Ceph 3**)] *Dosage: see footnote¹*		See Comments under Amnionitis, septic abortion, above
Late postpartum (48 hrs to 6 wks) (usually after vaginal delivery	Chlamydia trachomatis, M. hominis	**Doxy** 100 mg IV or po q12h times 14 days		Tetracyclines not recommended in nursing mothers; discontinue nursing. M. hominis sensitive to tetra, clinda, not erythro (CCTID 17:5200, 1993).
Fitzhugh-Curtis syndrome	C. trachomatis, N. gonorrhoeae	Treat as for pelvic inflammatory disease immediately below		Perihepatitis (violin-string adhesions)
Pelvic Inflammatory Disease (PID), salpingitis, tubo-ovarian abscess				
Outpatient rx: limit to pts with temp <38° C, WBC <11,000 per mm³, minimal evidence of peritonitis, active bowel sounds & able to tolerate oral nourishment	N. gonorrhoeae, chlamydia, bacteroides, Enterobacteria- ceae, streptococci	**Outpatient rx:** [(**Oflox** 400mg po bid or **Levo** 500mg po q24h)] ± **metro** 500 mg po bid x 14 days] **OR** [(**ceftriaxone** 250 mg IM or IV x 1) + **metro** 500mg po bid x 14 days) + **doxy** 100mg po bid x 14 days)]	**Ingatient regimens:** [(**cefotetan** 2gm IV q12h or **cefoxitin** 2gm IV q6h) + **doxy** 100mg IV/po q12h] **OR** [**Clinda** 900mg IV q8h + **gentamicin** 2mg/kg loading dose, then 1.5mg/kg q8h or 4.5mg/kg once per day), then **doxy** 100mg po bid x 14 days	Alternative parenteral regimens: 1. **Oflox** 400mg IV q12h or **Levo** 500mg IV q24h) + **metro** 500mg IV q8h 2. **AM-SB** 3gm IV q6h + **doxy** 100mg IV/po q12h] + Another alternative: **Moxi** 400mg po q24h + **metro** 500mg po bid x 14 d (Sex Trans Dis 2006, e-pub) Note: Remember increasing prevalence of fluroquinolone-resistant N. gonorrhoeae

¹ **P Ceph 2** (**cefotetan** 2gm IV q6-8h, **cefotetan** 2gm IV q12h, **cefuroxime** 750mg IV q8h). **TC-CL** 3.1gm IV q4-6h; **AM-SB** 3gm IV q6h; for nosocomial pneumonia: 4.5gm IV q8h; **PIP-TZ** 3.375gm q6h or for nosocomial pneumonia, 4.5gm IV q6h, **doxy** 100mg IV/po q12h; **clinda** 450-900mg IV q8h; **APAG** (gentamicin, see *Table 10D, page 100*), **P Ceph 3 (cefotaxime** 2gm IV q24h), **ceftriaxone** 2gm IV q24h), **cefotaxime** 2gm IV q24h); **ertapenem** 1gm IV q24h; **IMP** 0.5gm IV q6h; **MER** 1gm IV q8h; **azithro** 500mg IV q24h; **linezolid** 600mg IV/po q12h; **vanco** 1gm IV q12h.

NOTE: All dosage recommendations are for adults (unless otherwise indicated) and assume normal renal function.

Abbreviations on page 2.

TABLE 1 (20)

ANATOMIC SITE/DIAGNOSIS/ MODIFYING CIRCUMSTANCES	ETIOLOGIES (usual)	SUGGESTED REGIMENS* PRIMARY	ALTERNATIVE[1]	ADJUNCT DIAGNOSTIC OR THERAPEUTIC MEASURES AND COMMENTS
GENITAL TRACT/Women (continued)				
Vaginitis—*MMWR 51(RR-6), 2002 or CID 35 (Suppl.2):S135, 2002*				
Candidiasis Itching, thick, cheesy discharge, pH <4.5 See Table 11A, page 98	Candida albicans 80-90%, C. glabrata, C. tropicalis may be increasing—they are less susceptible to azoles	**Oral azoles:** Fluconazole 150mg po x 1: **Itraconazole** 200mg po bid x 1 day	**Intravaginal azoles:** variety of strengths—from 1 dose to 7-14 days. Drugs available (all end in -azole): butocon, clotrim, micon, ticocon, tercon (doses: Table 11A, footnote page 99)	Nystatin vag. tabs times 14 days less effective. Other rx for azole-resistant strains: gentian violet, boric acid. If recurrent candidiasis (4 or more episodes per yr): 6 mos. suppression with: fluconazole 150 mg po q week or itraconazole 100 mg po q24h or clotrimazole vag. suppositories 500 mg q week.
Trichomoniasis Copious, frothy discharge, pH >4.5 Treat sexual partners—see Comment	Trichomonas vaginalis	**Metro** 2gm as single dose or 500mg po bid x 7 days OR **Tinidazole** 2gm po single dose **Pregnancy:** See Comment	**Rx of failure:** Re-treat with metro 500mg po bid x 7 days; if 2nd failure: metro 2gm po q24h x 3-5 days. If still failure, suggest ID consultation and/or contact CDC: 770-488-4115 or www.cdc.gov/std.	**Treat male sexual partners (2 gm metronidazole as single dose)** Nearly 20% men with NGU are infected with trichomonas (JID 188:465, 2003). Another option if metro-resistant: **Tinidazole** 500mg po bid x 14 days. Ref. CID 33:1341, 2001. **Pregnancy:** No data indicating metro teratogenic or mutagenic [MMWR 51(RR-6), 2002].
Bacterial vaginosis Malodorous vaginal discharge, pH >4.5 Date on recurrence & review: JID 193:1475,2006	Polymicrobic: associated with Gardnerella vaginalis, mobiluncus., Mycoplasma hominis, Prevotella sp., & Atopobium vaginae et al.	**Metro** 0.5gm po bid x 7 days or **metro vaginal gel** (1 applicator intra-vaginally) 1x/day bid x 5 days.	**Clinda** 0.3gm po bid x 7 days or 2% **clinda vaginal cream** 5gm intravaginally at bedtime x 7 days or **clinda ovules** 100mg intravaginally at bedtime x 3 days.	Rx of male sex partner **not** indicated unless balanitis present. **Metro 2gm po x 1 dose not as effective as 5-7 day course** (JAMA 268:92, 1992). Metro extended release tabs 750mg po q24h x 7 days available; no published data. **Pregnancy:** Rx same as non-pregnancy, except avoid clindamycin cream (↑ risk premature birth). Atopobium resistant to metro in vitro; suscept. To clinda (BMC Inf Dis 6:51, 2006)
Men:				
Balanitis	Candida 40%, Group B strep, gardnerella	Oral azoles as for vaginitis		Occurs in 1/4 of male sex partners of women infected with candida. Exclude circinate balanitis (Reiter's syndrome). Plasma cell balanitis (non-infectious) responds to hydrocortisone cream.
Epididymo-orchitis				
Age < 35 years	N. gonorrhoeae, Chlamydia trachomatis	**Ceftriaxone** 250mg IM x 1 + **doxy** 100mg po bid x 10 days		Also: bedrest, scrotal elevation, and analgesics.
Age > 35 years or homosexual men (insertive partners in anal intercourse)	N. gonorrhoeae, Enterobacteriaceae (coliforms)	**FQ: CIP-ER** 500mg po 1x/day or **CIP** 400mg IV 1x/day or **Levo** 750mg IV/po 1x/day x10-14 days	**AM-SB**, **P Ceph 3**, **TC-CL**, **PIP-TZ** (Dosage: see footnote page 22)	Midstream pyuria and scrotal pain and edema. Also: bedrest, scrotal elevation, and analgesics.
Non-gonococcal urethritis—See Chlamydia et al; Non-gonococcal urethritis, Table 1(16), page 19				
Prostatitis—Review: AJM 106:327, 1999				
Acute ≤ 35 years of age	N. gonorrhoeae, C. trachomatis	**Oflox** 400mg po x 1 then 300mg po bid x 10 days or **ceftriaxone** 250mg IM x 1 then **doxy** 100mg bid x 10 days		Oflox effective vs gonococci & C. trachomatis and penetrates prostate. In AIDS pts, prostate may be focus of Cryptococcus neoformans.

[1] 1 applicator contains 5 gm of gel with 37.5 mg metronidazole
Abbreviations on page 2.   *NOTE: All dosage recommendations are for adults (unless otherwise indicated) and assume normal renal function.*

TABLE 1 (21)

ANATOMIC SITE/DIAGNOSIS/ MODIFYING CIRCUMSTANCES	ETIOLOGIES (usual)	SUGGESTED REGIMENS*		ADJUNCT DIAGNOSTIC OR THERAPEUTIC MEASURES AND COMMENTS
		PRIMARY	ALTERNATIVE†	
GENITAL TRACT/Men/Prostatitis (continued)				
≥35 years of age	Enterobacteriaceae (coliforms)	**FQ** (dosage: see Epididymo-orchitis, >35 yrs., above) or **TMP-SMX** 1 DS tablet (160mg TMP) po bid x 10–14 days	**TMP-SMX-DS** 1 tab po bid x 1–3mo	Treat as acute urinary infection, 14 days (not single-dose regimen). Some authorities recommend 3–4wk rx (IDCP 4:325, 1995).
Chronic bacterial	Enterobacteriaceae 80%, enterococci 15%, P. aeruginosa	**FQ** (**CIP** 500mg po bid x 4wk; **Levo** 750mg po q24h x 4wk—see **Comment**)		With rx failures consider infected prostatic calculi
Chronic prostatitis/chronic pelvic pain syndrome (New classification, JAMA 282:236, 1999)	Etiology is unknown; molecular probe data suggest infectious etiology (Clin Micro Rev 11:604, 1998)	**α-adrenergic blocking agents are controversial** (AnIM 133:367, 2000).		Pt has six of prostatitis but negative cultures and no cells in prostatic secretions. Rev: JAC 46:157, 2000. In randomized double-blind study, CIP and an alpha-blocker of no benefit (AnIM 141:581 & 639, 2004).
HAND (Bites: See Skin)				
Paronychia				
Nail biting, manicuring	Staph. aureus (maybe MRSA)	I&D; db culture	**TMP-SMX-DS** 2 tabs po bid while waiting for culture result.	See Table 6 for alternatives
Contact with oral mucosa—dentists, anesthesiologists, wrestlers	Herpes simplex (Whitlow)	**Acyclovir** 400mg tid po x 10 days	**Famciclovir** or **valacyclovir** should work; see **Comment**	Gram stain and routine culture negative. Famciclovir/valacyclovir doses used for primary genital herpes should work; see Table 14, page 138.
Dishwasher (prolonged water immersion)	Candida sp.	**Clotrimazole** (topical)		Avoid immersion of hands in water as much as possible.
HEART				
Infective endocarditis—Native valve—empirical rx awaiting cultures—No IV illicit drugs Valvular or congenital heart disease including mitral valve prolapse but no modifying circumstances See Table 15C, page 162 for prophylaxis	NOTE: Diagnostic criteria include evidence of continuous bacteremia (multiple positive blood cultures), definite emboli, and echocardiographic (transthoracic or transesophageal) evidence of valvular vegetations. Viridans strep 30–40%, 'other' strep 15–25%, enterococci 5–18%, staphylococci 20–35%	(Pen G 20 million units IV q24h, continuous iv div. q4h) or (AMP 12gm IV q24h, continuous iv div. q4h) + (nafcillin or oxacillin 2gm IV q4h) + gentamicin 1mg/kg IM or IV q8h (see Comment)	(Vanco 15mg/kg† IV q12h (not to exceed 2gm q24h unless serum levels monitored) + gentamicin 1mg/kg† IM or IV q8h) OR dapto 6mg/kg IV q24h	If patient not acutely ill and not in heart failure, we prefer to wait for blood culture results. If initial 3 blood cultures neg. after 24–48 hrs, obtain 2–3 more blood cultures before empiric rx started. Nafcillin/oxacillin + gentamicin may not be adequate coverage of enterococci, hence addition of penicillin G pending cultures. When blood cultures +, modify regimen from empiric to specific based on organism in vitro susceptibilities, clinical experience. **Gentamicin** used for synergy; peak levels need not exceed 4 mcg per mL.
Infective endocarditis—Native valve—IV illicit drug use ± evidence rt-sided endocarditis—empiric rx	S. aureus All others rare	**Vanco** 1gm IV q12h	**Dapto** 6mg/kg IV q24h. Approved for right-sided endocarditis.	Quinupristin-dalfopristin cidal vs S. aureus if both constituents active. In controlled clinical trial, dapto equivalent to vanco plus initial gentamicin for right-sided endocarditis.

---

* Assumes estimated creatinine clearance ≥80 mL per min., see Table 17.
Abbreviations on page 2.   NOTE: All dosage recommendations are for adults (unless otherwise indicated) and assume normal renal function.

† Assumes estimated creatinine clearance ≥80 mL per min (unless otherwise indicated) and assume normal renal function.

TABLE 1 (22)

ANATOMIC SITE/DIAGNOSIS/ MODIFYING CIRCUMSTANCES	ETIOLOGIES (usual)	SUGGESTED REGIMENS* PRIMARY	ALTERNATIVE¹	ADJUNCT DIAGNOSTIC OR THERAPEUTIC MEASURES* AND COMMENTS
HEART *(continued)*				
Infective endocarditis—Native valve—culture positive *(NEJM 345:1318, 2001; CID 36:615, 2003; JAC 54:971, 2004¹)*				
Viridans strep, S. bovis. Viridans strep, S. bovis (S. gallolyticus) with **penicillin G MIC <0.1mcg/mL**. **Note:** New name for S. bovis; biotype 1 is S. gallolyticus.	Viridans strep, S. bovis	[(Pen G 12–18 million units/day IV (divided q4h) **x 2wks**) PLUS **gentamicin** 1mg/kg IV q8h **x2wks)]** **OR** (Pen G 12–18 million units/day IV (divided q4h) **x 4wks)** OR **ceftriaxone** 2gm IV q24h x 4wks]	[(Ceftriaxone 2gm IV q24h + **gentamicin** 1mg per kg IV q8h) x 2wks, or (ceftriaxone 2gm IV q24h). If very obese pt, recommend consultation for dosage adjustment. Infuse vanco over >1 hr to avoid "red man" syndrome. Since relapse rate may be greater in pts ill for >3 mos. prior to start of rx, the pen G or ceftriaxone; use **vanco** 15mg/kg IV q12h to 2gm/day max unless serum levels measured] **x 4 wks**	Also effective: (ceftriaxone 2gm IV q24h) + (netilmicin[NUS] 4mg/kg q24h) x2 wks (CID 21:1406, 1995). Target gent levels: peak 3mcg/mL, trough <1 mcg/mL. If penicillinase-producing or dosage adjustment. **S. bovis suggests occult bowel pathology (new name: S. gallolyticus).** relapse rate may be greater in pts ill for > 3 mos. prior to start of rx, the penicillin-gentamicin synergism theoretically may be advantageous in this group. **Dropped option of continuous infusion of Pen G due to instability in acidic IV fluids, rapid renal clearance and rising MICs (AAC 48:4463, 2004).** **NOTE: If necessary to remove infected valve & valve culture neg., 2 weeks antibiotic treatment post-op sufficient (CID 41:187, 2005).**
Viridans strep, S. bovis, nutritionally variant streptococci, (e.g. abiotrophia) tolerant strep.	Viridans strep, S. bovis (S. gallolyticus) with **penicillin G MIC >0.1 to <0.5mcg/mL**	Pen G 18 million units/day x 4 wks PLUS **gentamicin** 1 mg/kg IV q8h **x 2 wks** **NOTE: Low dose of gentamicin**	**Vanco** 15 mg/kg IV q12h to max 2 gm/day unless serum levels documented **x 4 wks**	Can use cefazolin for pen G in pt with allergy, that is not IgE-mediated (e.g., anaphylaxis). Alternatively, can use vanco. (See Comment above on gent and vanco)
For viridans strep or S. bovis with **pen G MIC >0.5** and enterococci (see below), all enterococci causable to AMP/pen G/ampi, and endocarditis (see below), all enterococci variant strep (new names are: Abiotrophia sp. & Granulicatella sp.).	For viridans strep or S. bovis with **pen G MIC >0.5** and enterococci susceptible to AMP/pen G. NOTE: Inf. Dis. consultation suggested	[(Pen G 18–30 million units per 24h IV, divided q4h **x 4–6 wks)** PLUS (gentamicin 1.5 mg/kg IV q8h)] OR [(**AMP** 12 gm/day IV, divided q4h + **gent** as above **x 4–6 wks)**	**Vanco** 15 mg/kg IV q12h to max of 2 gm/day unless serum levels measured **x 4–6 wks** PLUS 1.5 mg/kg q8h IV x **4–6 wks** **NOTE: Low dose of gent**	4 wks of rx if symptoms <3 mos.; 6 wks of rx if symptoms >3 mos. Vanco for pen-allergic pts; do not use cephalosporins. Do not give gent once-q24h for enterococcal endocarditis. Target gent levels: peak 3 mcg/mL, trough 1 mcg/mL. Vanco target serum levels: peak 20–50 mcg/mL, trough 5–12 mcg/mL. **NOTE: Because of ↑ frequency of resistance (see below), all enterococci causing endocarditis should be tested in vitro for susceptibility to penicillin, β-lactamase production, gent susceptibility and vanco susceptibility.** 10–25% E. faecalis and 45–50% E. faecium resistant to high gent levels. May be sensitive to streptomycin, check MIC. (Case report of success with combination of AMP, IMP, and vanco (Scand J Inf Dis 23:628, 1997).
Enterococci, high-level aminoglycoside resistance	Enterococci, high-level aminoglycoside resistance	Pen G or AMP IV as above **x 8–12 wks** (approx. 50% cure)	If prolonged pen G/AMP fails, consider surgical removal of infected valve. See Comment.	
Enterococci: MIC streptomycin >2000 mcg/mL, MIC gentamicin >500–2000 mcg/mL, no resistance to penicillin	Enterococci, penicillin resistance	**AM-SB** 3gm IV q6h PLUS **gentamicin** 1–1.5mg/kg q8h IV x **4–6 wks. Low dose of gent**	**AM-SB** 3 gm IV q6h PLUS **vanco** 15 mg/kg IV q12h (check levels if >2 gm) **x 4–6 wks**	β-lactamase not detected by MIC tests with standard inocula. Detection requires testing with the chromogenic cephalosporin in an animal model of E. faecalis endocarditis (JAC 49:437, 2002). **Once-q24h gentamicin rx** is not recommended.
Enterococci: β-lactamase production positive & no penicillin resistance.	Enterococci, penicillin resistance	**AM-SB** 3gm IV q6h PLUS **gentamicin** 1.5mg/kg q8h IV x **4–6 wks. Low dose of gent**	**Vanco** 15mg/kg IV q12h PLUS **gent** 1–1.5mg/kg q8h x **4–6 wks**	Desired vanco serum levels: peak 20–50 mcg/mL, trough 5–12 mcg/mL. **Gentamicin** used for synergy; peak levels need not exceed 4 mcg/mL.
Enterococci: β-lactamase test neg., pen G MIC >16 mcg/mL, no gentamicin resistance	Enterococci, intrinsic pen G/AMP resistance	**Vanco** 15mg/kg IV q12h PLUS **gent** 1–1.5mg/kg q8h x **4–6 wks** (see Comment)		

¹ Ref. for Guidelines of British Soc. for Antimicrob. Chemother. Includes drugs not available in U.S.: flucloxacillin IV, teicoplanin IV, rifampin IV./renal renal/renal function.

² Tolerant streptococci = MBC/MIC-32-fold greater than MIC
    NOTE: All dosage recommendations are for adults (unless otherwise indicated) and assume normal renal/renal function.
Abbreviations on page 2.

TABLE 1 (23)

ANATOMIC SITE/DIAGNOSIS/ MODIFYING CIRCUMSTANCES	ETIOLOGIES (usual)	SUGGESTED REGIMENS* PRIMARY	ALTERNATIVE†	ADJUNCT DIAGNOSTIC OR THERAPEUTIC MEASURES AND COMMENTS
HEART/Infective endocarditis—Native valve culture positive *(continued)*				
Enterococci: Pen/AMP resistant + high-level gent/strep resistant + vanco OR vanco-resistant; usually VRE. **Consultation suggested**	**Enterococcal, vanco-resistant, usually E. faecium**	No reliable effective rx. Can try **quinupristin-dalfopristin (Synercid)** or **linezolid**—see **Comment**, footnote†, and **Table 5**	**Teicoplanin** active against a subset of vanco-resistant enterococci. Teicoplanin is not available in U.S. **Dapto** is an option.	Synercid activity limited to E. faecium and is usually bacteriostatic, therefore expect high relapse rate. Dose: 7.5 mg per kg IV (via central line) q8h. **Linezolid** active most enterococci, but bacteriostatic. Dose: 600 mg IV or po q12h. Linezolid failed in pt with E. faecalis endocarditis (CID 37:e29, 2003). **Dapto** is bactericidal in vitro; clinical experience in CID 41:1134, 2005.
Staphylococcal endocarditis Aortic &/or mitral valve infection—MSSA	**Staph. aureus, methicillin-sensitive** **Note: Low dose of gentamicin for 3-5 days**	**Nafcillin (oxacillin) 2gm IV q4h x 4-6 wks** **PLUS gentamicin 1mg/kg IV q8h x 3-5 days**	**(Cefazolin 2gm IV q8h x 4-6 wks PLUS gentamicin 1mg/kg IV q8h x3-5 days)** **Low dose of gent OR** **Vanco 15mg/kg IV q12h (check levels if >2 gm per day) x 4-6 wks**	If IgE-mediated penicillin allergy: 10% cross-reactivity to cephalosporins (AHM 61:164, 2004). Vanco failures are common; avoid if possible for S. aureus endocarditis. No definitive data, pro or con on once-q24h gentamicin for S. aureus endocarditis. At present, favor q8h dosing times 3-5 days. Recognition of IV catheter-associated S. aureus endocarditis. May need TEE to detect endocarditis (CID 115:106 & 115, 1999). If TEE neg., may only need 2 wks of therapy.
Tricuspid valve infection (usually IVDUs): MSSA	**Staph. aureus, methicillin-sensitive**	**Vanco 1gm IV q12h (V q12h) x 4-6 wks**	**Dapto** not FDA-approved for left-sided endocarditis.	(NEJM 355:653, 2006); high failure rate with both vanco and dapto in clinical trial (NEJM 355:653, 2006). For other alternatives, see Table 6, pg 73. **2-week regimen not recommended if metastatic infection (e.g., osteo) or left-sided endocarditis.**
	Staph. aureus, methicillin-sensitive	**Nafcillin (oxacillin) 2gm IV q4h PLUS gentamicin 1mg/kg IV q8h x 2 wks. NOTE: low dose of gent**	**If penicillin allergy: Vanco 15mg/kg IV q12h + low-dose gent IV q8h x 2 wks** **OR** **Dapto 6mg/kg IV q24h (avoid if concomitant left-sided endocarditis) See Comment**	Success with **4-week oral regimen:** CIP 750 mg bid + RIF 300 mg bid. Less than 10% pts had MRSA (Ln 2:1071, 1989; AJM 101:68, 1996). High failure rate with <2 wks of vanco + gentamicin (CID 33:120, 2001). Can try longer duration rx of **vanco ± RIF (if sensitive). Daptomycin.** Approved for bacteremia and **right-sided** endocarditis based on randomized study (NEJM 355:653 & 727, 2006). **Note:** 1/3 of microbiological failures due to dapto resistance that developed during therapy.
Methicillin resistant (MRSA)	**Staph. aureus, methicillin-resistant**	**Vanco 15mg/kg IV q12h (check levels if >2 gm/day) x 4-6 wks**	**Dapto 6 mg/kg IV q24h x 4-6wk equiv to vanco for rt-sided endocarditis, both vanco & dapto did poorly if lt-sided endocarditis (NEJM 355:653, 2006). (See Comments & table 6, pg 73)**	For MRSA, no difference in duration of bacteremia or fever between pts rx with **vanco or vanco + RIF** (AHM 115:674, 1991). Quinupristin-dalfopristin another option. See Table 6, page 73. **Linezolid:** Limited experience (see JAC 58:273, 2006) in patients with few treatment options; 64% cure rate; clear failure in 21%; thrombocytopenia in 31%.
Slow-growing fastidious Gm-neg. bacilli	**HACEK group** (see Comments). Change to HABCEK if add Bartonella.	**Ceftriaxone 2gm IV q24h x 4 wks**	**AMP 12 gm q24h (continuous or div q4h) x 4 wks + gentamicin 3 mg/kg IV once q24h x 14 days + doxy 100 mg bid x 4-6 wks.**	**HACEK (acronym for Haemophilus parainfluenzae, H. aphrophilus, Actinobacillus, Cardiobacterium, Eikenella, Kingella).** H. aphrophilus resistant to vanco, clinda and methicillin. Penicillinase-positive HACEK organisms should be susceptible to AM-SB + gentamicin. **Dx:** Immunofluorescent antibody titer ≥1:800; blood cultures only occ. positive, or PCR of tissue from surgery. **Surgery:** Over ½ pts require valve surgery; relation to cure unclear.
Bartonella species (for bacteremia, see page 53—Urban trench fever) AAC 48:1921, 2004	**B. henselae, B. quintana**	**Ceftriaxone 2gm IV q24h x 4 wks + gentamicin 3 mg/kg IV q24h x 14 days + doxy 100 mg bid x 4-6 wks**	Optimal rx evolving. Retrospective & open prospective trials support **gentamicin** (see below).	B. quintana transmitted by body lice among homeless; asymptomatic colonization of RBCs described (Ln 360:226, 2002).

---

† Three interesting recent reports: (1) Successful rx of vanco-resistant E. faecium prosthetic valve endocarditis with Synercid without change in MIC (CID 25:163, 1997); (2) resistance to Synercid emerged during therapy of E. faecium bacteremia (CID 24:90, 1997); and (3) super-infection with E. faecalis occurred during Synercid rx of E. faecium (CID 24:91, 1997).

NOTE: All dosage recommendations are for adults (unless otherwise indicated) and assume normal renal function.

Abbreviations on page 2.

TABLE 1 (24)

ANATOMIC SITE/DIAGNOSIS/ MODIFYING CIRCUMSTANCES	ETIOLOGIES* (usual)	SUGGESTED REGIMENS*		ADJUNCT DIAGNOSTIC OR THERAPEUTIC MEASURES AND COMMENTS
		PRIMARY	ALTERNATIVE[1]	
Infective endocarditis—"culture negative" Fever, valvular disease, and ECHO vegetations ± emboli and neg. cultures. Rev. *Medicine 84:162, 2005*	Etiology in 348 cases studied by serology, culture, histopath, & molecular detection: C. burnetii 48%, Bartonella sp. 28%, and rarely, (Abiotrophia elegans (nutritionally variant strep), Mycoplasma hominis, Legionella pneumophila, Tropheryma whipplei—together only 1%), & rest without etiology identified (most on antibiotic).			
Infective endocarditis—Prosthetic valve—empiric therapy (cultures pending)				
Early (<2mo post-op)	S. epidermidis, S. aureus. Rarely, Enterobacteriaceae, diphtheroids, fungi.	**Vanco** 15 mg/kg IV q12h + **gentamicin** 1 mg/kg IV q8h + **RIF** 600 mg po q24h		Early surgical consultation advised. Watch for evidence of heart failure.
Late (>2mo post-op)	S. epidermidis, viridans strep, enterococci, S. aureus.			
Infective endocarditis—Prosthetic valve—positive blood cultures	Staph. aureus	**(Vanco** 15 mg/kg IV q12h + RIF 300 mg po q8h) **x 6 wks + gentamicin** 1 mg/kg IV q8h **x 14 days.**		If S. epidermidis is susceptible to nafcillin/oxacillin in vitro (not common), then substitute nafcillin (or oxacillin) for vanco.
Surgical consultation advised: retrospective analysis shows ↓ mortality of pts with S. aureus endocarditis if valve replaced during antibiotic rx (*CID 26:1302 & 1310, 1998*); also, retrospective study showed ↑ risk of death 2° neuro events in assoc. with Coumadin rx (*AfIM 159:473, 1999*)	Methicillin sensitive: Methicillin resistant:	**Nafcillin** 2 gm IV q4h + **RIF** 300 mg po q8h **times 6 wks + gentamicin** 1 mg/kg IV q8h **times 14 days.**[1] **(Vanco** 1 gm IV q12h + **RIF** 300 mg po q8h) **times 6 wks + gentamicin** 1 mg/kg IV q8h **times 14 days.**[1]		
	Viridans strep, enterococci	See *Infective endocarditis, native valve, culture positive page 25*		
	Enterobacteriaceae or P. aeruginosa	**Aminoglycoside (tobra** IV if P. aeruginosa) + **(AP Pen** or **P Ceph 3 AP** or **P Ceph 4)**		In theory, could substitute CiP for APAG, but no clinical data.
	Candida, aspergillus	**Ampho B** ± an azole, e.g., fluconazole (*Table 11, page 97*)		High mortality. Valve replacement plus antifungal therapy standard therapy but some success with antifungal therapy alone (*CID 22:262, 1996*).
Infective endocarditis—Q fever *LnID 3:709, 2003*	Coxiella burnetii	**Doxy** 100 mg po bid + **hydroxychloroquine** 600 mg/day x 1.5–3 yrs		**Dx:** Complement-fix or ELISA IgG antibody to phase II antigen diagnostic of acute Q fever. IgG antibody of ≥ to phase I antigen diagnostic of chronic Q fever. (*JCM 43:4238, 2005; 44:2283, 2006*) Want doxy serum conc. >5 mcg/mL (*IJID 18:1322, 2004*)
Pacemaker/defibrillator infections Rev. *Medicine 82:385, 2003*	S. aureus, S. epidermidis, rarely others	**Device removal + RIF** 300 mg IV/po q12h	**Device removal + dapto** 6 mg/kg IV q24h[AM-SB] no data.	**Duration of rx after device removal:** For "pocket" or subcutaneous infection, 10–14 days; if lead-assoc. endocarditis, 4–6 wks depending on organism. Refs: *Circulation 108:2015, 2003; NEJM 350:1422, 2004*
Pericarditis, purulent—empiric rx	Staph. aureus, Strep, pneumoniae, Group A strep, Enterobacteriaceae	**Vanco + CIP** (Dosage, see footnote[2])	**Vanco** 1 gm IV q12h + **CFP** (see footnote[2])	Drainage required if signs of tamponade. Forced to use empiric vanco due to high prevalence of MRSA.
Rheumatic fever with carditis Ref.: *Ln 366:155, 2005*	Post-infectious sequelae of Group A strep infection (usually pharyngitis)	**ASA** and usually prednisone 2 mg/kg po q24h for symptomatic treatment of fever, arthritis, arthralgia. May not influence carditis.		Clinical features: Carditis, polyarthritis, chorea, subcutaneous nodules, erythema marginatum. For Jones criteria: *Circulation 87:302, 1993. Prophylaxis; see page 54*
Ventricular assist device-related infection Ref: *LnID 6:426, 2006*	S. aureus, S. epidermidis, aerobic gn-neg bacilli, Candida sp	After culture of blood, wounds, drive line, device pocket and maybe pump. **Vanco** 1 gm IV q12h + **CIP** 750 mg po bid or 400 mg IV q12h. With fungemia: **vanco** 1 gm IV q12h, CIP as above + **fluconazole** 800mg IV q24h.		Can substitute **daptomycin** 6 mg/kg/d for **vanco, cefepime** 2 gm IV q12h for FQ, and (**vori, caspo, micafungin or anidulafungin** for **fluconazole.**

[1] Case report of dapto success: *Heart & Lung 34:69, 2005.*

APAG (see Table 10D, page 100); **IMP** 0.5 gm IV q6h; **MER** 1 gm IV q8h; **nafcillin** or **oxacillin** 2 gm IV q4h; **TC-CL** 3.1 gm IV q6h; **PIP-TZ** 3.375 gm IV q6h or 4.5 gm IV q8h; **AM-SB** 3 gm IV q6h, **P Ceph 3** (cephalothin 2 gm IV q4h or ceftazidim 2 gm IV q8h or cefotaxime 2 gm IV q4h); **CiP** 750 mg po bid or 400 mg IV q12h; **vanco** 1 gm IV q12h; **CFP** (cefepime) 2 gm IV q12h

Abbreviations on page 2. *NOTE: All dosage recommendations are for adults (unless otherwise indicated) and assume normal renal function.*

TABLE 1 (25)

ANATOMIC SITE/DIAGNOSIS/ MODIFYING CIRCUMSTANCES	ETIOLOGIES (usual)	SUGGESTED REGIMENS*		ADJUNCT DIAGNOSTIC OR THERAPEUTIC MEASURES AND COMMENTS
		PRIMARY	ALTERNATIVE†	
JOINT—Also see Lyme Disease, page 52				
Reactive arthritis Reiter's syndrome (See Comment for definition)	Occurs wks after infection with C. trachomatis, Campylobacter jejuni, Yersinia enterocolitica.	Only treatment is non-steroidal anti-inflammatory drugs		Definition: Urethritis, conjunctivitis, arthritis, and sometimes uveitis and rash. Arthritis: asymmetrical oligoarthritis of ankles, knees, feet, sacroiliitis. Rash: palms and soles—keratoderma blennorrhagia; circinate balanitis of glans penis. HLA-B27 positive predisposes to Reiter's.
Poststreptococcal reactive arthritis (See Rheumatic fever, above)	Strep. pyogenes, Sabella sp.	Treat strep pharyngitis and then NSAIDs (prednisone needed in some pts)		A reactive arthritis after a β-hemolytic strep infection in absence of sufficient Jones criteria for acute rheumatic fever. Ref. Mayo Clin Proc 75:144, 2000.
Septic arthritis: Treatment requires both adequate drainage of purulent joint fluid and appropriate antimicrobial therapy. Empiric therapy after collection of blood and joint fluid for culture; review Gram stain of joint fluid. For full differential, see LN 351:197, 1998.				**There is no need to inject antimicrobials into joints**
Infants <3mo (neonate)	Staph. aureus, Enterobacteriaceae, Group B strep, N. gonorrhoeae	**If MRSA no concern:** (Nafcillin or oxacillin) + P Ceph 3	**If MRSA concern: Vanco** + P Ceph 3	Blood cultures frequently positive. Adjacent bone involved in 2/3 pts. Group B strep and gonococcal most common community-acquired etiologies.
		Dosage, see Table 16, page 168		
Children (3mo–14yr)	Staph. aureus 27%, S. pyogenes & S. pneumo 14%, H. influenzae 3%, Gm-neg. bacilli 6%, other (GC, N. meningitidis) 14%, unknown 36%	**Vanco + P Ceph 3** (until culture results available) See Table 16 for dosage Steroids—see Comment		Marked ↓ in H. influenzae since use of conjugate vaccine NOTE: Septic arthritis due to salmonella has no association with sickle cell disease, unlike salmonella osteomyelitis. Duration of treatment varies with specific microbial etiology. Short-course steroid. Benefit reported (PIDJ 22:883, 2003)
Adults (review Gram stain) See page 52 for Lyme Disease				
Acute monoarticular		**Gram stain negative:**	If Gram stain shows Gm+ cocci in clusters: **vanco** 1 gm IV q12h	
At risk for sexually-transmitted disease	N. gonorrhoeae (see page 20), S. aureus, streptococci, rarely aerobic Gm-neg. bacilli	**Ceftriaxone** 1gm IV q24h or **cefotaxime** 1gm IV q8h or **ceftizoxime** 1gm IV q8h		For rx comments, see Disseminated GC, page 20
Not at risk for sexually-transmitted disease	S. aureus, streptococci, Gm-neg. bacilli	**All empiric choices guided by Gram stain Vanco + P Ceph 3** For treatment duration, see Table 3, page 64 For dosage, see Table 2, Table 11, & Table 12	**(CIP or Levo)**	Differential includes gout and chondrocalcinosis (pseudogout). **Look for crystals in joint fluid.** **NOTE:** See Table 6 for MRSA treatment.
Chronic monoarticular	Brucella, nocardia, mycobacteria, fungi			If GC, usually associated petechiae and/or pustular skin lesions and tenosynovitis. Consider Lyme disease if exposure areas known to harbor infected ticks. See Lyme page 52.
Polyarticular, usually acute	**Gonococcal:** N.gonorrhoeae acute rheumatic fever, rubella/live vaccine, parvo B19, hepatitis B. MSSE/MRSE 40%, MSSA/MRSA 20%, P. aeruginosa, Propionibacteria	Gram stain usually negative for GC. If usually active, culture urethra, cervix, anal canal, throat, blood, joint fluid, and then: **ceftriaxone** 1gm IV q24h		Expanded differential incl gout, pseudogout, reactive arthritis (HLA-B27 pos.). Treat based on culture and sensitivity.
Septic arthritis, post intra-articular injection		**NO empiric therapy.** Arthroscopy for culture/sensitivity, incl crystals, washout		Treat based on culture results x 14 days (assumes no foreign body present).

Abbreviations on page 2. NOTE: All dosage recommendations are for adults (unless otherwise indicated) and assume normal renal function.

TABLE 1 (26)

ANATOMIC SITE/DIAGNOSIS/ MODIFYING CIRCUMSTANCES	ETIOLOGIES (usual)	SUGGESTED REGIMENS*		ADJUNCT DIAGNOSTIC OR THERAPEUTIC MEASURES AND COMMENTS
		PRIMARY	ALTERNATIVE†	
JOINT (continued)				
Infected prosthetic joint CID 36:1157, 2003; JAC 53:127, 2004; NEJM 351:1645, 2004 See surgical options in Comments **Drug dosages in footnote¹** **For dental prophylaxis, see Table 15B**	See below S. pyogenes; Gps A, B, or G; viridans strep in MSSE/MRSA MRSE/MRSA P. aeruginosa	**No empiric therapy.** Need culture & sens. results. Surgical options in Comment. Debridement & prosthesis retention: (**Pen G** or **ceftriax** IV x 4 wks. Cured 17/19 pts (CID 39:847, 2003) **Nafcillin/oxacillin + RIF** po) x 6 wks (**Vanco** IV + **RIF** po) x 6 wks **Ceftaz** IV + (**CIP** or **Levo** po)	(**Vanco** IV + **RIF** po) x 6wk [(**CIP** or **Levo** po) if suscepti-ble—po) + (**RIF** po)] OR (**Dapto** IV + **RIF** po) OR **RIF** x6wk	**Surg.** options: 1, 2-stage: Remove infected prosthesis & leave spacer, anti-microbics, then new prosthesis. Highest cure rate (CID 42:216, 2006). **2. 1-stage:** Remove infected prosthesis, debride, new prosthesis, then antimicro-bics. **3. Extensive debridement & leave prosthesis in place** plus antimicro-bics. 53% failure rate, esp. if ≥8 d of symptoms (CID 42:471, 2006). Other—Remove prosthesis & treat ± bone fusion of joint. Last: Chronic antimicrobial suppression. **RIF** bactericidal vs surface-adhering, slow-growing, & biofilm-producing bacteria. Never use **RIF** alone due to rapid development of resistance (JAMA 279:1537, 1575, 1998). **RIF + Fusidic acid** another option (Cl. Micro. &Inf. Table 10C, page 89. **Dapto** experience: JDCP 14:144, 2006.) Limited linezolid experience favorable (JAC 55:387, 2005). Watch for toxicity, AAC 39:2423, 1995
Rheumatoid arthritis	TNF inhibitors (adalimumab, etanercept, infliximab) ↑ risk of TBc; fungal infection and malignancy (CID 38:1261, 2004; JAMA 295:2275, 2006). Treat latent TBc first (MMWR 53:683, 2004).			
Septic bursitis; Olecranon bursitis; prepatellar bursitis	Staph. aureus >80%, M. tuberculosis (rare), M. marinum (rare)	**Naficillin** or **oxacillin** 2 gm IV q4h or **dicloxacillin** 500 mg po q6h if **MSSA**	**Vanco** 1 gm IV q12h or line-zolid 600 mg po bid) if **MRSA**	**Initially aspirate q24h and treat for a minimum of 2-3 weeks.** Surgical excision of bursa/hand not be necessary if treated for at least 3 weeks Ref.: Semin Arth & Rheum 24:391, 1995
KIDNEY, BLADDER AND PROSTATE [For review, see AJM 113(Suppl 1A):1S, 2002 & NEJM 349:259, 2003]				
Acute uncomplicated urinary tract infection (cystitis-urethritis) in females [NOTE: Routine urine culture not necessary; self-pay Rx works (AnIM 135:9, 2001)]. Try to spare FQs.				
NOTE: Resistance of E. coli to TMP-SMX approx. 15-20% (CID 36:183, 2003) & correlates with microbiological/clinical failure (CID 34:1061 & 1165, 2002). **Recent reports of E. coli resistant to CIP & Levo as well**	Enterobacteriaceae (E. coli), Staph. saprophyticus, enterococci	Local E. coli resist <20%: **TMP-SMX** <20% & no allergy: **TMP-SMX-DS** bid x 3 days; if sulfa allergy: **fosfomycin** single dose	Local E. coli resistant ≥20% (TMP-SMX) or resist 5 days of **CIP** 250 mg bid, **Levo** 250 mg q24h. **Do not use Moxi** or **Gemi.** Due to low urine concentrations.	7-day Rx recommended in pregnancy [discontinue or do not use sulfonamides (2/3 trimester, term (2 weeks before EDC) because of potential ↑ in kernicterus]. If failure on 3-day course, culture and rx 2 weeks. **Fosfomycin** 3 gm po times 1 less effective vs E. coli than multi-dose TMP-SMX or FQ (Med Lett 39:66, 1997). Foslo active vs E. faecalis; poor activity vs other coliforms. **Moxifloxacin & gemifloxacin:** Neither approved for UTIs. Do not use. **Phenazopyridine (Pyridium)**—non-prescription—may relieve dysuria; inadequate urine concentration. **Phenazopyridine (Pyridium),** 200 mg po tid times 2 days. Hemolysis (if G6PD deficient). Pelvic exam for vaginitis & herpes simplex, urine LCR/PCR for GC and C. trachomatis
Risk factors for STD. Dipstick: positive leukocyte esterase or hemoglobin; neg. Gram stain	C. trachomatis	**Doxy** 100 mg po bid x 7 days	**Azithro** 1 gm po single dose	
Recurrent (3 or more episodes/ year) in young women	Any of the above bacteria	Eradicate infection, then **TMP-SMX** 1 single-strength tab po q24h long term		A cost-effective alternative to continuous prophylaxis is self-administered single dose of **TMP-SMX-DS,** 2 tabs, 320/1600 mg) at symptom onset. Another alternative: 1 DS tablet TMP-SMX post-coitus.
Child ≤5 yrs old & grade 3-4 reflux	Coliforms	**TMP-SMX** (2 mg TMP/10 mg SMX) per kg po q24h) or (**nitrofurantoin** 2 mg per kg po q24h)		**CIP** approved as alternative drug ages 1-17 yrs.

---

¹ **Aqueous Pen G** 2 million units IV q4h, **ceftriaxone** 2 gm IV q24h, **nafcillin** or **oxacillin** 2 gm IV q4h, **vancomycin** 1 gm IV q12h, **vancomycin** 2 gm IV q4h; **ceftazidime** 2 gm IV q8h; **ciprofloxacin** 400 mg IV q12h, **RIF** 300 mg IV q24h, RIF 300 mg IV/po q24h, **CIP** 750 mg IV/po bid, **Levo** 750 mg IV/po q24h; **ceftazidime** 2 gm IV/po q24h. **Daptomycin** 6mg/kg IV q24h; RIF 300 mg IV/po bid, **CIP** 750 mg IV/po bid

Abbreviations on page 2.   NOTE: All dosage recommendations are for adults (unless otherwise indicated) and assume normal renal function.

TABLE 1 (27)

ANATOMIC SITE/DIAGNOSIS/ MODIFYING CIRCUMSTANCES	ETIOLOGIES (usual)	SUGGESTED REGIMENS* PRIMARY	ALTERNATIVE¹	ADJUNCT DIAGNOSTIC OR THERAPEUTIC MEASURES AND COMMENTS
KIDNEY, BLADDER AND PROSTATE *(continued)*				
Recurrent UTI in postmenopausal women See CID 30:152, 2000	E. coli & other Enterobacteriaceae, enterococci, S. saprophyticus	Treat as for uncomplicated UTI. Evaluate for potentially correctable urologic factors—see Comment. NF more effective than vaginal cream in decreasing frequency, but Editors worried about pulmonary fibrosis with long-term use (Ln ID 4:1, 2003)		Definition: ≥3 culture + symptomatic UTIs in 1 year or 2 UTIs in 6 months. Urologic factors: (1) cystocele, (2) incontinence, (3) ↑ residual urine volume (≥50 mL).
Acute uncomplicated pyelonephritis (usually women 18–40 yrs., hemolytic uremic syndrome as result of toxin-producing E. coli UTI (NEJM 335:635, 1996)). If male, look for obstructive **uropathy or complicating pathology.** Report of definite costovertebral tenderness and temperature >102°F: definite costovertebral tenderness)				
Moderately ill (outpatient) **NOTE:** May need one IV dose due to nausea	Enterobacteriaceae (most likely E. coli), enterococci (Gm stain of uncentrifuged urine may allow identification of Gm-neg. bacilli vs Gm+ cocci).	An **FQ** po times 7 days: **CIP** 500 mg bid or CIP-**ER** 1000 mg q24h, **Levo** 250 mg q24h, **Oflox** 400 mg bid	**AM-CL**, **1 O Ceph**, or **TMP-SMX-DS p.o.** Treat for 14 days. Beta-lactams not as effective as FQs JAMA 293:949, 2005)	In randomized double-blind trial, bacteriologic and **clinical success higher for 7 days of CIP than for 14 days of TMP-SMX** failures correlated with in-vitro resistance (JAMA 283:1583, 2000). Since CIP worked with 7-day rx, suspect other FQs effective with 7 d. of rx. Do not use Moxi or Gem due to low urine concentrations. **NOTE:** Increasing resistance of E. coli to both TMP-SMX & FQs a concern.
Hospitalized	E. coli most common, enterococci 2° in frequency	**FQ** IV (or (**AMP + gentamicin**) or **P Ceph 3a** or **PIP-TZ Pen**. Treat for 14 days. Do not use cephalosporins for suspect or proven enterococcal infection	**TC-CL** or **AM-SB** or **PIP-TZ** or **ERTA**. Treat for 14 days. Dosages in footnote¹	Treat IV until pt afebrile 24–48 hrs, then complete 2-wk course with oral drugs (as Moderately ill, above). If no clinical improvement in 3 days, we recommend imaging. On CT, if single focal mass-like lesion, avg. response requires 6.1, if lesions diffuse, avg. response 13 days (AJM 93:289, 1992). **If hypotensive, prompt imaging (Echo or CT) is recommended to ensure absence of obstructive uropathy.** **NOTE: Cephalosporins & ertapenem not active vs enterococci.**
Complicated UTI/catheters Obstruction, reflux, azotemia, transplant, **Foley catheter-related. R/O obstruction**	Enterobacteriaceae, P. aeruginosa, enterococci, rarely S. aureus (CID 42:46, 2006)	(**AMP + gent**) or **PIP-TZ** or **TC-CL** or **IMP** or **MER** Switch to **po FQ** or **TMP-SMX** when possible	IV (or **FQ, CIP, Gati, Levo**), x 2–3 wks Dosages in footnote¹ For dosages, see footnote¹	Not all listed drugs predictably active vs enterococci or P. aeruginosa. **Cip** approved in children (1–17 yrs) as alternative. Not 1st choice secondary to ↑ incidence joint adverse effects. Peds dose: 6–10 mg/kg (400 mg max) **IV** q8h or 10-20 mg/kg (750 mg max) **po** q12h.
Asymptomatic bacteriuria. IDSA Guidelines: CID 40:643, 2005				Diagnosis requires ≥10⁵ CFU/mL per mL urine of same bacterial species in 2 specimens, obtained 3–7 days apart.
Preschool children		Base regimen on C&S, not empirical		Screen monthly for recurrence. Some authorities treat continuously until delivery (stop TMP-SMX 2 wks before EDC). ↑ resistance of E. coli to TMP-SMX.
Pregnancy		Screen 1st trimester. If positive, rx 3–7 days with **amox. NF, O Ceph, TMP-SMX,** or **TMP** alone		In one study, single dose 2-TMP-SMX DS 80% effective (AnIM 114:713, 1991).
Before and after invasive urologic intervention, e.g., Foley catheter		Obtain urine culture and then rx 3 days with TMP-SMX DS, bid		Antimicrobial-coated Foley catheters may ↓ risk of clinically significant bacteriuria (AnIM 144:116, 2006).

¹ **AM-CL** 875/125 mg q12h or 500/125 mg tid or 2000/125 mg po bid; **aztreonam** 2 gm IV q8h; **FQ** IV q8h; **CIP** 400 mg po q24h for mild uncomplicated disease. 750 mg IV q24h for hospital pts, **Cip**-ER 500 & 1000 mg (once daily); **cefotaxime** 2 gm IV q8h; **P Ceph 3 cefotaxime** 1 gm IV q12h for uncomplicated disease, up to 2 gm IV q8h for life-threatening infections; **Levo** (250 mg po q24h for uncomplicated, up to 2 gm IV q8h; **ceftazidime** 2 gm IV q8h, **cefazolin** 2 gm IV q8h (cefazolin) (see Table 10C/D, page 65); **AP Pen** (PIP 3 gm IV q6h), **AM-SB 3** gm IV q6h, **TC-CL** 3.1 gm IV q6h, **PIP-TZ** 3.375 gm IV q6h or for nosocomial pneumonia 4.5 gm IV q6h, **gentamicin** (see Table 10D, page 100); **TMP-SMX** 2.0 mg per kg (TMP) IV q6h; **P Ceph 4 CFP 2** gm IV q12h, **ERTA** 1 gm IV q24h; **IMP** 0.5 gm IV q8h; **MER 1** gm IV q8h. **Nafcillin** 2 gm IV q4h. For oral cephalosporin dosages, see Table 10C, page 93. **Dicloxacillin** 500 mg po q6h. **Metronidazole** 500 mg po q6h or 15 mg per kg IV q12h (max. 4 gm per day), **Vanco** 1 gm IV q12h, **linezolid** 600 mg IV/po q12h

NOTE: All dosage recommendations are for adults (unless otherwise indicated) and assume normal renal function.

Abbreviations on page 2.

TABLE 1 (28)

ANATOMIC SITE/DIAGNOSIS/ MODIFYING CIRCUMSTANCES	ETIOLOGIES (usual)	SUGGESTED REGIMENS*		ADJUNCT DIAGNOSTIC OR THERAPEUTIC MEASURES AND COMMENTS
		PRIMARY	ALTERNATIVE†	
KIDNEY, BLADDER AND PROSTATE/ Asymptomatic bacteriuria (continued)				
Neurogenic bladder – see "spinal cord injury" below		No rx in asymptomatic; intermittent catheterization if possible		Ref.: AJM 113(1A):67S, 2002—Bacteriuria in spinal cord injured patient.
Asymptomatic advanced age, male or female Ref. CID 40:643, 2005	E. coli	No rx indicated unless in conjunction with surgery to correct obstructive uropathy; measure residual urine vol. in females, prostate exam/PSA in males.		
Malacoplakia		Bethanechol chloride → CIP or TMP-SMX		Chronic pyelo with abnormal inflammatory response. See CID 29:444, 1999
Perinephric abscess Associated with staphylococcal bacteremia	Staph. aureus	If MSSA, Nafcillin, oxacillin or P Ceph 1 (Dosage, see footnote page 29)	If MRSA: Vanco 1 gm IV q12h OR dapto 6mg/kg IV q24h	Drainage, surgical or image-guided aspiration
Associated with pyelonephritis	Enterobacteriaceae	See pyelonephritis, complicated UTI, above		Drainage, surgical or image-guided aspiration
Prostatitis		See prostatitis, page 23		
Spinal cord injury pts with UTI	E. coli, Klebsiella sp. entero-cocci	CIP 250 mg po bid x 14 days		Suspect assoc. pyelonephritis. In RDBPC* trial microbiologic cure greater after 14 vs 3 days of CIP (CID 39:658 & 665, 2004).
LIVER (for spontaneous bacterial peritonitis, see page 42)				
Cholangitis		See Gallbladder, page 15		
Cirrhosis & UGI bleeding	Meta-analysis of 8 RCTs of cirrhosis with variceal bleeding (Cochrane database 2: CD 022907, 2002). Mostly FQs. Decreased mortality 6.5% and bacterial infection 26%. No blinded studies, rare placebo control. Needs more study.			
Hepatic abscess Pyogenic abscess ref.: CID 39:1654, 2004	Enterobacteriaceae (esp. Klebsiella sp.), bacteroides, enterococci, Entamoeba histolytica, Yersinia entero-colitica (rare) For echinococcus, see Table 13, page 128. For cat-scratch disease (CSD), see pages 40 & 51.	Metro + (P Ceph 3 or cefotetin or TC-CL or PIP-TZ) → AMP + MTR or levo	Metro (for amoebiasis) + either IMP or MER (Dosage, see footnote page 32)	Serological tests for amebiasis should be done on all patients; if neg., surgical drainage or percutaneous aspiration. In pyogenic abscess, ½ have identifiable GI source or underlying biliary tract disease. If amoeba serology positive, treat with metro alone without surgery. Empiric Metro included for both E. histolytica & bacteroides.
		AMP + APAG + metro traditional & effective but AMP-resistant Gm-neg. bacilli ↑ and APAG toxicity an issue.		Hemochromatosis associated with Yersinia enterocolitica liver abscess (CID 18:938, 1994); regimens listed are effective for yersinia.
Leptospirosis	Leptospirosis, see page 54			
Peliosis hepatis in AIDS pts	Bartonella henselae and B. quintana	See page 51		
Post-transplant infected biloma (CID 39:517, 2004)	Enterococci (incl. VRE), candida, Gm-neg. bacilli (P. aeruginosa 8%), anaerobes (5%)	Linezolid 600 mg IV bid + CIP 400 mg IV q12h + flu-conazole 400 mg IV q24h	Dapto 6 mg/kg per day + Levo 750 mg IV q24h + fluconazole 400 mg IV q24h.	Suspect if fever & abdominal pain post-transplant. Exclude hepatic artery throm-bosis. Presence of candida and/or VRE bad prognosticators.
Viral hepatitis	Hepatitis A, B, C, D, E, G	See Table 14, page 135		

NOTE: bid = twice a day, tid = 3 times a day, qid = 4 times a day.

NOTE: All dosage recommendations are for adults (unless otherwise indicated) and assume normal renal function.

Abbreviations on page 2.

* RDBPC = Randomized double-blind placebo-controlled

TABLE 1 (29)

ANATOMIC SITE/DIAGNOSIS/ MODIFYING CIRCUMSTANCES	ETIOLOGIES (usual)	SUGGESTED REGIMENS*		ADJUNCT DIAGNOSTIC OR THERAPEUTIC MEASURES AND COMMENTS
		PRIMARY	ALTERNATIVE[1]	
LUNG/Bronchi				
Bronchitis				
Bronchiolitis/wheezy bronchitis Infants/children (≤ age 5) See RSV, Table 14B page 145 Ref.: Ln 368:312, 2006	**(expiratory wheezing)** **Respiratory syncytial virus** (RSV) 50%, parainfluenza 25%, other viruses 20%	Antibiotics not useful, mainstay of rx is oxygen. Ribavirin of no benefit (AJRCCM 160:829, 1999). For prevention & treatment, humanized mouse monoclonal antibody (palivizumab). See Table 14, page 145. RSV immune globulin is no longer available.		RSV most important. Rapid dx with antigen detection methods. Ribavirin: No data on effect on long-term pulmonary function; IV ribavirin but little enthusiasm. Emphasis now on oxygen, decongestant and preventive modulation with immunoglobulins. Reviews: PIDJ 19:773, 2000; Red Book of Peds 2006, 27th Ed.
Bronchitis Infants/children (≤ age 5)	< Age 2. Adenovirus; age 2–5: Respiratory syncytial virus, parainfluenza 3 virus. Usually viral. M. pneumoniae 5%, C. pneumoniae 5%. See Persistent cough, below	Respiratory syncytial Antibiotics not indicated. Antitussive± inhaled bronchodilators	strep, H. influenzae only with associated sinusitis or heavy growth on throat culture for S. pneumo.. Group A strep, H. influenzae rx is symptomatic. Otherwise rx is symptomatic.	Purulent sputum alone not an indication for antibiotics. Azithro vs no better than 2 wks low-dose vitamin C in a controlled trial (Ln 359:1648, 2002). Expect cough to last 2 weeks. If fever/rigors, get chest x-ray. M. pneumoniae ref. LnID 1:334, 2001. Rare pt with true C. pneumo infection may require 6 wks of clarithro to clear organism (J Med Micro 52:265, 2003).
Adolescents and adults with acute tracheobronchitis (Acute bronchitis) Ref.: NEJM 355:2125, 2006				
Persistent cough (>14 d.), afebrile Pertussis (whooping cough) Rx: adults with cough >14 d. have pertussis (MMWR 54 (RR-14), 2005	Bordetella pertussis & occ. Bordetella parapertussis Also consider asthma, gastroesophageal reflux, post-nasal drip	**Peds doses: Azithro/ clarithro OR erythro estolate[2]** OR **TMP-SMX** (doses in footnote 1&2)	**Adult doses: Azithro** po 500 mg (day 1), 250 mg q24h x 4 days OR **erythro esto-late** 500 mg po qid times 14 days OR **TMP-SMX-DS** 1 tab po bid times 14 days OR **clarithro** 500 mg po bid or 1 gm ER q24h times 7 days).	**3 stages of illness:** catarrhal (1–2 wks), paroxysmal coughing (2–4 wks), and convalescence (1–2 wks). Treatment may shorten early stage. **Diagnosis:** PCR on nasopharyngeal secretions or [1] pertussis-toxin antibody. **Azithro** works fastest (PIDJ 22:847, 2003). Hypertrophic pyloric stenosis reported in infants under 6 wks of age given erythro (MMWR 48:1117, 1999).
Prophylaxis of household contacts		Drugs and doses as per treatment immediately above		Recommended by Am. Acad. Ped. Red Book 2006 for all household or close contacts of a case. Chemoprophylaxis not recommended.
Acute bacterial exacerbation of chronic bronchitis (ABECB), adults (almost always smokers with COPD) Pertinent refs.: Chest 118: 193, 2000; NEJM 347:465, 2002; CID 39:960 & 987, 2004; AJM 116:5915, 2005; Thorax 61:535, 2005.	Viruses 20–50%, C. pneumoniae 5%, M. pneumoniae <1%; role of S. pneumo, H. influenzae & M. catarrhalis controversial. Tobacco use, air pollution contribute.	**Severe ABECB:** (1) dyspnea, (2) sputum viscosity/purulence, febrile &/or low O₂, sat.; (2) inhaled anticholinergic bronchodilator; (3) oral corticosteroid; taper over 2 wks(Cochrane Library 3, 2006); (4) D/C tobacco use; (5) non-invasive positive pressure ventilation. **Role of antimicrobial rx debated even for severe disease. For mild or moderate disease, no antimicrobial treatment** or maybe amox, doxy, TMP-SMX, or O Ceph. For more resistant strains, use drug-resistant S. pneumo (Gemi, Levo, or Moxi). **For severe disease,** AM-CL, azithro/clarithro, or O Ceph or FQs with enhanced activity vs drug-resistant S. pneumo Placebo-controlled studies: Pul Pharm & Therap 14:449, 2001.		**Severe ABECB:** (1) consider chest x-ray, esp. if higher fever. **For severe ABECB:** (1) consider chest x-ray, esp. if higher volume. For severe disease, therapies with drug, range 3–10 d. Limit Gemi to 5 d to decrease risk of rash (Ln 358:2020, 2001.

---

[1] **TMP-SMX** 1 double-strength tab (160 mg TMP) po bid, peds (>6 mo of age) 8 mg/kg/d TMP component, div bid x 14 d.   **doxy** 100 mg po bid, **amox** 500 mg po tid, **AM-CL** 875/125 mg po bid or 500/125 mg po tid or 2000/125 mg po bid, adult dose of 3 cephalosporins, **cefprozil** 500 mg q8h or 500 mg q12h, **cefdinir** 300 mg q12h or 600 mg q24h, **cefixime** 400 mg po q24h, **cefpodoxime proxetil** 200 mg po q12h, **cefprozil** 500 mg q12h, **ceftibuten** 400 mg q24h, **cefuroxime axetil** 250 or 500 mg po q12h, **cefdinir** 300 mg q12h or 600 mg po q24h, **azithro** 500 mg po initial dose then 250 mg q24h times 3 days, **clarithro** 500 mg po q12h or **clarithro ER** 1000 mg po q24h times 7 days, **dirithromycin** 500 mg po q24h, **erythro estolate** 40 mg/kg/d po div. q6h x 14 d, **erythro estolate** 40 mg/kg/d po q8h x 14 d, **Oflox** 400 mg or **CIP** 750 mg po q8-12h x 14 d, **Levo** 500 mg po q24h, **Gemi** 320 mg po q24h times 5 days, **Moxi** 400 mg po q24h.

NOTE: CIP and ceftibuten have relatively poor in vitro activity vs S. pneumo.

[2] Abbreviations on page 2.   NOTE: All dosage recommendations are for adults (unless otherwise indicated) and assume normal renal function.

TABLE 1 (30)

ANATOMIC SITE/DIAGNOSIS/ MODIFYING CIRCUMSTANCES	ETIOLOGIES (usual)	SUGGESTED REGIMENS*		ADJUNCT DIAGNOSTIC OR THERAPEUTIC MEASURES AND COMMENTS
		PRIMARY	ALTERNATIVE†	
LUNG/Bronchi (continued)				
Fever, cough, myalgia during influenza season	Influenza A & B	**Oseltamivir** 75 mg po bid x 5 d (see Table 14A)		**Complications: Influenza pneumonia, secondary bacterial pneumonia** (S. pneumo., S. aureus, S. pyogenes, H. influenzae), S. aureus TSS. Ref: LnID 6:296, 2006.
Bronchiectasis. Ref: NEJM 346:1383, 2002	H. influ, P. aeruginosa, and rarely S. pneumo.	**Gemi, levo, or moxi** x 7-10 d (dosage in footnote 11)		Many potential etiologies: obstruction, ↓ immune globulins, cystic fibrosis, dyskinetic cilia, tobacco, prior severe or recurrent necrotizing bronchitis; e.g. pertussis.
Acute exacerbation				
Prevention	Not applicable	**One option: Erythro** 500 mg po bid **or azithro** 250 mg q24h x 8 wks (AMA 290:1749, 2003; Eur Resp J 13:361, 1999)		
Specific organisms	Aspergillus (see Table 11) MAI (Table 12) and P. aeruginosa (Table 5)			
Pneumonia				
Neonatal: Birth to 1 month	Viruses: CMV, rubella, H. simplex viruses, Group B strep, listeria, coliforms, S. aureus, P. aeruginosa **Other:** Chlamydia trachomatis, syphilis	**AMP + gentamicin ± cefotaxime** Add **vanco** if MRSA a concern. For chlamydia rx, **erythro** 12.5 mg per kg po or IV qid times 14 days.		Blood cultures indicated. Consider C. trachomatis if afebrile pneumonia. If MRSA documented, **vanco**. **TMP-SMX**, **& linezolid** alternatives. **Linezolid** dosage birth to age 11 yrs is **10 mg per kg q8h**. Ref: PIDJ 22(Suppl):S158, 2003.
CONSIDER TUBERCULOSIS IN ALL PATIENTS; ISOLATE ALL SUSPECT PATIENTS				
Age 1–3 months Usually afebrile	C. trachomatis, RSV, parainfluenza virus 3, Bordetella, S. pneumoniae. S. aureus (rare)	**Outpatient: po** **erythro** 12.5 mg/kg q6h x 14 days or po **azithro** 10 mg/kg x dose, then 5 mg/kg qd	**Inpatient: If afebrile erythro** 10 mg/kg IV q6h or **azithro** 2.5 mg/kg IV q12h (see Comment) **if febrile**, add **cefotaxime 200** mg per day div q8h	Pneumonia syndrome: cough, tachypnea, dyspnea, diffuse infiltrates, afebrile. Usually requires hospital care. Reports of hypertrophic pyloric stenosis after erythro under age 6 wks; not sure about azithro, but both could theoretically might ↑ risk of hypertrophic pyloric stenosis. If lobar pneumonia, give AMP 200-300 mg per kg per day for S. pneumoniae. No empiric coverage for S. pneumoniae as it is rare etiology.
Age 4 months–5 years For RSV, see bronchiolitis, page 32, & Table 14 Refs: NEJM 346:429, 2002; Ln 364:1141, 2004		For RSV, see bronchiolitis		
	RSV, other resp. viruses, S. pneumo., H. flu, mycoplasma, S. aureus (rare), M. tbc	**Outpatient: Amox** 100 mg/kg/day po q8h. **Inpatient (not ICU):** No antibiotic if viral or **AMP** 200 mg/kg per day div q6h	**Outpatient: Amox** 100 mg/kg/day (max 1 gm bid) if pt >8 yrs old) **or erythro** 500 mg/day po then 250 mg/day q6h]	Common "other" viruses: rhinovirus, influenza, parainfluenza, adenovirus (PIDJ 19:293, 2000). Often of mild to moderate severity; S. pneumo, non-type B H. flu in 4–20%. Treat times 10–14 days. NOTE: High frequency of resistance of DRSP to cefuroxime. See footnote 1 page 29, footnote 1 page 29, footnote 2 page 34, and Table 5, page 71, for drug-resistant S. pneumo.
Age 5 years–15 years, Non-hospitalized, immuno-competent NEJM 346:429, 2002; PIDJ 21:592, 2002	Mycoplasma, Chlamydophila pneumoniae, S. pneumoniae, H. flu, myco-plasma, S. pneumo-niae, Mycobacterium tuberculosis Respiratory viruses: mixed, e.g. influenza Bacterial/viral mixed in 23% (Peds 113:701, 2004) Legionella: especially in pts with malignancy Ln Inf Dis 6:529, 2006	**Inpatient (ICU):** **Cefotaxime** 200 mg per kg per day IV div q8h or **ceftriaxone** 50–75 mg per kg per day IV once per day	**Inpatient (ICU): Amox** 100 mg/kg (max 1 gm per pt) bid if pt >8 yrs old) **Clarithro** 500 mg po bid or 1 gm ER q24h; **(azithro** 0.5 gm po x1, then 0.25 gm/day, max. 10 mg/kg per day, max. of 500 mg po, then 5 mg/kg per day, max. 250 mg)	If otherwise healthy and if not concomitant with (or post-) influenza, S. pneumoniae & S. aureus uncommon in this subset; suspect S. pneumo if sudden onset and large amount of purulent sputum. **Macrolide-resistant S. pneumo** an issue. Higher prevalence of macrolide-resistant S. pneumo in pts <5 yrs old (JAMA 286:1857, 2001). **Mycoplasma** requires 2–3 wks of rx, C. pneumoniae up to 6 wks. (LnID 1:334, 2001; J Med Micro 55:225, 2002). Macrolide-resistant M. pneumo reported (AAC 50:709, 2006). **Linezolid** approved for pts use for pen-susceptible & multi-drug resistant S. pneumo (including bacteremia) & methicillin-sensitive S. aureus.

Abbreviations on page 2.

NOTE: All dosage recommendations are for adults (unless otherwise indicated) and assume normal renal function.

TABLE 1 (31)

ANATOMIC SITE/DIAGNOSIS/ MODIFYING CIRCUMSTANCES	ETIOLOGIES (usual)	SUGGESTED REGIMENS*		ADJUNCT DIAGNOSTIC OR THERAPEUTIC MEASURES AND COMMENTS
		PRIMARY	**ALTERNATIVE[1]**	
			See Comment regarding macrolide resistance	
LUNG/Pneumonia/Age 5 years–15 years (continued) **Children, hospitalized, immunocompetent— 2–18 yrs**	S. pneumoniae, viruses, mycoplasma, consider S. aureus if abscesses or necrotizing, esp. during influenza season	**Ceftriaxone** 50 mg per kg per day IV (to max. 2 gm per day) + **azithro** 10 mg per kg per day up to 500 mg IV div q12h. Add anti-staph drug if evidence of lung necrosis: **vanco** 40mg/kg/day divided q8h.		**Alternatives are a problem in children:** If proven S. pneumo resistant to azithro & ceftriaxone (or severe ceftriaxone allergy): IV vanco, linezolid, or off-label respiratory FQ. No doxy under age 8. Linezolid reported efficacious in children (PIDJ 22:677, 2003). Cefuroxime failures vs drug-resistant S. pneumo (CID 29:482, 1999).
Adults (over age 18)—New IDSA Guidelines in Jan 2007—see www.idsociety.org (CID 37:1405, 2003; Chest 125:1888 & 1913, 2004; AJM 117(3A):39S, 2004; Thorax 56(Suppl.1):1, 2001) Varies with clinical setting. Guidelines reflect variable approaches: **1.** Focus on S. pneumo, ignore atypicals, & emphasize **high dose amox or AM-CL 2.** If no comorbidity, focus on atypicals, & emphasize **macrolides** that are still active vs majority of S. pneumo **3.** Focus on both S. pneumo & atypicals by combining (**high dose amox + a macrolide**) OR suggesting a **respiratory FQ or telithromycin**				
No co-morbidity: Azithro 0.5 gm q24h po times 1, then 0.25 gm po times 1 then 0.25 gm per day or **azithro-ER** 2 gm times 1 **OR clarithro** 500 mg po bid or **clarithro-ER** 1 gm po bid **OR** if prior antibiotic within 3 months: (**azithro** or **clarithro**) + (**amox** 1 gm po q8h) or high dose (**AM-CL**) OR **Respiratory FQ**	**No co-morbidity present:** **Respiratory FQ** (see footnote[2]) OR (**azithro** or **clarithro**) + (**high dose amox**, high dose **AM-CL, cefdinir, cefpodoxime, cefprozil**) OR **telithromycin**—**status unclear, see comment, page 35** Doses in footnote[3]	**No co-morbidity: Pro:** Active vs S. pneumo at 3–4 gm per day **Con:** Appropriate spectrum of action; more in vitro resistance than clinical failure (CID 34(Suppl.1):S27, 2002); q24h dosing; better tolerated than erythro **Con:** Overall S. pneumo resistance in vitro 20–30% (CID 34(Suppl.1):S4, 2002); it pen G resist. S. pneumo, up to 50%+ resistance to azithro/clarithro. Breakthrough infections reported (NEJM 346:630, 2002; CID 35:556, 2002) **Amoxicillin: Pro:** Active 90–95% S. pneumo at 3–4 gm per day **Con:** No activity atypicals or β-lactamase + bacteria. Need 3–4 gm per day **AM-CL: Pro:** Spectrum includes β-lactamase + H. influenzae, M. catarrhalis, MSSA, & Bacteroides sp. **Con:** No activity atypicals **Cephalosporins**—po: Cefdinir, cefpodoxime, cefprozil, cefuroxime & others—see footnote[3]. **Pro:** Active 75–85% S. pneumo & H. influenzae. Cefuroxime least active & higher mortality rate when S. pneumo resistant (CID 37:230, 2003). **Con:** Inactive vs atypical pathogens	
Prognosis prediction: CURB-65 (AJM 118:384, 2005): C: confusion = 1 pt U: BUN >19 mg/dl = 1 pt R: RR >30/min = 1 pt B: BP <90/60 = 1 pt Age ≥65 = 1 pt If score = 1, ok or outpt therapy; if >1, hospitalize	**Co-morbidity:** COPD—M. pneumoniae, C. psittaci, Legionella sp., M. pneumoniae, C. burnetii (Q fever) **Alcoholism:** S. pneumo, anaerobes, coliforms **Aspiration:** S. pneumo, M. pneumoniae, coliforms **Bronchiectasis:** see Cystic fibrosis, page 39 COPD: H. influenzae, S. pneumo, M. catarrhalis, S. pneumo **IVDU:** Hematogenous: S. aureus **Post-CVA aspiration:** Oral flora, incl. S. pneumo **Post-obstruction of bronchi:** S. pneumo, anaerobes **Post-influenza:** S. pneumo, and S. aureus	**Co-morbidity present: Gati** 400 mg IV/po q24h (no longer marketed in US due to hypo- and hyperglycemic reactions), **Moxi** 400 mg IV/po q24h, **Levo** 750 mg IV/po q24h. Ketolide: **telithro** 800 mg po q24h(physicians warned about rare instances of hepatotoxicity). Duration of rx: S. pneumo—Not bacteremic: until afebrile 3 days —Bacteremic: 10–14 days reasonable C. pneumoniae—Unclear. Some reports suggest 21 days. Some bronchitis pts required 5–6 wks of clarithro (J Med Micro 52:265, 2003) Legionella—10–21 days Necrotizing pneumonia due to coliforms, S. aureus, anaerobes: ≥2 weeks **Cautions:** **1.** If local macrolide resistance to **S. pneumoniae >25%**, use alternative empiric therapy. **2.** Esp. during influenza season, look for **S. aureus.**		**Doxycycline: Pro:** Active vs S. pneumo (DMID 49:147, 2004) but resistance may be increasing. Active vs H. influenzae, atypicals, & bioterrorism agents (anthrax, plague, tularemia). **Con:** Resistance of S. pneumo (CID 35:633, 2002). Sparse clinical data (AJM 159:266, 1999; CID 37:870, 2003).

(continued on next page)

[1] Atypical pathogens: Chlamydophila pneumoniae, C. psittaci, Legionella sp., M. pneumoniae, C. burnetii

[2] Respiratory FQs with enhanced activity vs S. pneumo with HLR to penicillin: **Gati** 400 mg IV/po q24h (no longer marketed in US due to hypo- and hyperglycemic reactions), **Gemi** 320 mg po q24h, **Levo** 750 mg IV/po q24h, **Moxi** 400 mg IV/po q24h.

[3] **O Ceph doses: Cefdinir** 300 mg po q12h; **cefditoren pivoxil** 200 mg, 2 tabs po bid; **cefpodoxime proxetil** 200 mg po q12h; **high dose amox** 1 gm po tid; **high dose cefprozil** 500 mg po q12h. **AM-CL**—use **AM-CL-ER** 1000/62.5 mg, 2 tabs po bid, **telithromycin** 800 mg po q24h times 7–10 days.

Abbreviations on page 2.   NOTE: All dosage recommendations are for adults (unless otherwise indicated) and assume normal renal function.

TABLE 1 (32)

ANATOMIC SITE/DIAGNOSIS/ MODIFYING CIRCUMSTANCES	ETIOLOGIES (usual)	SUGGESTED REGIMENS*		ADJUNCT DIAGNOSTIC OR THERAPEUTIC MEASURES AND COMMENTS
		PRIMARY	ALTERNATIVE†	
LUNG/Pneumonia/Adult (continued)				(continued from page 34)
Community-acquired, hospitalized—NOT in the ICU Empiric therapy	Etiology by co-morbidity & risk factors as above. Culture sputum & blood. S. pneumo, urine antigen reported helpful (CID 40:16/08, 2005). Legionella urine antigen indicated. In general, the sicker the pt, the more valuable culture data.	Ceftriaxone 2 gm IV q24h (1 gm IV q24h > age 65) + azithro 500 mg IV q24h	Levo 750 mg IV (q24h or Moxi 400 mg IV q24h Gati 400 mg IV q24h (gati no longer marketed in US due to hypo- and hyperglycemic reactions) po.	**FQs—Respiratory** FQs: Moxi, levo & gemi Pro: In vitro & clinically effective vs pen-sensitive & pen-resistant S. pneumo. Gemi only available po. **NOTE: dose of Levo is 750 mg q24h.** Q24h dosing. Con: Geographic pockets of resistance with clinical failure (NEJM 346:747, 2002). Important Drug-drug interactions (see Table 22A, page 184). Reversible rash in young females given Gemi for > 7 days. **Ceftriaxone/cefotaxime:** Pro: Drugs of choice for pen-sens. S. pneumo, active H. influenzae. M. catarrhalis, & MSSA Con: Not active atypicals or pneumonia due to bioterrorism pathogens. Add macrolide for atypicals.
Community-acquired, hospitalized—IN ICU Empiric therapy	**Severe COPD** pt with pneumonia. S. pneumoniae, H. influenzae, Moraxella sp., Legionella sp.	Levo 750 mg IV q24h or Moxi 400 mg IV q24h. Gati not available in US due to hypo- and hyperglycemic reactions	[Ceftriaxone 2 gm IV q24h (1 gm IV q24h > age 65) + azithro 500 mg IV q24h] or ERTA 1 gm q24h IV + azithro 500 mg IV q24h (see Comment)	**Telithromycin:** Pro: Virtually no resistant S. pneumo. Active vs atypical pathogens. Con: Concern of severe hepatotoxicity (AnIM 244:415, 2006; NEJM 355:2260, 2006). Only available po. Transient reversible blurry vision due to paralysis of lens accommodation; avoid in myasthenia gravis pts (Black Box Warning). **Various studies** indicate improved outcome when azithro added to a β-lactam (CID 36:389 & 1239, 2003; AnIM 164:1807, 2001 & 159:2562, 1999). Similar results in prospective study of critically ill pts with pneumococcal bacteremia (AJRCCM 170:440, 2004). **Ertapenem** could substitute for ceftriaxone. Need azithro for atypical pathogens. Do not use if suspect P. aeruginosa. **Legionella:** Not all Legionella species detected by urine antigen; if suspicious culture or PCR on airway secretions.
Community-acquired, hospitalized—IN ICU Empiric therapy	Culture sputum, blood and maybe pleural fluid. Look for respiratory viruses. Urine antigen for both Legionella and S. pneumoniae. Sputum PCR for Legionella.			In patients with normal sinus rhythm and not receiving beta-blockers, relative bradycardia suggests Legionella, psittacosis, Q-fever, or typhoid fever (Clin Micro Infect 6:633, 2000).
Community-acquired, hospitalized—IN ICU If concomitant with or post-influenza. S. aureus and S. pneumoniae possible	If concomitant with or post-influenza. S. aureus and S. pneumoniae possible	Vanco 1 gm IV q12h + (Levo 750 mg IV q24h or moxi 400 mg IV q24h)	Linezolid 600 mg IV bid + (levo or moxi)	Sputum gram stain may help. S. aureus post-influenza ref: EID 12:894, 2006 Empiric therapy vs MRSA decreases risk of mortality (CCM 34:2069, 2006)

NOTE: q24h = once q24h; bid = twice q24h; tid = 3 times a day; qid = 4 times a day.

NOTE: All dosage recommendations are for adults (unless otherwise indicated) and assume normal renal function.

Abbreviations on page 2.

TABLE 1 (33)

ANATOMIC SITE/DIAGNOSIS/ MODIFYING CIRCUMSTANCES	ETIOLOGIES (usual)	SUGGESTED REGIMENS* PRIMARY	ALTERNATIVE†	ADJUNCT DIAGNOSTIC OR THERAPEUTIC MEASURES AND COMMENTS
LUNG/Pneumonia/Adult *(continued)*				
	Suspect aerobic gm-neg bacilli: esp. P. aeruginosa and/or life-threatening infection (see comment). Hypoxic and/or hypotensive	Anti-pseudomonal beta-lactam¹ + (respiratory FQ or aminoglycoside)	If beta-lactam allergy: FQ + or aminoglycoside) (aztreonam + aminoglycoside + azithro)	At risk for gm-neg rod pneumonia due to: alcoholism with necrotizing pneumonia, underlying chronic bronchiectasis (e.g. cystic fibrosis), chronic tracheostomy and/or mechanical ventilation, febrile neutropenia and pulmonary infiltrates, septic shock, or underlying malignancy. Microbiologic documentation of pneumonia due to an aerobic gm-neg rod acquired in the community and admitted to the ICU is an uncommon event (AnIM 162:1849, 2002; CID 16:135, 2003; AJRCCM 160:397, 1999).
	If increased risk of drug-resistant S. pneumoniae.	High dose IV amp + azithro + respiratory FQ	Beta-lactam allergy: vanco + respiratory FQ	
Hospital-acquired—usually with mechanical ventilation (empiric therapy) Diagnosis confirmed by quantitative cultures (see Comment) Vent-Assoc. Pneumonia Guidelines: AJRCCM 171:388, 2005. Review: Chest 130:597, 2006	Highly variable depending on clinical setting: S. pneumo, S. aureus, Legionella, coliforms, P. aeruginosa, stenotrophomonas, acinetobacter,² anaerobes all possible	(IMP 0.5 gm IV q6h or MER 1 gm IV q8h) plus, if suspect legionella or bioterrorism (Levo or Moxi) FQ **NOTE:** Regimen not active vs **MRSA**—see specific rx See Comment regarding diagnosis Dosages: See footnotes pages 22, 30, 32, & 34 Duration depends on specific organism (see below) and host response.	(Cefepime or high-dose PIP-TZ³) + tobra. Add resp. FQ if suspect legionella or bioterrorism.	**Dx of ventilator-associated pneumonia:** Fever & lung infiltrates often **not** pneumonia (Chest 106:221, 1994). Quantitative cultures helpful: bronchoalveolar lavage (> 10⁴ per mL pos.) or protected spec. brush (>10³ per mL pos.) Ref.: AJRCCM 165:867, 2002; AnIM 132:621, 2000. **Microbial etiology:** No empiric regimen covers all possibilities. Regimens listed above majority of S. pneumo, legionella, & most coliforms. Regimens not active vs MRSA, Stenotrophomonas & others; see below. Specific rx when culture results known. **Ventilator-associated pneumonia—Prevention:** If possible, keep head of bed elevated 30° or more. Remove N-G, endotracheal tubes as soon as possible. If available, continuous subglottic suctioning. Chlorhexidine paste may help. Refs.: Chest 130:251, 2006; CCM 32:1396, 2004; AJRCCM 173:1297, 1949, 2006.
Hospital- or community-acquired, neutropenic pt (<500 neutrophils per mm³)	Any of organisms listed under community-, & hospital-acquired + fungi (aspergillus). See Table 1	See Hospital-acquired; immediately above + vanco n.b. included in initial rx unless low suspicion of infected IV access or drug-resistant S. pneumo. Ampho not used unless still febrile after 3 days or high clinical likelihood See Comment		See consensus document on management of febrile neutropenic pt: CID 34:730, 2002.
Adults—Selected specific rx when culture results (sputum, blood, pleural fluid, etc.) available. Also see Table 2, page 61				
Burkholderia (Pseudomonas) pseudomallei (etiology of melioidosis) Ref.: Ln 361:1715, 2003	Gram-negative	Initial parenteral rx: Ceftazidime 30-50 mg per kg IV q6h or IMP 20 mg per kg IV q6h Rx minimum 10 days & improving, then po therapy.	Post-parenteral po rx: Adults (see Comment for peds dose) TMP-SMX 10 mg per kg (TMP component) bid times 20 wks: **Doxy** 2 mg per kg bid times 20 wks; **TMP-SMX** 5 mg per kg (TMP component) bid times 20 wks.	**Children <8 yrs old & pregnancy:** For oral regimen, use **AM-CL-ER** 1000/62.5, 2 tabs po bid times 20 wks. Even with compliance, relapse rate is 10%. Max. daily ceftazidime dose 6 gm.
				Tigecycline: No clinical data but active in vitro (AAC 50:1555, 2006).

---

¹ Antipseudomonal beta-lactams: **Aztreonam** 2 gm IV q6h; **piperacillin** 3 gm IV q4h; **piperacillin/tazobactam** 3.375 mg IV q4h (high dose for Pseudomonas); **cefepime** 2 gm IV q12h; **ceftazidime** 2 gm IV q8h; **imipenem/cilastatin** 500 mg IV q6h; **meropenem** 1 gm IV q8h; **gentamicin** or **tobramycin** (see Table 10D, pg 93). Respiratory FQs: **levofloxacin** 750 mg IV q24h or **moxifloxacin** 400 mg IV q24h; **high-dose ampicillin** 2 gm IV q4h; **azithromycin** 500 mg IV q24h; **vanco** 1 gm IV q12h.

² If Acinetobacter sp., susceptibility to IMP & MER may be discordant (CID 41:758, 2005).

³ **PIP-TZ** dose: 4.5 gm IV q6h or 3.375 gm IV q6h   NOTE: All dosage recommendations are for adults (unless otherwise indicated) and assume normal renal function.

Abbreviations on page 2.

TABLE 1 (36)

ANATOMIC SITE/DIAGNOSIS/ MODIFYING CIRCUMSTANCES	ETIOLOGIES (usual)	SUGGESTED REGIMENS*		ADJUNCT DIAGNOSTIC OR THERAPEUTIC MEASURES AND COMMENTS
		PRIMARY	ALTERNATIVE[1]	
LUNG/Other (continued) **Cystic fibrosis** **Acute exacerbation of pulmonary symptoms** Refs.: Ln 361:681, 2003; AJRCCM 168:918, 2003; J.Peds&Child-Health 42:601, 2006.	S. aureus or H. influenzae early in disease. P. aeruginosa later in disease	**For P. aeruginosa:** **Tobra** 3.3 mg/kg q8h or tobra 12 mg/kg q24h (See footnote 6). Combine tobra with (**PIP** or **ticarcillin** 100 mg/kg q8h) or **ceftaz** 50 mg/kg IV q8h to max of 6 gm per day. See footnote6	**For S. aureus: (1) MSSA—oxacillin/nafcillin**,2 gm IV q4h; **penicillin-allergic: (2) MRSA—vanco**—see Comment	Other options: **Clarithro** synergistic with tobra vs P. aeruginosa (AAC 46: 1105, 2002) + anti-inflammatory properties (Pharmacotherapy 22:227, 2002). **Azithro** 1x/day for pts chronically infected with P. aeruginosa (JAMA 290: 1749, 2003) 1x/day **tobra** reported less nephrotoxic (Ln 365:573, 2005). For pharmacokinetics of aminoglycosides in CF, J.Peds&Child-Health 42:601, 2006. For chronic suppression of P. aeruginosa, **inhaled phenol-free tobra** 300 mg bid x 28 d., then no rx x 28 d., then repeat cycle (AJRCCM 167:841, 2003).
			(2) MRSA—vanco 15-20 mg per kg q12h & check serum levels. See Comment	
	Burkholderia (Pseudomonas) cepacia	**TMP-SMX** 5 mg per kg (TMP) IV q6h	**Chloro** 15-20 mg per kg IV/po q6h	B. cepacia has become a major pathogen. Patients develop progressive respiratory failure, 62% mortality at 1yr. **Fail to respond to APAG**, piperacillin, & ceftazidime. Patients with B. cepacia should be isolated from other CF pas. **NOTE:** 3- & 4-drug combos under study in refractory pts (AAC 43:213, 1999).
Empyema. Ref.: CID 22:747, 1996.	Pleural effusion review: NEJM 346:1971, 2002		*For other alternatives, see Table 2*	
Neonatal	Staph. aureus	See Pneumonia, neonatal, page 33		Drainage indicated.
Infants/children (1 month–5 yrs)	Staph. aureus, Strep. pneumoniae, H. influenzae	See Pneumonia, age 1 month–5 years, page 33		Drainage indicated.
Child ~5 yrs to ADULT—Diagnostic thoracentesis; chest tube for empyemas				
Acute, usually parapneumonic For dosage, see Table 10 or footnote page 30	Strep. pneumoniae, Group A strep	**(Cefotaxime or ceftriaxone)** (Dosage, see footnote 1, page 30)	Vanco	In large multicenter double-blind trial, intrapleural streptokinase did not improve mortality, reduce the need for surgery or the length of hospitalization (NEJM 352:865, 2005).
Microbiologic diagnosis: CID 42:1135, 2006.	Staph. aureus: Check for MRSA H. influenzae	**Nafcillin or oxacillin** if MSSA **Ceftriaxone**	Vanco if MRSA TMP-SMX or AM-SB	Usually complication of S. aureus pneumonia &/or bacteremia. Pleomorphic Gm-neg. bacilli. ↑ resistance to TMP-SMX.
Subacute/chronic	Anaerobic strep, Strep. milleri, also M. tbc, fungi, Kaposi's sarcoma, & lymphoma. NOTE: AIDS pts may develop pneumonia due to DRSP or other pathogens—see next box below	**Clinda** 450–900 mg IV q8h + **ceftriaxone**	**Cefoxitin** or **IMP** or **TC-CL** or **PIP-TZ** or **AM-SB** (Dosage, see footnote 1 page 30)	If organisms not seen, treat as subacute. Drainage. R/O tuberculosis or tumor. Pleural biopsy with culture for mycobacteria and histology if Tbc suspected (CID 22:747, 1996).
Human immunodeficiency virus infection (HIV+): See SANFORD GUIDE TO HIV/AIDS THERAPY **CD4 T-lymphocytes <200 per mm³ or clinical AIDS** Dry cough, progressive dyspnea, & diffuse infiltrate **Prednisone first if suspect pneumocystis (see Comment)**	Pneumocystis carinii most likely; also M. tbc, fungi, Kaposi's sarcoma, & lymphoma	Rx listed here is for **severe** pneumocystis; page 125 for po regimens for **mild** disease. **Prednisone 1st (see Comment)**, then: **TMP-SMX** (IV 15 mg per kg per day q8h (TMP component) or po 2 DS tabs q8h), total of 21 days	For listed here is for severe pneumocystis, page 125 for po regimens for mild disease. **Prednisone** (po) 40 mg 2x/day times 5 days, then 40 mg q24h po times 5 days, then 20 mg q24h po times 11 days if **indicated** (see Comment). then: **(Clinda** 600 mg IV q8h + **primaquine** 30 mg (base) po q24h) or **(pentamidine isethionate** 4 mg per kg per day IV) times 21 days See Comment	Diagnostic procedure if po or IV. If negative, bronchoscopy. Pts with PCP and <200 CD4 cells per mm³ should be on anti-PCP prophylaxis for life. **Prednisone 40 mg bid po times 5 days then 40 mg q24h po times 5 days then 20 mg q24h po times 11 days is indicated when PCP (pO₂ <70 mmHg) should be given at initiation of anti-PCP rx; don't wait until pt's condition deteriorates** (Table 13, page 125). If PCP studies negative, consider bacterial pneumonia, Tbc, cocci, histo, crypto, Kaposi's sarcoma or lymphoma. **Pentamidine not active vs bacterial pathogens. NOTE:** Pneumocystis resistant to TMP-SMX, albeit rare, does exist.

[1] Other options: (Tobra + aztreonam 50 mg per kg IV q8h); (IMP 15-25 mg per kg IV q6h + tobra); **CIP commonly used in children**. e.g. CIP IV/po + ceftaz IV (LnID 3:537, 2003). Abbreviations on page 2. NOTE: All dosage recommendations are for adults (unless otherwise indicated) and assume normal renal function.

TABLE 1 (37)

ANATOMIC SITE/DIAGNOSIS/ MODIFYING CIRCUMSTANCES	ETIOLOGIES (usual)	SUGGESTED REGIMENS*		ADJUNCT DIAGNOSTIC OR THERAPEUTIC MEASURES AND COMMENTS
		PRIMARY	ALTERNATIVE†	
LUNG/Other (continued) **CD4 T-lymphocytes normal** Acute onset, purulent sputum & pulmonary infiltrates ± pleuritic pain. **Isolate pt until TBc excluded: Adults**	Strep. pneumoniae, H. influenzae, aerobic Gm-neg. bacilli (including P. aeruginosa), Legionella rare, M. tbc	Ceftriaxone 2 gm IV q24h (over age 65 1 gm IV q24h) + azithro (500 mg IV q24h use, **Levo**, or **Moxi** IV as alternative (see Comment)		In Gram stain of sputum shows Gm-neg. bacilli, options include **P. Ceph 3 AP**, TC pen, **PIP-TZ**, **IMP**, **MER**. **FQs: Levo** 750 mg po/IV q24h; **Moxi** 400 mg po/IV q24h. Gati not available in US due to hypo- & hyperglycemic reactions.
As above: Children	Same as adult with HIV + lymphoid interstitial pneumonia (LIP)	As for HIV + adults with pneumonia. If diagnosis is LIP rx with steroids.		In children with AIDS, LIP responsible for 1/3 of pulmonary complications, usually >1 yr of age. In contrast to PCP, which is seen at <1 yr of age. Clinically: clubbing, hepatosplenomegaly, salivary glands enlarged (take up gallium), lymphocytosis.
Viral (interstitial) pneumonia suspected (See Table 14, page 134)	Consider: Adenovirus, coronavirus (SARS), hantavirus, influenza, metapneumovirus, parainfluenza virus, respiratory syncytial virus	**For Influenza A: rimantadine** 100 mg po q12h or **amantadine** 100 mg po q12h		No known efficacious drugs for adenovirus, coronavirus (SARS), hantavirus, metapneumovirus, parainfluenza or RSV. Need travel (SARS) & exposure (Hanta) history. RSV as serious as influenza in the elderly (NEJM 352:1749 & 1810, 2005).
		For Influenza A or B: oseltamivir 75 mg po bid x 5 d or **zanamivir** 10 mg inhaled bid x 5 d. Start within 48 hrs of symptom onset.		
LYMPH NODES (approaches below apply to lymphadenitis without an obvious primary source)				
Lymphadenitis, acute Generalized	Etiologies: EBV, early HIV infection, syphilis, toxoplasma, tularemia, Lyme disease, sarcoid, lymphoma, systemic lupus erythematosus, and **Kikuchi-Fujimoto** disease (CID 39:138, 2004). Complete history and physical examination followed by appropriate serological tests. Treat specific agent (s).			
Regional				
Cervical—see cat-scratch disease (CSD), below	CSD (B. henselae), Grp A strep, Staph. aureus, anaerobes, M. TBc (scrofula), M. avium, M. scrofulaceum, M. malmoense, toxo, tularemia	History & physical exam directs evaluation. If nodes fluctuant, aspirate and base rx on Gram & acid-fast stains. Review of mycobacterial etiology: CID 20:954, 1995. **Kikuchi-Fujimoto** disease causes fever and benign self-limited adenopathy; the etiology is unknown (AJM 171:401, 1996; CID 39:138, 2004).		
Inguinal	HSV, chancroid, syphilis, LGV			
Sexually transmitted	GAS, SA tularemia, CSD			
Not sexually transmitted	GAS, SA, CSD, tularemia, Y. pestis, sporotrichosis			
Axillary	Sporotrichosis, leishmania, Mycobacterium marinum, Nocardia brasiliensis, tularemia			
Extremity, with associated nodular lymphangitis (For full discussion: AnIM 118:883, 1993)	Sporotrichosis, leishmania, Mycobacterium marinum, Mycobacterium chelonae, tularemia	Treatment varies with specific etiology		A distinctive form of lymphangitis characterized by subcutaneous swellings along inflamed lymphatic channels. Primary site of skin invasion usually present; regional adenopathy variable.
Cat-scratch disease— immunocompetent patient Axillary/epitrochlear nodes 46%, neck 26%, inguinal 17%	Bartonella henselae Reviews: AAC 48:1921, 2004; PIDJ 23:1161, 2004	No rx; resolves in 2–6 mos. Needle aspiration relieves pain in suppurative nodes. Avoid I&D	**Azithro** dosage— **Adults** (>45.5 kg): 500 mg po x 1 then 250 mg/day x4 days; **Children** (<45.5 kg) liquid azithro 10 mg/kg x 1 then 5 mg/kg per day x 4 days. Rx is controversial —see Comment	**Clinical:** Approx. 10% nodes suppurate. Atypical presentation in <5% pts, i.e. lung nodules, liver/spleen lesions, Parinaud's oculoglandular syndrome, CNS manifestations in 2% of pts (encephalitis, peripheral neuropathy, retinitis), FUO. **Dx:** Cat exposure. Positive IFA serology. Rarely need biopsy. **Rx:** Only 1 prospective randomized blinded study; used azithro with ↑ rapidity of resolution of enlarged lymph nodes (PIDJ 17:447, 1998). **Note:** In elderly, endocarditis less frequent; lymphadenitis more frequent (CID 41:969, 2005).

NOTE: All dosage recommendations are for adults (unless otherwise indicated) and assume normal renal/renal function.

Abbreviations on page 2.

TABLE 1 (38)

ANATOMIC SITE/DIAGNOSIS/ MODIFYING CIRCUMSTANCES	ETIOLOGIES (usual)	SUGGESTED REGIMENS*		ADJUNCT DIAGNOSTIC OR THERAPEUTIC MEASURES AND COMMENTS
		PRIMARY	ALTERNATIVE†	
MOUTH				
Odontogenic infection, including Ludwig's angina. Can result in more serious para- pharyngeal space infection (see page 44)	Oral microflora: infection polymicrobial	**Clinda** 300–450 mg po q6h or 600 mg IV q6-8h	**AM-CL** 875/125 mg po bid or 500/125 mg tid or 2000/125 mg bid) or **cefotetan** 2 gm IV q12h	Surgical drainage & removal of necrotic tissue essential. β-lactamase pro- ducing organisms are ↑ in frequency. Ref.: Canad Dental Assn J 64:508, 1998 Other parenteral alternatives: AM-SB, PIP-TZ, or TC-CL. For Noma (cancrum oris) see Ln 368:147, 2006.
Buccal cellulitis Children <5 yrs	H. influenzae	**Cefuroxime** or **ceftriaxone**	**AM-CL** or **TMP-SMX** Dosage: see Table 16, page 168	With Hib immunization, invasive H. influenzae infections have ↓ by 95%. Now occurring in infants prior to immunization.
Herpetic stomatitis	Herpes simplex virus 1 & 2	See Table 14		
Aphthous stomatitis, recurrent, HIV-neg	Etiology unknown	Topical steroids (Kenalog in Orabase) may ↓ pain and swelling. If AIDS, see SANFORD GUIDE TO HIV/AIDS THERAPY.		
MUSCLE				
"Gas gangrene" Contaminated traumatic wound Can be spontaneous without trauma (CID 28:159, 1999)	Cl. perfringens, other histo- toxic Clostridium sp.	**(Clinda** 900 mg IV q8h) + **(pen G** 24 million units/day div q4-6h IV)	**Ceftriaxone** 2 gm IV q12h or **erythro** 1 gm q6h IV (not by bolus)	Surgical debridement primary rx. Hyperbaric oxygen adjunctive efficacy debated, consider if debridement not complete or possible (NEJM 334:1642, 1996). Clinda decreases toxin production.
Pyomyositis Review: AJM 117:420, 2004	Staph. aureus, Group A strep, (rarely Gm-neg. bacilli), variety of anaerobic organisms	**(Nafcillin** or **oxacillin** 2 gm IV q4h) or **(P Ceph 1 (cefazolin** 2 gm IV q8h)) if **MSSA**	**Vanco** 1 gm IV q12h if **MRSA**	Common in tropics; rare, but occurs, in temperate zones (IDCP 7:265, 1998). Follows exercise or muscle injury; see Necrotizing fasciitis. Now seen in HIV/AIDS. Add **metro** if anaerobes suspected/proven (IDCP 8:252, 1999).
PANCREAS: Reviews—Ln 361:1447, 2003; JAMA 291:2865, 2004; NEJM 354:2142, 2006.				
Acute alcoholic (without necrosis) (idopathic) pancreatitis	Not bacterial	None CT-diagnosed		1–9% become infected most prospective studies show no advantage of prophylactic antimicrobials (Ln 346:652, 1995). Observe for pancreatic abscesses or necrosis which require rx.
Pancreatic abscess, infected pseudocyst, post-necrotizing pancreatitis	Enterobacteriaceae, entero- cocci, S. aureus, S. epider- midis, anaerobes, candida	Need culture of abscess/infected pseudocyst to direct therapy		Can often get specimen by fine-needle aspiration.
Antimicrobic prophylaxis, necrotizing pancreatitis	As above	Controversial: Cochrane Database 2: CD 002941, 2004 supports prophylaxis. Subsequent, double-blind, randomized, controlled study, showed no benefit (Gastroenterol 126:997, 2004). Consensus conference voted against prophylaxis (CCM 32:2524, 2004)		
PAROTID GLAND				
"Hot" tender parotid swelling	S. aureus, oral flora, & aerobic Gm-neg. bacilli (rare), mumps, rarely enteroviruses/ influenza. **Nafcillin** or **oxacillin** 2 gm IV q4h			Predisposing factors: stone(s) in Stensen's duct, dehydration. Rx depends on ID of specific etiologic organism.
"Cold" non-tender parotid swelling	Granulomatous disease (e.g., mycobacteria, fungi, sarcoidosis, Sjögren's syndrome), drugs (iodides, et al.), diabetes, cirrhosis, tumors			History/lab results may narrow differential; may need biopsy for dx

Abbreviations on page 2.

NOTE: All dosage recommendations are for adults (unless otherwise indicated) and assume normal renal function.

TABLE 1 (39)

ANATOMIC SITE/DIAGNOSIS/ MODIFYING CIRCUMSTANCES	ETIOLOGIES (usual)	SUGGESTED REGIMENS*		ADJUNCT DIAGNOSTIC OR THERAPEUTIC MEASURES AND COMMENTS
		PRIMARY	ALTERNATIVE*	
PERITONEUM—PERITONITIS: Reference—CID 31:997, 2003 **Primary (spontaneous bacterial peritonitis, SBP)** Rev. CID 27:669, 1998 ESBL see CID 28:683, 1999 Microbiology: CID 33:1513, 2001	Enterobacteriaceae 63%, S. pneumo 15%, enterococci 6–10%, anaerobes <1%. Extended β-lactamase (ESBL) positive Klebsiella species.	**Cefotaxime** 2 gm IV q8h (↑ if life-threatening, q4h) or **TC-CL** or **AM-SB** or **(ceftriaxone** 2 gm IV q24h) or **ERTA** 1 gm IV q24h) If resistant Gm-neg or Klebsiella with ESBL(+), then: **IMP** or **MER** or **(FQ: Levo, Moxi)** (Dosage in footnote[1])		One-year **risk of SBP** in pts with ascites and cirrhosis as high as 29% (Gastro 104:1133, 1993). 30–40% of pts have neg. cultures of blood and ascitic fluid. % pos. cultures ↑ if 10 mL of pt's ascitic fluid added to blood culture bottles. **Duration of rx unclear:** Suggest 2wks if blood culture +. One report suggests repeat paracentesis after 48 hrs of rx to confirm <250/mm3 & ascitic fluid sterile, success with 5 days of rx (AJM 97:169, 1994). IV albumin (1.5gm/kg at dx & 1gm/kg day 3) may ↓ frequency of renal impairment (p 0.002) & ↓ hospital mortality (p 0.01) (NEJM 341:403, 1999). Ref. for CIP: Hpt
Prevention of SBP: Cirrhosis & ascites For prevention see Liver, page 31		**TMP-SMX-DS** 1 tab po 5 days/wk or **CIP** 750 mg po q.wk.	**TMP-SMX** ↓ peritonitis or spontaneous bacteremia from 27% to 3% (AnIM 122:595, 1995).	
Secondary (bowel perforation, ruptured appendix, ruptured diverticuli) Refs.: NEJM 338:1521, 1998 & CID 37:997, 2003	Enterobacteriaceae, Bacteroides sp., enterococcus, P. aeruginosa (3–15%)	**Mild-moderate disease—Inpatient—parenteral rx:** (e.g., focal perityphlitis/appendiceal peritonitis, peridiverticular abscess, endomyometritis) **PIP-TZ** 3.375 gm IV q6h or 4.5 gm IV q8h, **OR AM-SB** 3 gm IV q6h OR **(ceftriaxone 2 gm IV q24h + metro)** or **ERTA** 1 gm IV q24h OR **MOXI** 400 mg IV q24h **Severe life-threatening disease—ICU patient:** **IMP** 500 mg IV q6h or **MER** 1 gm IV q8h	**[CIP** 400 mg IV q12h or **Levo** 750 mg IV q24h] **+ metro** 1 gm IV loading then 0.5 gm q6h or 1 gm q12h **[CFP/CPZ** or **Ceft** 2 gm IV q12h + **metro)** or **tigecycline** 100 mg IV times 1 dose, then 50 mg q12h. **[AMP + metro + (CIP** 400 mg IV q12h or **Levo** 750 mg IV q24h)] OR **[AMP** 2 gm IV q6h + **metro** 500 mg IV q6h + **APAG** [see Table 10D, page 93]	Must "cover" both Gm-neg. aerobic & Gm-neg. anaerobic bacteria. **Drugs active only vs anaerobic Gm-neg. bacilli:** clinda, metro. **Drugs active only vs aerobic Gm-neg. bacilli:** APAG, P Ceph 2/3/4, aztreonam, AP Pen, CIP, Levo. **Drugs active vs both aerobic/anaerobic Gm-neg. bacteria:** cefoxitin, cefotetan, TC-CL, PIP-TZ, AM-SB, IMP, MER, Gati, Moxi. Increasing resistance (%) of B. fragilis to some drugs:
				Cefoxitin Clindamycin
				% R 4–25 17–87
				Cefotetan Clindamycin
				4–25 16–44
				Essentially no resistance: **metro**. **PIP-TZ** (CID 35(Suppl.1):S126, 2000). Case reports of metro resistance (CID 40:e67, 2005; JCM 43:4127, 2004. Mechanisms of resistance: CID 39:92, 2004. **Ertapenem** not active vs P. aeruginosa/Acinetobacter species. If absence of ongoing focal contamination, aerobic/anaerobic culture of peritoneal exudate/abscess of help in guiding specific therapy. Less need for aminoglycosides. **With severe pen allergy, can "cover" Gm-neg. aerobes with CIP or aztreonam. Remember IMP/MER are β-lactams.**
		Concomitant surgical management important. If of moderate severity, can rx by adding drug to dialysis fluid—see Table 10D for dosage. Reasonable empiric combinations: **(vanco + ceftazidime)** or **(vanco + APAG)** IP severely ill, IV with same drug (+ adjust dose for renal failure). See Table 10D, page 93, and in addition for dialysis.		For diagnosis: concentrate several hundred mL of removed dialysis fluid by centrifugation. Gram stain concentrate and then inject into aerobic/anaerobic blood culture bottles. A positive Gram stain will guide initial therapy. If culture shows Staph. epidermidis, good chance of "saving" dialysis catheter; if multiple Gm-neg. bacilli cultured, consider bowel perforation and catheter removal.
Associated with chronic ambulatory peritoneal dialysis (defined as ≥100 WBC per mcL, >50% PMNs)	Staph. aureus (most common), Staph. epidermidis, Gm-neg. bacilli 7%, P. aeruginosa 7%, sterile 20%, M. fortuitum (rare)			

---

[1] Parenteral IV therapy for peritonitis: **TC-CL** 3.1 gm q6h; **PIP-TZ** 3.375 gm q6h or 4.5 gm q8h; **AM-SB** 3 gm q6h; **IMP** 0.5 gm q6h; **MER** 1 gm q8h; **FQ** [**CIP** 400 mg q12h; **Oflox** 400 mg q12h; **Levo** 750 mg q24h; **Moxi** 400 mg q24h]; **AMP** 1 gm q6h; **APAG** [see Table 10D, page 93]; **cefotetan** 2 gm q12h; **cefotaxime** 2 gm q4–8h; **ceftriaxone** 1–2 gm q6h; **PIP** 4 gm q6h; **ceftizoxime** 2 gm q4–8h); **P Ceph 3** [**cefotaxime** 2 gm q12h, ceftazidime 2 gm q8h]; **clinda** 450–900 mg q8h; **metro** 1 gm loading then 0.5 gm q6h or 1 gm q12h; **AP Pen** [**ticarcillin** 4 gm q6h, **PIP** 4 gm q6h, aztreonam 2 gm q8h) Abbreviations on page 2.   NOTE: All dosage recommendations are for adults (unless otherwise indicated) and assume normal renal function.

43

TABLE 1 (40)

ANATOMIC SITE/DIAGNOSIS/ MODIFYING CIRCUMSTANCES	ETIOLOGIES (usual)	SUGGESTED REGIMENS*		ADJUNCT DIAGNOSTIC OR THERAPEUTIC MEASURES AND COMMENTS
		PRIMARY	ALTERNATIVE†	
PHARYNX				
Pharyngitis/Tonsillitis—Reviews: NEJM 344:205, 2001; *AnIM* 139:113, 2003. Guideline for Group A strep: *CID* 35:113, 2002				
Exudative or diffuse erythema For relationship to acute rheumatic fever, see footnote[1] Rheumatic fever[2] *Ln* 366:155, 2005	Group A,C,G strep, "viral," infectious mononucleosis diphtheriae, see footnote[1] C. diphtheriae, A. haemolyticum, Mycoplasma pneumoniae. In adults, only 10% pharyngitis due to Group A strep	**Pen V** po x 10 days or (if compliance unlikely) **benzathine pen** IM times 1 dose See footnote[2] for adult and pediatric dosages	**O Ceph 2** or **4–6 days** (*CID* 38:1526 & 1535, 2004) or **azithro** x 10 days or **dirithro** x 10 days or **erythro** x 10 days Up to 35% of isolates resistant to erythro, azithro, clarithro, clinda (*AAC* 48:473, 2004)	**Dx:** Rapid strep test or culture. (*JAMA* 291:1587, 2004, & 292:167, 2004). Rapid strep test valid in adults: *An IM* 166:640, 2006. **Pen allergy & macrolide resistance:** No penicillin or cephalosporin-resistant S. pyogenes, but now **macrolide-resist. S. pyogenes** (7%, 2000–2003). Culture & susceptibility testing if clinical failure with azithro/clarithro (*CID* 41:599, 2005) **S. pyogenes Groups C & G cause pharyngitis but not a risk for post-strep rheumatic fever.** To prevent rheumatic fever, eradicate Group A strep. Requires 10 days of pen V po, 4–6 days of po O Ceph 2, 5 days of po azithro. 10 days of dirithro. In controlled trial, better eradication rate with 10 days clarithro (91%) than 5 days azithro (82%)(*CID* 32: 1798,2001) Because of risk of concomitant genital C. trachomatis, add either (azithro 1 gm po times 1) or (doxy 100 mg po q12h times 7 days). See page 20 for more options.
	Gonococci	**Ceftriaxone** 125 mg IM x 1 dose+ (**azithro** or **doxy**) (see Comment)	**CIP** 500 mg po x 1) or **Levo** 250 mg po x 1) + (**azithro** or **doxy**) (see Comment)	
Asymptomatic post-rx carrier Multiple repeated culture-positive episodes (*CID* 25:574, 1997)	Group A strep	**No rx required** Clinda or AM-CL po	Parenteral **benzathine pen G** + **RIF** (see Comment) Dosages in footnote[3]	Routine post-rx throat culture not advised. Small % of pts have recurrent culture-pos. Group A strep with symptomatic tonsillo-pharyngitis. Hard to tell if true Group A strep carrier or new active viral infection in carrier of Group A strep. Addition of **RIF** may help: 20 mg per kg per day times 4 days to max. of 300 mg (*J Ped* 106:481 & 876, 1985)
Whitish plaques, HIV+, (thrush)	Candida albicans (see *Table 11, page 98*)	Antibacterial agents not indicated. For HSV-1/2:		
Vesicular, ulcerative	Coxsackie A9, B1-5, ECHO (multiple types), Enterovirus 71, Herpes simplex 1,2	**acyclovir** 400 mg tid po x 10 days.		

Abbreviations on page 2.

---

[1] Primary rationale for rx is eradication of Group A strep (GAS) and prevention of acute rheumatic fever (ARF). Benzathine penicillin G has been shown in clinical trials to ↓ rate of ARF from 2.8 to 0.2%. This was associated with clearance of GAS on pharyngeal cultures (*CID* 19:1110, 1994). Subsequent studies have been based on cultures, not actual prevention of ARF. Treatment decreases duration of symptoms.

[2] Treatment of Group A strep: **All po unless otherwise indicated. PEDIATRIC DOSAGE: Benzathine penicillin** 25,000 units per kg IM to max. 1.2 million units; **Pen V** 25–50 mg per kg per day div. q8h times 10 days; **AM-CL** 45 mg per kg per day div. q12h times 10 days; **erythro estolate** 20 mg per kg per day div. bid times 10 days; **cefuroxime axetil** 20 mg per kg per day div. bid for 4–10 days (*Peds* 105:19, 2000); **cefpodoxime proxetil** 10 mg per kg IM to max. 1 gm IM to max.—otherwise rel; see footnote 1 see footnote 1 times 10 days; **cefdinir** 7 mg per kg q24h times 10 days or 14 mg per kg q24h times 10 days; **cefprozil** 15 mg per kg per day div. bid times 10 days; **azithro** 12 mg per kg per day times 5 days; **clinda** 20–30 mg per kg per day div. q8h times 10 days. **ADULT DOSAGE: Benzathine penicillin** 1.2 million units IM times 1; **Pen V** 500 mg bid times 10 days; dosage varies—**azithro** 500 mg po times 1, then 250 mg per day times 4 days; **cefuroxime axetil** 250 mg po bid times 10 days; **cefpodoxime proxetil** 100 mg bid times 4 days; **cefdinir** 300 mg q12h times 5–10 days or 600 mg q24h times 10 days; **cefditoren** 200 mg bid; **cefprozil** 200 mg bid times 10 days; **NOTE: All O Ceph 2 drugs** approved for 10-day rx of strep. pharyngitis, increasing number of studies show efficacy of 4–6 days; **clarithro** 250 mg bid times 10 days; **azithro** 500 mg times 1 and then 250 mg q24h times 4 days or 500 mg q24h times 3 days; **dirithromycin** 500 mg q24h times 10 days.

NOTE: All dosage recommendations are for adults (unless otherwise indicated) and assume near-normal renal function.

TABLE 1 (41)

ANATOMIC SITE/DIAGNOSIS/ MODIFYING CIRCUMSTANCES	ETIOLOGIES (usual)	SUGGESTED REGIMENS* PRIMARY	SUGGESTED REGIMENS* ALTERNATIVE†	ADJUNCT DIAGNOSTIC OR THERAPEUTIC MEASURES AND COMMENTS
PHARYNX / Pharyngitis/Tonsillitis *(continued)*				
Membranous—diphtheria or Vincent's angina	C. diphtheriae	**[Antitoxin** 20-25 mg/kg IV q12h times 7-14 days (*JAC 35:717, 1995*)] or **[benzyl pen G** 50,000 units/kg per day x 5 days, then po **pen VK** 50 mg/kg per day]	Diphtheria occurs in immunized individuals. Antibiotics may ↓ toxin production, ↓ spread of organisms. Penicillin superior to erythro in randomized trial (*CID 27:845, 1998*).	
Vincent's angina (anaerobes/spirochetes)	Vincent's angina (anaerobes/spirochetes)	**Pen G** 4 million units IV q4h	**Clinda** 600 mg IV q8h	May be complicated by F. necrophorum bacteremia, *see jugular vein phlebitis (Lemierre's), page 44.*
Epiglottitis				
Children	H. influenzae (rare), S. pyogenes, S. pneumoniae, S. aureus	**Peds dosage: Cefotaxime** 50 mg per kg IV q8h **or ceftriaxone** 50 mg per kg IV q24h	**Peds dosage: AM-SB** 50-200 mg/kg per day div q6h or **TMP-SMX** 8-12 mg/kg per day TMP component /kg per day div q12h	Have tracheostomy set "at bedside." Chloro is effective, but potentially less toxic alternative agents available. Review (adults). *JAMA 272:1358, 1994*)
Adults	Group A strep), H. influenzae (rare)	**Adult dosage:** See footnote†		
Parapharyngeal space infection	Spaces include: sublingual, submandibular, submaxillary (Ludwig's angina, used loosely for these), lateral pharyngeal, retropharyngeal, pretracheal]	**[Clinda** 600-900 mg IV q8h] or **[pen G** 24 million units by cont. infusion or div q4-6h IV + **metro** 1 gm load and then 0.5 gm IV q6h]	**Cefoxitin** 2 gm IV q8h or **clinda** or **TC-CL** or **PIP-TZ** or **AM-SB** (*Dosage, see footnote†*)	Close observation of airway, 1/3 require intubation. MRI or CT to identify abscess; if present, surgical drainage. **Metro** may be given 1 gm IV q12h.
Jugular vein septic phlebitis (Lemierre's disease) (*PIDJ 22:921, 2003; CID 31:524, 2000*)	Fusobacterium necrophorum in vast majority	**[Clinda** 600-900 mg IV q8h] or **[pen G** 24 million units q24h by cont. infusion or div q4-6h]	**Clinda** 600-900 mg IV q8h	Usual rx includes external drainage of lateral pharyngeal space. Emboli, pulmonary and systemic common. Erosion into carotid artery can occur.
Larynchitis (hoarseness)/tracheitis	Viral (90%)	Not indicated		
Sinusitis, acute; current terminology: acute rhinosinusitis Obstruction of sinus ostia, viral infection, allergens Refs.: *Otolaryng--Head & Neck Surgery 130:51, 2004; AnIM 134:495 & 498, 2001.* For rhinovirus infections (common cold), see *Table 14, page 145* Pediatric Guidelines: *Peds 108:798, 2001*	**Acute rhinosinusitis** S. pneumoniae 31%, H. influenzae 21%, M. catarrhalis 2%, Group A strep 2%, Staph. aureus 4%, viruses 15%, By CT scans, sinus mucosa inflamed in 87% of viral URIs; only 2% develop bacterial rhinosinusitis	Reserve antibiotic rx for pts given decongestants/ analgesics for 7 days who have (1) maxillary/facial pain & (2) purulent nasal discharge; if severe illness (pain, fever), treat sooner—usually require hospitalization. By CT scans, sinus mucosa inflamed in 87% of viral URIs; only 2% develop bacterial rhinosinusitis	**For pts with pen/cephalosporin allergy:** Ask if antibiotics in prior month	Rx goals: (1) Resolve infection, (2) prevent complications, e.g., meningitis, brain abscess, (3) avoid chronic sinus disease, (4) avoid unnecessary antibiotic rx. High rate of spontaneous resolution. **For pts with pen/cephalosporin allergy, esp. severe IgE-mediated allergy—e.g., hives, anaphylaxis; treatment options: clarithro, azithro, TMP-SMX, doxy or FQs. Avoid FQs if under age 18. Dosages in footnote 2 page 43.** If allergy just skin rash, po cephalosporin OK. (*continued on next page*)

† **Ceftriaxone** 2 gm IV q24h; **cefotaxime** 2 gm IV q4-8h; **AM-SB** 3 gm IV q6h; **PIP-TZ** 3.375 gm IV q6h; **TC-CL** 3.1 gm IV q4-6h; **TMP-SMX** 8-10 mg per kg per day (based on TMP component) div q6h, q8h, or q12h. *NOTE: All dosage recommendations are for adults (unless otherwise indicated) and assume normal renal function.*

Abbreviations on page 2.

(continued on next page)

TABLE 1 (42)

ANATOMIC SITE/DIAGNOSIS/ MODIFYING CIRCUMSTANCES	ETIOLOGIES (usual)	SUGGESTED REGIMENS*		ADJUNCT DIAGNOSTIC OR THERAPEUTIC MEASURES AND COMMENTS
		PRIMARY	ALTERNATIVE†	
PHARYNX/Sinusitis, acute; current terminology: acute rhinosinusitis (continued)				
	As above, consider diagnostic tap/aspirate	**NO:** Amox-HD or AM-CL-ER or cefpodoxime or cefprozil	**YES:** AM-CL-ER (adults) or FQ (adults). For pen. allergy, see AM-CL-ER comments. Use AM-CL susp. in peds.	**Usual rx 10 days.** Results of 3 & 10 d. of TMP-SMX the same (*JAMA 273:1015, 1995*). Telithro. FDA's often given for 5 days (see NOTE below). Watch for pts with fever & fascial erythema; ↑ risk of S. aureus infection, requires IV **nafcillin/oxacillin** (antistaphylococcal penicillin, penicillinase-resistant for MSSA or vanco for MRSA).
Clinical failure after 3 days		In general, treat 10 days (see Comment). Adult and pediatric doses, footnote¹ and footnote to page 2 (Otitis). **Mild/Mod. Disease:** AM-CL-ER OR (cefpodoxime, cefprozil) or cefdinir	**Severe Disease:** Gati[NUS], Gemi, **Levo, Moxi**. Treat 10 days. Adult doses in footnote 2 & Comment See Table 11, pages 94 & 103. Ref: *NEJM 337:254, 1997*.	Pts aged 1–18 yrs with **clinical diagnosis** of sinusitis randomized to placebo, amox, or AM-CL for 14 d. **No difference** in multiple measures of efficacy (*Peds 107:619, 2001*). Similar study in adults: *AiM 163:1793, 2003*. Hence, without bacteriologic endpoints, data are hard to interpret. NOTE: **Levo** 750 mg q24h x 5 d vs **levo** 500 mg q24h x 10 d: equivalent microbiologic and clinical efficacy (*Otolaryngo Head Neck Surg 134:10, 2006*)
Diabetes mellitus with acute ketoacidosis, neutropenia, ceforoxamine rx	Rhizopus sp. (mucor), aspergillus			
Hospitalized + nasotracheal or nasogastric intubation	Gm-neg. bacilli 47% (pseudomonas, acinetobacter, E. coli common), Gm+ = (S. aureus) 35%, yeasts 18%. Polymicrobial in 80%	Remove nasotracheal tube and if fever persists, recommend sinus aspiration for C/S prior to empiric Rx. **IMP** 0.5 gm IV q6h or **MER** 1 gm IV q8h. Add vanco for MRSA if Gram stain suggestive.	(**Ceftaz** 2 gm IV q8h + **vanco**) or (**CFP** 2 gm IV q12h + **vanco**). Vanco if possible MRSA	After 7 d of nasotracheal or gastric tubes, 95% have x-ray "sinusitis" (fluid in sinuses), but on transnasal puncture only 38% culture +. (*ARCM 150:776, 1994*). For pts requiring mechanical ventilation for ≥1 wk, bacterial sinusitis occurs in <10% (*CID 27:851, 1998*). May need bicarbonate if yeast on Gram stain of aspirate. Review *CID 25:1441, 1997 and 27:463, 1998*
Sinusitis, chronic Adults	Prevotella, anaerobic strep, H. fusobacterium—common anaerobes. Strep sp. haemophilus, P. aeruginosa, S. aureus, & moraxella—aerobes. (*CID 35:428, 2002*)	Antibiotics usually not effective	Otolaryngology consultation. If acute exacerbation, rx as acute	Pathogenesis unclear and may be polyfactorial: damage to ostiomeatal complex during acute bacterial disease; allergy ± polyps; occult immunodeficiency, and/or odontogenic disease (periodontitis in maxillary teeth).
SKIN				
Acne vulgaris (*JAMA 292:726, 2004; NEJM 352:1463, 2005; Ln 364:2188, 2004; Cochrane Database Syst Rev 2000, 2:CD002086*)				
Comedonal acne, "blackheads," "whiteheads," earliest form, no inflammation	Excessive sebum production & gland obstruction. No Propionibacterium acnes	Topical **tretinoin** (cream 0.025 or 0.05%) or (gel 0.01 or 0.025%)	All once-q24h: tretinoin-like **adapalene** 0.1% gel or **azelaic acid** 20% cream or **tazarotene** 0.1% cream	Goal is prevention, ↓ number of new comedones and create an environment unfavorable to P. acnes. Adapalene causes less irritation than tretinoin. Azelaic acid is less potent but less irritating than retinoids. Expect 40–70% ↓ in comedones in 12 weeks.

---

¹ **Pediatric doses for sinusitis (all oral): Amoxicillin** high dose 90 mg per kg per day times 1, then 5 mg per kg per day times 3 days, **clarithro** 15 mg per kg per day div. q12h, **cefpodoxime** 10 mg per kg per day (max. 400 mg) div. q12-24h; **cefdinir** 14 mg per kg per day div q24h or divided bid, **TMP-SMX** 8-12 mg TMP/40-60 mg SMX per kg per day div. q12h.

Adult doses for sinusitis (all oral): AM-CL-ER (Augmentin XR) 2000/125 mg bid, **amox high-dose (HD)** 1 gm tid, **clarithro** 500 mg bid or **clarithro ext. release** 1 gm q24h, **doxy** 100 mg bid, **axeth** 30 mg per kg per day div. q12h, **cefdinir** 14 mg per kg per day once q24h or divided bid, **TMP-SMX** 1 double-strength (TMP 160 mg) bid (results after 3- and 10-day rx similar)

² **Levo** 500 mg or 750 mg q24h, **Gati** 400 mg q24h, **Gemi** 320 mg q24h (not FDA indication but should work), **Levo** 750 mg q24h x 5 d, **Moxi** 400 mg q24h, **O Ceph** (**cefdinir** 300 mg q12h or 600 mg q24h). NOTE: All dosage recommendations are for adults (unless otherwise indicated) and assume normal renal function.

Abbreviations on page 2.

TABLE 1 (43)

ANATOMIC SITE/DIAGNOSIS/ MODIFYING CIRCUMSTANCES	ETIOLOGIES (usual)	SUGGESTED REGIMENS* PRIMARY	ALTERNATIVE†	ADJUNCT DIAGNOSTIC OR THERAPEUTIC MEASURES AND COMMENTS
SKIN/Acne vulgaris *(continued)* Mild inflammatory acne: small papules or pustules	Proliferation of *P. acnes* + abnormal desquamation of follicular cells	Topical **erythro** 3% + **benzoyl peroxide** 5%, bid.	Can substitute **clinda** 1% gel for erythro	In random. controlled trial, topical benzoyl peroxide + erythro of equal efficacy to oral minocycline & tetracycline and not affected by antibiotic resistance of propionibacteria (*Ln* 364:2188, 2004).
Inflammatory acne: comedones, papules & pustules. Less common: deep nodules (cysts)	Progression of above events	Topical **erythro** 3% + **benzoyl peroxide** 5% bid ± oral antibiotic. See Comment for mild acne	Oral drugs: (**doxy** 100 mg bid) or (**minocycline** 50 mg bid). Others: **tetracycline**, **erythro**, **TMP-SMX, clinda**	Systemic **isotretinoin** reserved for pts with severe widespread nodular cystic lesions that fail oral antibiotic rx. 4–5 mo. course of 0.1–1 mg per kg per day. Aggressive/violent behavior reported. Doxy can cause photosensitivity. Minocycline side-effects: urticaria, vertigo, pigment deposition in skin or oral mucosa.
Acne rosacea	Skin mite: Demodex folliculorum	**Azelaic acid gel** bid, topical	**Metro** topical cream bid	Generally poor quality studies: *Cochrane Database CD003262, Vol 4, 2005*)
Anthrax, cutaneous, inhalation (pulmonary, mediastinal) **To report bioterrorism event: For info: www.bt.cdc.gov** **For info:** 770-488-7100; Refs.: *JAMA 281:1735, 1999; & MMWR 50:909, 2001*	B. anthracis See *Lung, page 38, and Table 1B, page 39*	**Adults (including pregnancy):** CIP 500mg po bid or **Levo** 500mg IV/po q24h x 60 days. **Children:** CIP 20–30 mg/kg/day div q12h po to max. 1 gm po q24h) x 60 days	**Adults (including pregnancy):** Doxy 100 mg po bid x 60 days. **Children:** Doxy > 8 y/o & >45kg: 100 mg po bid; > 8 y/o & <45kg: 2.2 mg/kg po bid; ≤8 y/o: 2.2mg/kg po bid All for 60 days.	1. If penicillin susceptible, then: **Adults: Amox** 500 mg po q8h times 60 days. **Children: Amox** po 80 mg per kg per day div q8h (max. 500 mg q8h) 2. Usual treatment of cutaneous anthrax is 7–10 days; 60 days in setting of bioterrorism with presumed aerosol exposure 3. Other **FQs** (Levo, Moxi) should work based on in vitro susceptibility data
Bacillary angiomatosis: For other Bartonella infections, see *Cat-scratch disease lymphadenitis, page 40, and Bartonella, page 51* In immunocompromised patients HIV/AIDS THERAPY	Bartonella henselae and quintana	**Clarithro** 500mg po bid or ext release (gm po q24h or **azithro** 500 mg po q24h or **CIP** 500–750mg po bid (see	**Erythro** 500mg po bid or **doxy** 100 mg po bid	In immunocompromised pts with severe disease, doxy 100 mg po/IV bid + RIF 300 mg po bid reported effective (*IDC No. Amer 12:37, 1998; Adv PID 11:1, 1996*).
Bite: Remember tetanus prophylaxis—see Table 20. See Table 20F for rabies prophylaxis				page 51
Bat, raccoon, skunk	Strep & staph from skin; rabies	**AM-CL** 875/125 mg po bid or 500/125 mg po tid	Doxy 100 mg po bid	In Americas, **antirabies rx indicated**, rabies immune globulin + vaccine. (See Table 20D)
Cat: 80% get infected, culture & treat empirically.	*Pasteurella multocida*, Staph. aureus	**AM-CL** 875/125 mg po bid or 500/125 mg po tid	**Cefuroxime axetil** 0.5 g po q12h or **doxy** 100 mg po bid. **Do not use cephalexin.** Sens. to FQs in vitro.	*P. multocida* resistant to dicloxacillin, cephalexin, clinda; many strains resistant to erythro (most sensitive to azithro but no clinical data). If culture multocida infection develops within 24 hrs. Observe for osteomyelitis. If culture + for only *P. multocida*, can switch to pen G IV or pen VK po.
Cat-scratch disease: *page 40* Catfish sting		See Comments		Presents as immediate pain, erythema and edema. Resembles strep cellulitis. May become secondarily infected; AM-CL is reasonable choice for prophylaxis
Dog: Only 5% get infected; treat only if bite severe or bad co-morbidity (e.g. diabetes).	Toxins *P. multocida*, S. aureus, Fusobacterium sp., EF-4, Capnocytophaga	**AM-CL** 875/125 mg po bid or 500/125 mg po tid	**Clinda** 300 mg po qid + FQ (adults) or **clinda + TMP-SMX** (children)	Consider antirabies rx, rabies immune globulin + vaccine (*Table 20C*). Usual therapy with decolonized local swab, local cleaning, debridement, if needed. DiCP. **P. multocida resistant to diclox, cephalexin, clinda and erythro**, sensitive to FQs in vitro (*AAC 43:1475, 1999*).

Abbreviations on page 2. NOTE: All dosage recommendations are for adults (unless otherwise indicated) and assume normal renal function.

TABLE 1 (44)

ANATOMIC SITE/DIAGNOSIS/ MODIFYING CIRCUMSTANCES	ETIOLOGIES (usual)	SUGGESTED REGIMENS*		ADJUNCT DIAGNOSTIC OR THERAPEUTIC MEASURES AND COMMENTS
		PRIMARY	**ALTERNATIVE†**	
SKIN (continued)				
Human For bacteriology, see CID 37:1481, 2003	Viridans strep 100%, Staph epidermidis 53%, corynebacterium 41%, **eikenella 15%**, **Staph. aureus =9%, eikenella 15%**, Bacteroides 82%, peptostrep 26%	**Early** (not yet infected) **AM-CL 875/125 mg po bid** times 5 days. **Later:** Signs of infection (usually in 3–24 hrs). **[AM-SB 1.5 gm IV q6h or cefoxitin 2 gm IV q8h) or (TC-CL 3.1 gm IV q6h or (PIP-TZ 3.375 gm IV q6h or 4.5 gm q8h)**	(either **CIP** or **TMP-SMX**) + (either **P Ceph 3** or **TC-CL** or **AM-SB** or **IMP**	Cleaning, irrigation and debridement most important. For clenched fist injuries, x-rays should be obtained. Bites inflicted by hospitalized pts, consider aerobic gm-neg. bacilli. **Eikenella resistant to clinda, nafcillin/oxacillin, metro, P Ceph 1, and erythro; susceptible to FQs and TMP-SMX.**
			Pen allergy: **Clinda** + (either **CIP** or **TMP-SMX**)	
Pig (swine)	Polymicrobic: Gm+ cocci, Gm-neg. bacilli, anaerobes, *Pasteurella* sp.	**AM-CL 875/125 mg po bid**	**P Ceph 3** or **TC-CL** or **AM-SB** or **IMP**	Information limited but infection is common and serious (Ln 348:888, 1996)
Prairie dog **Primate, non-human**	Monkeypox Herpesvirus simiae	See Table 14A, page 143. No rx recommended **Acyclovir.** See Table 14B, page 140		CID 20:421, 1995
Rat	Spirillum minus & Strepto-bacillus moniliformis	**AM-CL 875/125 mg po bid.**	**Doxy**	Antibacks rx not indicated
Seal **Snake: viper** (Ref.: NEJM 347:347, 2002)	Mimivirus mycoplasma *Pseudomonas* sp. *Enterobacteriaceae*, Staph. epider-midis, *Clostridium* sp.	Tetracycline times 4 wks **Primary therapy is antivenom.** Penicillin generally used but would not be effective vs organisms isolated. Ceftriaxone the more effective. Tetanus prophylaxis indicated. Ref. CID 43:1309, 2006.		Can take weeks to appear (after the bite (Ln 364:448, 2004)
Spider bite: Most necrotic ulcers attributed to spiders are probably due to another cause, e.g. cutaneous anthrax (Ln 364:549, 2004) or **MRSA infection** (spider bite painful; anthrax not painful)				
Widow (Latrodectus)	Not infectious	None	May be confused with "acute abdomen." Diazepam or calcium gluconate helpful to control pain, muscle spasm. Tetanus prophylaxis.	
Brown recluse (Loxosceles) NEJM 352:700, 2005	Not necrotic. Overdiag-nosed! Spider identification limited to U.S. Central & Southwest SW of US	Bite usually self-limited & self-healing. No therapy of proven efficacy.	Dapsone 50 mg po q24h often used despite marginal supportive data	Dapsone causes hemolysis (check for G6PD deficiency). Can cause hepatitis; baseline & weekly liver panels suggested.
Boils—Furunculosis—Subcutaneous abscesses ("skin poppers"), Carbuncles = multiple connecting furuncles				
Active lesions See Table 6, page 73 Community-acquired MRSA widespread. I&D mainstay of rx. Refs: NEJM 355:666, 2006 & http://www.cdc.gov/ncidod/dhqp/ar_mrsa_ca_clinicians.html ccra.com/english/pdfs/CAMRS-A-ExpMgStrategies.pdf	Staph aureus, both MSSA & MRSA—concern for community-acquired MRSA (See Comments)	**If afebrile & abscess <5 cm in diameter: I&D** drugs. **If ≥5 cm in diameter: TMP-SMX-DS** 2 tabs po bid times 5–10 days. **Doxy/mino** alternatives.	**Febrile, large &/or multiple abscesses: outpatient care: I&D** culture abscess & maybe blood, hot packs. (**TMP-SMX 2** bid times 5–10 days. **RIF** 300 mg bid) times 10 days. **Incision and Drainage** mainstay of therapy)	Why 2 **TMP/SMX-DS**? 1) To ensure adequate serum levels with respect to MIC. 2) Optimize concentration-dependent killing. 3) No definitive clinical trials; animal studies underway. **TMP/SMX** activity vs streptococcal of strep cellulitis (erysipelas) from S. aureus abscess. If unclear or strep, use **clinda** or **TMP/SMX** plus **beta-lactam**. **Rifampin** Consider with severe infection after I&D, and in combination with **TMP/SMX** (or other drugs). Other options: 1) If compliance an issue, **dalbavancin** 1000 mg IV x 1 then, if necessary, 500mg IV on day 8, CID 41:1407, 2005); 2) **Linezolid** 600 mg p.o. b.i.d. x 10 d. 3) **Fusidic acid**‡‡ 500 mg p.o. q12h (CID 42:394, 2006), 4) **FQs** only if in vitro suscept. Known.

Abbreviations on page 2.   NOTE: All dosage recommendations are for adults (unless otherwise indicated) and assume normal renal function.

TABLE 1 (45)

ANATOMIC SITE/DIAGNOSIS/ MODIFYING CIRCUMSTANCES	ETIOLOGIES (usual)	SUGGESTED REGIMENS*		ADJUNCT DIAGNOSTIC OR THERAPEUTIC MEASURES AND COMMENTS
		PRIMARY	ALTERNATIVE*	
SKIN/Boils—Furunculosis/Active Lesions (continued) **to lesser number of recurrences** MSSA & MRSA		Guided by in vitro susceptibilities: **Diclox-** 500mg po qid or **TMP-SMX-DS** 2 tabs po bid) + **RIF** 600mg po qid, all x 10 days		Plus: Shower with Hibiclens q24h times 3 days & then 3 times per week. Others have tried 5% povidone-iodine cream intranasal qid times 5 days. Reports of S. aureus resistant to mupirocin. Triple antibiotic ointment active vs S. epidermidis and S. aureus (DMID 54:63, 2006). Mupirocin prophylaxis of non-surgical hosp. pts had no effect on S. aureus infections in placebo-controlled study (AJM 140:419 & 494, 2004).
Hidradenitis suppurativa	Lesions secondarily infected: S. aureus, Enterobacteriaceae, pseudomonas, anaerobes	Aspirate, base rx on culture	Many pts ultimately require surgical excision.	Caused by keratinous plugging of apocrine glands of axillary and/or inguinal areas.
Burns. For overall management: Initial burn wound care (CID 37:543, 2003& BMJ 332:649, 2006)	Not infected	Early excision & wound closure; shower hydrotherapy. Role of topical antimicrobics unclear.	**Silver sulfadiazine** cream, 1%, apply 1-2 times per day or **0.5% silver nitrate** solution or **mafenide acetate** cream. Apply bid.	Marrow-induced neutropenia can occur during 1st wk. of sulfadiazine but reaches even if use is continued. Silver nitrate leaches electrolytes from wounds & stains everything. Mafenide inhibits carbonic anhydrase and can cause metabolic acidosis.
Burn wound sepsis Variety of skin grafts and skin substitutes, see JAMA 283:717, 2000 & Adv Skin Wound Care 18:323, 2005.	Strep. pyogenes, Enterobacter sp., S. aureus, S. epidermidis, E. faecalis, E. coli, P. aeruginosa. Fungi rare. Herpesvirus rare.	**(Vanco** 1 gm IV q12h) + **(amikacin** 10 mg per kg loading dose then 7.5 mg per kg q24h or **PIP** 4 gm IV q4h (give ½ q24h dose of piperacillin or **PIP** 4 gm IV tissues with surgical removal as needed [q12h] + **PIP-TZ** PIP not available	See Comment	Monitor serum levels, ½ of most antibiotics ↓. Staph. aureus tend to remain localized to burn wound; if toxic, consider toxic shock syndrome. Candida sp. colonize but seldom invade. Pneumonia as the major infectious complication. Other staph complications include septic thrombophlebitis. Dapto (4 mg per kg IV q24h) alternative for vanco.
Cellulitis, erysipelas: Be wary of macrolide (erythro)-resistant) **Extremities**, not associated with venous catheter (see Comments); non-diabetic For diabetes, see below	S. pyogenes. Review NEJM 350:904, 2004. **NOTE:** Consider diseases that masquerade as cellulitis (AJM 142:47, 2005) Strep. pyogenes, Group A strep, occ. Group B, C, G; Staph. Aureus, including MRSA reported.	**Pen G** 1-2 million units IV q6h or **(Nafcillin** or **oxacillin** 2 gm IV q4h). If not severe, **dicloxacillin** 500 mg po qid or **cefazolin** 1 gm IV q8h.	**Erythro** 1 gm IV q12h) or **P Ceph 1** or **AM-CL** or **azithro** or **clarithro** or **dirithro** or **tigecycline** or **dapto** 4 mg/kg IV. See page 32 or **Dapto IOD**	**"Spontaneous" erysipelas** of leg in non-diabetic is usually due to strep. **Gps A,B,C or G.** Hence OK to **start with IV pen G 1-2 million units q6h** & observe for localized S. aureus infection. Look for tinea pedis with fissures, a common portal of entry; can often culture strep from between toes. For prophylaxis of recurrent erysipelas in treatment, See page 15. Reports of CA-MRSA presenting as erysipelas rather than furunculosis. If a concern, use empiric dapto or linezolid.
Facial, adult (erysipelas)	Group A strep, Staph. aureus (to include MRSA), S. pneumo	**Vanco** 1 gm IV q12h	**Dapto** 4 mg/kg IV q24h or **Linezolid 600mg** IV q12h	**Choice of empiric therapy must have activity vs S. aureus.** S. pyogenes erysipelas of an extremity. Forced to treat empirically for MRSA until in vitro susceptibilities available.
Diabetes mellitus and Erysipelas (See Foot, "Diabetic", page 14)	Group A strep, Staph. aureus, Enterobacteriaceae, clostridia (rare)	**Early mild: TMP-SMX-DS** 2 tabs po bid + **RIF** 300 mg bid po. **For severe disease:** **IMP** or **MER** or **ERTA** IV (dose, 600 mg IV) po or **(vanco IV)** or **dapto 4mg/kg IV** q4h.		Prompt surgical debridement indicated to rule out necrotizing fasciitis and to obtain cultures. If septic, consider x-ray of extremity to assess arteries. See diabetic foot, **(linezolid** 600 mg **Prog-nosis dependent on blood supply; assess arteries.** See diabetic foot, page 14.
Erysipelas 2° to lymphedema (congenital) = Milroy's disease); post-breast surgery with lymph node dissection	S. pyogenes, Groups A, C, G	**Benzathine pen G** 1.2 million units IM q4 wks (at Dosage, see page 14)		Indicated only if pt is having frequent episodes of cellulitis. Pen V 250 mg po bid should be effective but most are not aware of clinical trials. In pen-allergic pts: erythro 500 mg po q24h, azithro 250 mg po q24h, or clarithro 500 mg po q24h.
Dandruff (seborrheic dermatitis)	Malassezia species	**Ketoconazole shampoo** 2% or **selenium sulfide** 2.5% (see page 9, chronic external otitis)		

TABLE 1 (46)

ANATOMIC SITE/DIAGNOSIS/ MODIFYING CIRCUMSTANCES	ETIOLOGIES (usual)	SUGGESTED REGIMENS* PRIMARY	ALTERNATIVE†	ADJUNCT DIAGNOSTIC OR THERAPEUTIC MEASURES AND COMMENTS
SKIN *(continued)*				
Decubitus or venous stasis or arterial insufficiency ulcers: with sepsis	Polymicrobic: S. pyogenes (Grps A,C,G), enterococci, anaerobic strep, Enterobacteriaceae, Pseudomonas sp., Bacteroides sp., Staph. aureus	IMP or MER or TC-CL or PIP-TZ or ERTA *Dosages, see footnotes pages 14, 22, 27, 55*	(CIP, Levo, or Moxi) + (clinda or metro)	Without sepsis or extensive cellulitis local care may be adequate. Debride as needed. Topical mafenide or silver sulfadiazine adjunctive. R/O underlying osteomyelitis. May need wound coverage with skin graft or skin substitute (*JAMA 283:716, 2000*).
Erythema multiforme	H. simplex type 1, mycoplasma, Strep. pyogenes, drugs (sulfonamides, phenytoin, penicillins)			**Rx: Acyclovir** if due to H. simplex
Erythema nodosum	Sarcoidosis, inflammatory bowel disease, M. tbc, coccidioidomycosis, yersinia, sulfonamides			**Rx: NSAIDs; glucocorticoids** if refractory.
Erythrasma	C. corynebacterium minutissimum	Erythro 250 mg po q6h times 14 days		Coral red fluorescence with Wood's lamp. Alt: 2% aqueous clinda topically.
Folliculitis	Many etiologies: S. aureus, candida, P. aeruginosa, malassezia, demodex	*See individual entities. See Whirlpool folliculitis, page 50.*		
Furunculosis	Staph aureus	*See Boils, page 47*		
Hemorrhagic bullous lesions	Vibrio vulnificus, V. damsela (*CID 37:272, 2003*)	Ceftazidime 2 gm IV q8h + doxy 100 mg IV/po bid	Either cefotaxime 2 gm IV q8h or (CIP 750 mg po bid or 400 mg IV bid)	⅓ pts have chronic liver disease with mortality in 50% (*NEJM 312:343, 1985*). In Taiwan, where a number of cases are seen, the impression exists that ceftazidime is superior to tetracyclines (*CID 15:271, 1992*) hence both
Impetigo, ecthyma—usually children			*page 16B for children*	
"Honey-crust" lesions (non-bullous)	Group A strep Impetigo, crusted lesions can be Staph. aureus + streptococc	Mupirocin ointment 2% tid or fusidic acid cream^NUS 2% times 3-5 days *For dosages, see Table 10C*	Azithro or clarithro or erythro or O Ceph 2 *For dosages, see Table 16, page 168 for children*	In meta-analysis that combined strep & staph impetigo, mupirocin had higher cure rates than placebo. Mupirocin superior to oral erythro. Penicillin inferior to erythro. Few placebo-controlled trials. Ref.: *Cochrane Database Systemic Reviews, 2004 (2): CD003261.*
Bullous (if ruptured, thin "varnish-like crust)	Staph. aureus impetigo MSSA & MRSA	For MSSA: po therapy with dicloxacillin, oxacillin, cephalexin, AM-CL, azthro, clarithro, or mupirocin ointment	For MRSA: Mupirocin ointment, TMP-SMX-DS, minocycline *For dosages, see Table 10C*	46% of USA-300 CA-MRSA isolates carry gene encoding resistance to Mupirocin (*Ln 367:731, 2006*). **Note**: While resistance to Mupirocin continues to evolve, over-the-counter triple antibiotic ointment (Neomycin, polymyxin B, Bacitracin) remains effective (*DMID 54:63, 2006*).

Abbreviations on page 2.   *NOTE: All dosage recommendations are for adults (unless otherwise indicated) and assume normal renal function.*

TABLE 1 (47)

ANATOMIC SITE/DIAGNOSIS/ MODIFYING CIRCUMSTANCES	ETIOLOGIES (usual)	SUGGESTED REGIMENS* PRIMARY	ALTERNATIVE¹	ADJUNCT DIAGNOSTIC OR THERAPEUTIC MEASURES AND COMMENTS
Infected wound, extremity—Post-trauma (for bites, see page 46; for post-operative, see below)—**Gram stain negative**)				
Mild to moderate; uncomplicated	Polymicrobic; S. aureus (MSSA & MRSA), Group A & anaerobic strep, Enterobacteriaceae, Cl. Perfringens. Cl. tetani, if water exposure, Aeromonas sp. Acinetobacter in soldiers in Iraq EID 11:1218, 2005.	**TMP-SMX-DS** 2 tabs po bid or **clinda** 300–450 mg po bid (Dosage pg. See Comment)	**Minocycline** 100 mg po bid or **linezolid** 600 mg po bid (see Comment)	**Culture & sensitivity, check Gram stain. Tetanus toxoid if indicated. Mild infection:** Suggested drugs focus on S. aureus & Strep species. If suspect Gm-neg bacilli, add **AM-CL-ER** po or **ERTA** or **PIP-TZ** or **TC-CL** IV. **Severe infection:** add **AM-CL-ER** 1000/62.5 two tabs po bid. If MRSA in erythro-resistant, may have inducible resistance to clinda. **Fever—sepsis:** Another alternative is **linezolid** 600 mg IV/po q12h. If Gm-neg. bacilli & severe pen allergy, **CIP** 400 mg IV q12h or Levo 750 mg IV q24h. **TMP/SMX-DS?** (See Comment for Boils, pg 47) **TMP/SMX** not predictably active vs strep species.
Febrile with sepsis—hospitalized		**AM-SB** or **TC-CL** or **PIP-TZ** or **IMP** or **MER** or **ERTA** (Dosage, page 22) + **vanco** 1 gm IV q12h	**Vanco** 1 gm IV q12h or **dapto** 6mg/kg IV q24h + (**CIP** or **Levo** IV—dose in Comment)	
Infected wound, post-operative—Gram stain negative; for Gram stain positive cocci – see below				
Surgery not involving GI or female genital tract				Check Gram stain of exudate. If Gm-neg. bacilli, add β-lactam/β-lactamase inhibitor, AM-CL-ER po or ERTA or PIP-TZ or TC-CL IV (inexpensive) Why 2 **TMP/SMX-DS?** (See Comment for Boils, pg 47) **TMP/SMX** not predictably active vs strep species.
Without sepsis (mild)	Staph. aureus, Group A, (4), or G strep	**TMP-SMX-DS** 2 tabs po bid	**Clinda** 300–450 mg po bid	
With sepsis (severe)	MSSA/MRSA, coliforms, bacteroides & other anaerobes	**Vanco** 1 gm IV q12h	**Dapto** 6 mg per kg IV q24h	
Surgery involving GI (includes oropharynx, esophagus) or female genital tract—fever, neutrophilia		**PIP-TZ** or (**P Ceph 3** + **metro**) or **ERTA** or **IMP** or **MER**) + **vanco** 1 gm IV q24h; if severely ill, **MER**. **Mild infection: AM-CL-ER** 2 tabs po bid + Gram stain.	**Dapto** 6 mg per kg IV q24h + cocci ion **Mild infection: TMP-SMX-DS** 2 tabs po bid if Gm+ cocci on Gram stain.	For all treatment options, see Peritonitis, page 42. Most likely mixed. Drain wound & get cultures. Can sub **linezolid** for vanco. Can sub CIP or Levo for β-lactams. Why 2 **TMP-SMX-DS** (See Comment for Boils, pg 47).
Meleney's synergistic gangrene	See Necrotizing fasciitis, page 50			
Infected wound, febrile patient— Gram stain: Gram-positive cocci in clusters	S. aureus, possibly MRSA	Do culture & sensitivity **Oral: TMP-SMX-DS** 2 tabs po bid or **clinda** 300–450 mg po bid (see Comment)	**IV: Vanco** 1gm IV q12h or **dapto** 4mg/kg IV q24h or 6mg/kg q24h **dalbavancin** 1gm IV, then 0.5gm IV day 8	↑ in community-acquired MRSA (CA-MRSA). Need culture & sensitivity to verify. Other po options for CA-MRSA inc minocycline 100mg po q12h (inexpensive) & linezolid 600mg po q12h (expensive). If MRSA clinda-sensitive but erythro-resistant, watch out for inducible clinda resistance. IV alternative: **tigecycline** 100mg times 1 dose, then 50mg IV q12h.
Necrotizing fasciitis ("flesh-eating bacteria") Post-surgery, trauma, streptococcal skin infections See Gas gangrene, page 41, & Toxic shock, pages 56–57	4 types: (1) Streptococci Grp A, C, G, (2) Clostridia sp., (3) polymicrobic: aerobic sp. + anaerobic strep ± anaerobic strep = Meleney's synergistic gangrene), (4) Community-acquired MRSA	For treatment of clostridia, see Muscle, gas gangrene, page 41. The terminology of polymicrobic wound infections is not precise. Meleney's synergistic gangrene, Fournier's gangrene, necrotizing fasciitis have common pathophysiology. **All require prompt surgical debridement + antibiotics.** Dx of necrotizing fasciitis req incision & probing; subcut (fascial plane), dx = necrotizing fasciitis. **Need Gram stain/culture** to determine if etiology is strep, clostridia, polymicrobial, & S. aureus. **Treatment: Pen G** if strep or clostridia. IMP or **MER** if polymicrobial. add **vanco OR dapto** if MRSA suspected. NOTE: If strep necrotizing fasciitis, reasonable to treat with penicillin & clinda (SMJ 96:968, 2003). If clostridia ± gas gangrene, add clinda to penicillin (see page 41) MRSA ref.: NEJM 352:1445, 2005	
Puncture wound—nail	Through tennis shoe. P. aeruginosa	Local debridement to remove foreign body & tetanus prophylaxis		Osteomyelitis evolves in only 1–2% of plantar puncture wounds.
Staphylococcal scalded skin syndrome Ref.: PIDJ 19:819, 2000	Toxin-producing S. aureus	**Nafcillin** or **oxacillin** 2gm IV q4h (children: 150mg/kg/day div. q6h) x 5–7 days for MSSA. **Vanco** 1gm IV q12h (children 40–60mg/kg/day div. q6h) for MRSA		Toxin causes **intraepidermal split** and positive Nikolsky sign. Drugs cause epidermal/dermal split, called **toxic epidermal necrolysis**—more serious (Ln 351:1417, 1998). Biopsy differentiates.
Ulcerated skin lesions	Consider: anthrax, tularemia, P. aeruginosa (ecthyma gangrenosum), plague, blastomycosis, spider (rarely), mucormycosis, mycobacteria, leishmania, arterial insufficiency.	Usually self-limited, treatment not indicated		
Whirlpool (Hot Tub) folliculitis	Pseudomonas aeruginosa			Decontaminate hot tub: drain and chlorinate. Assume normal renal function. Also associated with exfoliative

TABLE 1 (48)

ANATOMIC SITE/DIAGNOSIS/ MODIFYING CIRCUMSTANCES	ETIOLOGIES (usual)	SUGGESTED REGIMENS*		ADJUNCT DIAGNOSTIC OR THERAPEUTIC MEASURES AND COMMENTS
		PRIMARY	ALTERNATIVE†	
SPLEEN. For post-splenectomy prophylaxis, see Table 15B, page 160; for Septic Shock Post-Splenectomy, see Table 1, pg 56.				
See Folliculitis, page 49				
Splenic abscess				beauty aids (loofah sponges) (*J Clin Micro 31:480, 1993*)
Endocarditis, bacteremia	Staph. aureus, streptococci	Nafcillin or oxacillin 2 gm IV q4h if MSSA	Vanco 1 gm IV q12h if MRSA	
Contiguous from intra-abdominal site	Polymicrobic	*treat as Peritonitis, secondary, page 42*		Burkholderia (Pseudomonas) pseudomallei is common cause of splenic abscess in SE Asia.
Immunocompromised	Candida sp.	Amphotericin B (Dosage, see Table 11, page 96)	Fluconazole, caspofungin	
SYSTEMIC FEBRILE SYNDROMES				
Spread by infected **TICK, FLEA, or LICE** (*CID 29:888, 1999*): Epidemiologic history crucial. **Babesiosis, Lyme disease, & granulocytic Ehrlichiosis** have same reservoir & tick vector.				
Babesiosis: see *CID 43:1089, 2006*. Do not treat if asymptomatic, young, has spleen, and immunocompetent	Etiol: B. microti et al. Vector: Usually ixodes ticks Host: White-looted mouse & others	[(Atovaquone 750 mg po q12h) + (azithro 500 mg po day 1, then 250 mg/day)] times 7 days	[(Clinda 1.2 gm IV bid or 600 mg po tid times 7 days) + quinine 650 mg po tid] times 7 days. **Ped. dosage Clinda** 20-40 mg per kg per day and **quinine** 25 mg per kg per day plus exchange transfusion	Exposure endemic areas May to Sept. Can result from blood transfusion (*JAMA 281: 927, 1999*). Usually subclinical. Illness likely in asplenic pts, pts with concomitant Lyme disease, older pts, pts with HIV. Dx: Giemsa-stained blood smear; antibody test available. PCR under study. **Rx: Exchange transfusions successful adjunct, used early, in severe disease.**
Bartonella infections: *CID 35:684, 2002*; for *B. Quintana – EID 12:217, 2006*; Review *EID 12:389, 2006*				
Asymptomatic bacteremia	B. quintana	Doxy 100 mg po/IV times 15 days		Can lead to endocarditis &/or trench fever: found in homeless, esp. lice/leg pain.
Cat-scratch disease	B. henselae	Azithro (if symptomatic only—see page 40		**Immunocompetent Patient:** Bacteremia/endocarditis/FUO)
Bacillary angiomatosis, Peliosis hepatis—pts with AIDS	B. henselae, B. quintana	(Clarithro 500 mg bid or clarithro ER 1 gm po q24h) or azithro 250 mg po q24h or CIP 500-750 mg po bid) times 8 wks	Erythro 500 mg po qid or doxy 100 mg po bid times 8 wks or if severe, combination of doxy 100 mg po/IV bid + RIF 300 mg po bid	**HIV/AIDS Patient:** Bacillary angiomatosis Bacillary peliosis Bacteremia/endocarditis/FUO
				encholbinitis Vertebral osteo Trench fever Parinaud's oculoglandular syndrome
Endocarditis (see page 24) (*AAC 47:2204, 2003*)	B. henselae, B. quintana	Gentamicin 3 mg (per kg) IV once q24h times minimum 14 days + doxy 200 mg po x once q24h times 6 wks	Doxy 100 mg po/IV bid times 6 wks	Hard to detect with automated blood cultures systems. Need lysis-centrifugation and/or blind subculture onto chocolate agar at 7, 8, 14 days. Diagnosis often by antibody titer ≥1:800. NOTE: Only aminoglycosides are bactericidal.
Trench fever (*page 53*)	B. quintana	Doxy 100 mg po bid (doxy alone if no endocarditis)		Same as Urban Trench Fever (*page 53*)
Ehrlichiosis*. CDC def. is one of (1) 4x ↑ IFA antibody, (2) detection of Ehrlichia DNA in blood or CSF by PCR, (3) visible morulae in WBC, and IFA ≥1:64 (*MMWR 46(RR-10):1-55, 1997*)				
Human monocytic ehrlichiosis (HME) (*MMWR 55(RR-4), 2006; CID 43:1089, 2006*)	Ehrlichia chaffeensis (Lone Star tick is vector)	Doxy 100 mg po/IV bid times 7-14 days	Tetracycline 500 mg po qid x7-14d. No current rec. for children or pregnancy	30 states: mostly SE of line from NJ to Ill. to Missouri to Oklahoma to Texas. History of outdoor activity and tick exposure. April-Sept. Fever, rash (36%), leukopenia and thrombocytopenia. Blood smears no help. PCR for early dx.
Human granulocytic ehrlichiosis (HGE) (*MMWR 55(RR-4), 2006; CID 43:1089, 2006*)	Anaplasma (Ehrlichia phagocytophilum (ixodes sp. ticks are vector). Dog variant is Ehrlichia ewingii (*NEJM 341:148 & 195, 1999*)	Doxy 100 mg po bid po or IV times 7-14 days	Tetracycline 500 mg po bid times 7-14 days. Not in children or pregnancy	Upper Midwest, NE, West Coast & Europe. Hx tick exposure. April-Sept. Febrile flu-like illness after outdoor activity. No rash. Leukopenia/thrombocytopenia common. Dx: Up to 80% have + blood smear. Antibody test for confirmation. Rx: RIF successful in pregnancy (*CID 27:213, 1998*) but worry about resistance developing. Based on in vitro studies, no clear alternative— Levo activity marginal (*AAC 47:413, 2003*)

† In endemic area (New York), high % of both adult ticks and nymphs were jointly infected with both HGE and B. burgdorferi (*NEJM 337:49, 1997*).
* Abbreviations on page 2.   NOTE: All dosage recommendations are for adults (unless otherwise indicated) and assume normal renal function.

TABLE 1 (49)

ANATOMIC SITE/DIAGNOSIS/ MODIFYING CIRCUMSTANCES	ETIOLOGIES (usual)	SUGGESTED REGIMENS*		ADJUNCT DIAGNOSTIC OR THERAPEUTIC MEASURES AND COMMENTS
		PRIMARY	ALTERNATIVE†	
Lyme Disease NOTE: Think about concomitant tick-borne disease—babesiosis (*JAMA 275:1657, 1996*) or ehrlichiosis. Bite by ixodes-infected tick in an endemic area **ISDA guideline *CID 43:1089, 2006***	*Borrelia burgdorferi*	**If endemic area**, if nymphal partially engorged. **If not endemic area**, not deer tick: No treatment	**If endemic area**, if nymphal partially engorged, not deer tick. No deer tick: **doxy** 200 mg po times 1 dose with food	Guideline *CID 43:1089, 2006.* Prophylaxis study in endemic area: erythema migrans developed in 3% of the control group and 0.4% doxy group (*NEJM 345:79 & 133, 2001*).
Early (erythema migrans) See Comment		**Doxy** 100 mg po bid, or **cefuroxime axetil** 500 mg po bid or **amoxicillin** 500 mg po tid or **cefuroxime axetil** 500 mg po bid or **erythro** 250 mg po tid. All regimens for 14-21 days. (10 days as good as 20: *AnIM 138:697, 2003*)	See Comment	High rate of clinical failure with azithro & erythro (*Drugs 57:157, 1999*). **Peds** (all po for 14-21 days): **Amox** 50 mg per kg per day in 3 div. doses or **cefuroxime axetil** 30 mg per kg per day in 2 div. doses or **erythro** 30 mg per kg per day in 3 div. doses.
Carditis See Comment		(**Ceftriaxone** 2 gm IV q24h) or (**cefotaxime** 2 gm IV q4h) or (**pen G** 24 million units IV q24h) times 14-21 days. See Comment for peds doses.	**Doxy** (see Comments) 100 mg po bid times14-21 days or **amoxicillin** 250-500 mg po tid times14-21 days.	Lesions usually homogenous—not target-like (*AnIM 136:423, 2002*). First degree AV block. Oral regimen. High degree AV block (PR >0.3 sec.). IV therapy—permanent pacemaker not necessary.
Facial nerve paralysis (isolated finding, early).		(**Doxy** 100 mg po bid or **amoxicillin** 500 mg po) tid times 14-21 days.	**Ceftriaxone** 2 gm IV times 14-21 days	LP suggested to exclude neurologic disease. If LP neg, oral regimen OK. If abnormal or not done, suggest parenteral regimen.
Meningitis, encephalitis For encephalopathy, see Comment		**Ceftriaxone** 2 gm IV q24h times 14-28 days	(**Pen G** 20 million units IV q24h in div dose) or (**cefotaxime** 2 gm IV q8h) times 14-28 days	Encephalopathy: memory difficulty, depression, somnolence, or headache. CSF abnormalities. 89% had objective CSF abnormalities. 18/18 pts improved with ceftriaxone 2 gm per day times 30 days (*JID 180:377, 1999*).
Arthritis		(**Doxy** 100 mg po bid or **amoxicillin** 500 mg po qid), both times 30 days	(**Ceftriaxone** 2 gm IV q24h) or (**pen G** 20-24 million units per day IV) times 14-28 days	
Pregnant women		Choice should **not** include doxy, **amoxicillin** 500 mg po tid times 21 days.	If pen. allergic: (**azithro** 500 mg po q24h times 7-10 days) or (**erythro** 500 mg po qid times 14-21 days)	
Asymptomatic seropositivity and symptoms post-rx		None indicated		No benefit from rx (*NEJM 345:85, 2001*)
Plague As a biological weapon: *JAMA 283:2281, 2000, and Table 1B, page 60*	*Yersinia pestis* Reservoir: rat Vector: rat flea	**Gentamicin** 2 mg/kg IV loading dose then 1.7 mg/kg IV q8h or **streptomycin** 1 gm IM/IV q12h	**Doxy** 100 mg IV/po bid or **chloro** 500 mg IV/po qid	Reference IV streptomycin (*DMID 19:1150, 1994.* Septicemic form can occur without buboes. **CIP** effective in vitro + in animal models (*JAC 41:301, 1998*); CIP success in 1 pt (*CID 36:521, 2003*). Monotherapy with either **gent** or **doxy** reported as efficacious. (*CID 42:614, 200*).
Relapsing fever *(EID 12:369, 2006)*	*Borrelia recurrentis,* B. hermsii, & other borrelia sp.	**Doxy** 100 mg po bid	**Erythro** 500 mg po qid	Jarisch-Herxheimer (fever, ↑ pulse, ↑ resp, ↓ blood pressure) in most patients (occurs in ~2 hrs). Not prevented by prior steroids. **Dx: Examine peripheral blood smear during febrile episode.** Can relapse up to 10 times. Post-exposure **doxy** pre-emptive therapy highly effective (*NEJM 355:148, 2006*).

Abbreviations on page 2.   NOTE: All dosage recommendations are for adults (unless otherwise indicated) and assume normal renal function.

TABLE 1 (50)

ANATOMIC SITE/DIAGNOSIS/ MODIFYING CIRCUMSTANCES	ETIOLOGIES (usual)	SUGGESTED REGIMENS*		ADJUNCT DIAGNOSTIC OR THERAPEUTIC MEASURES AND COMMENTS
		PRIMARY	ALTERNATIVE†	
SYSTEMIC FEBRILE SYNDROMES				
Rickettsial diseases. Review—Rickettsial Disease in travelers (CID 39:1493, 2004)				
Spotted fevers (NOTE: Ricketlsialpox and Q fever not included)				
Rocky Mountain spotted fever (RMSF) (AJM 63:21, 2000; AJM 163:769, 2003; MMWR 55(RR-4), 2006)	R. rifkettsii [*Dermacentor* ticks]	**Doxy** 100 mg po/IV bid times 7 days or for 2 days after temp. normal	**Chloro** use found as risk factor for fatal RMSF (JID 184:1437, 2001)	Fever, rash (95%), petechiae 40–60%. **Rash spreads from distal extremities to trunk.** Dx: Immunohistology on skin biopsy, confirmation with antibody titers. Highest incidence in Mid-Atlantic states; also seen in Oklahoma, S. Dakota, Montana. **NOTE: Only 3–18% of pts present with fever, rash, and hx of tick exposure; esp. in children many early deaths & empiric doxy reasonable** (MMWR 49: 888, 2000).
NOTE: Can mimic ehrlichiosis. Pattern of rash important—see Comment				
Other spotted fevers, e.g. Boutonneuse fever *R. africae* review: LnID 3:557, 2003	6 species: R. conorii et al. [multiple ticks]. In sub-Saharan Africa, R. africae	**Clarithro** 7.5 mg per kg q12h & azithro 10 mg per kg per day times 1 for 3 days equally efficacious in children with Mediterranean spotted fever (CID 34:154, 2002). R. africae review CID 36:1411, 2003. R. parkeri in U.S. CID 38:805, 2004		
Typhus group—Consider in returning travelers with fever				
Louse-borne	*R. prowazekii* (body louse)	**Doxy** 100 mg po/IV qid times 7 days	**Chloro** 500 mg IV/po qid times 7 days	**Brill-Zinsser disease** (Ln 357:1198, 2001) is a relapse of remote past infection, e.g. WW II. Truncal rash spreads centrifugally—opposite of RMSF. A winter disease.
Murine typhus (rat reservoir and flea vector)	*R. typhi* (rat reservoir and flea typhus similar)	**Doxy** 100 mg po/IV qid times 7 days	**Chloro** 500 mg IV/po qid times 7 days	Most U.S. cases south Texas and southern Calif. Flu-like illness. Rash in ~50%. Dx: based on suspicion, confirmed serologically.
Scrub typhus	*O. tsutsugamushi* [rodent reservoir, vector is larval stage of mites (chiggers)]	**Doxy** 100 mg po/IV bid times 7 days. NOTE: Reports of doxy & chloro resistance from northern Thailand. **RIF** alone 450 mg bid (or times 7 days reported effective (Ln 356:1057, 2000). Worry about RIF resistance.	single 500 mg dose of **azithro** effective as **doxy** (CID 39:1329, 2004)	Limited to Far East (Asia, India). Cases imported into U.S. Evidence of chigger bite, flu-like illness. Rash like louse-borne typhus.
Tularemia, typhoidal type Ref. bioterrorism: see Table 1B, page 60, & JAMA 285:2763, 2001	*Francisella tularensis.* [Vector depends on geography: ticks, biting flies, mosquitoes identified]	**Gentamicin or tobra** 5 mg per kg per day div. q8h IV times 7–14 days	Add **chloro** if evidence of meningitis. **CIP** reported effective in 12 children (PIDJ 19:449, 2000)	Typhoidal form in 5–30% pts. No lymphadenopathy. Diarrhea, pneumonia common. Dx: blood cultures. Antibody confirmation. Rx: Jarisch-Henheimer reaction may occur. Clinical failures with rx with P Ceph 3 (CID 17:976, 1993).
Urban trench fever (endocarditis) (AAC 47:2204, 2003)	*Bartonella quintana.* Vector: body louse	**Gentamicin** 3 mg per kg IV once q24h times min. of 14 days + **doxy** 200 mg po single q24h dose times 28 days		One of many Bartonella syndromes; see pages 26 & 51
Other Zoonotic Systemic Bacterial Febrile Illnesses: Obtain careful zoonotic epidemiologic history				
Brucellosis Review: NEJM 352:2325, 2005	Brucella sp. B. abortus—cattle B. suis—pigs B. melitensis—goats B. canis—dogs			**Clinical disease:** Protean. Fever in 91%. **Malodorous perspiration almost pathognomic.** Osteomyelitis: Osteoarticular disease in approx. 20%%, epididymitis/orchitis 6%. **Diagnosis:** Mild hepatitis. Leukopenia & relative lymphocytosis. Diagnosis: Serology. Blood cultures, bone marrow culture, real-time PCR if available. **Treatment:** Drugs must penetrate macrophages & act in acidic milieu. TMP-SMX-DS + RIF reasonable.
Adult or child >8 years		[**Doxy** 100 mg po times 6 wks + **gentamicin** times 7 days (see Table 1D, page 93)] or [**doxy** times 6 wks + **streptomycin** 1 gm IM q24h times 2–3 wks] See Comment	[**Doxy** + RIF 600–900 mg po q24h, both times 6 wks] or [**TMP-SMX** DS tab times 2 wks + **gentamicin** times 6 wks] or [**doxy** times 6 wks + **gentamicin** times 2]	**Pregnancy:** TMP-SMX-DS + RIF reasonable. Prospective random. Study documents **doxy** + 7 d of **gent** as effective as **doxy** + **streptomycin** x 14 d (CID 42:1075, 2006). Review of FQs (in combination) as alternative therapy. (AAC 50:22, 2006)
Child <8 years		**TMP-SMX** 5 mg per kg TMP po q12h times 6 wks + **gentamicin** 2 mg per kg IV/IM q8h times 2 wks		

Abbreviations on page 2. NOTE: All dosage recommendations are for adults (unless otherwise indicated) and assume normal renal function.

TABLE 1 (61)

ANATOMIC SITE/DIAGNOSIS/ MODIFYING CIRCUMSTANCES	ETIOLOGIES (usual)	SUGGESTED REGIMENS*		ADJUNCT DIAGNOSTIC OR THERAPEUTIC MEASURES AND COMMENTS
		PRIMARY	ALTERNATIVE†	
SYSTEMIC FEBRILE SYNDROMES/Rickettsial diseases *(continued)*				
Leptospirosis *(Ln 369:287 & 1514, 2003; LnID 3:757, 2003)*	Spread by infected TICK, **FLEA or LICE/Lyme Disease.** Leptospira—in urine of domestic animals, livestock, dogs, small rodents	**Pen G** 1.5 million units IV q6h or **ceftriaxone** 1 gm IV q24h. Duration: 7 days	**Doxy** 100 mg IV/po q12h or **AMP** 0.5–1 gm IV q6h	**Severity varies**. Two-stage mild anicteric illness to severe icteric disease (Weil's disease) with renal failure and myocarditis. **Rx:** Penicillin, doxy, & cefotaxime of equal efficacy in severe injdxn (CID 39:1417, 2004)
Salmonella bacteremia (enteric fever most often caused by S. typhi)	Salmonella enteritidis—a variety of serotypes	**CIP** 400 mg IV q12h times 14 days (switch to po 750 mg bid when clinically possible)	**Ceftriaxone** 2 gm IV q24h times 14 days (switch to po **CIP** when possible)	Usual exposure is contaminated poultry and eggs. Many others. Myriad of complications to consider, e.g., mycotic aneurysm (10% of adults over age 50. AJM 110:60, 2001), septic arthritis, osteomyelitis, septic shock. Sporadic reports of resistance to CIP. Ref. LnID 5:341, 2005
Miscellaneous Systemic Febrile Syndromes				
Kawasaki syndrome 6 weeks to 12 yrs of age; peak at 1 yr of age; 85% below age 5. *(Ln 364:533, 2004)*	Acute self-limited vasculitis with fever, rash, conjunctivitis, stomatitis, cervical adenitis, red hands/feet & coronary artery aneurysms (25% if untreated)	**IVIG** 2 gm per kg over 12 hrs + **ASA** 20-25 mg per kg qid THEN **ASA** 3–5 mg per kg per day po q24h times 6–8 wks	If still febrile after 1st dose of IVIG, some give 2nd dose	IV gamma globulin (2 gm per kg over 10 hrs) in pts rx before 10th day of illness ↓ IVIG. Some decrease coronary artery lesions (Ln 347:1128, 1996) See Table 14B, page 140 for IVIG adverse effects and expense.
Rheumatic Fever, acute Ref. *Ln 366:155, 2005*	Post-Group A strep pharyngitis (not Group B, C, or G). *See Pharyngitis, p. 43*	(1) Symptom relief: **ASA** 80–100 mg per kg per day in children; 4–8 gm per day in adults. (2) Eradicate Group A strep: **Pen** times 10 days (3). Start prophylaxis: see below.		
Prophylaxis Primary prophylaxis		**Benzathine pen G** 1.2 million units IM	**Penicillin** for 10 days, prevents rheumatic fever even when started 7–9 days after onset of illness. **Alternative: Penicillin V** 250mg po bid x 10 days or **erythro** 250mg po bid.	
Secondary prophylaxis (previous documented rheumatic fever)		**Benzathine pen G** 1.2 million units IM q3-4 wks	**Duration?** No carditis: 5 yr or age 21, whichever is longer. Carditis without residual valvular disease: 10 yr; carditis with residual valvular disease: 10 yr since last episode & at least age 40 (PEDS 96:758, 1995).	
Typhoid syndrome (typhoid fever, enteric fever) *(Ln 366:749, 2005; LnID 5:623, 2005)*	Salmonella typhi, S. para-typhi NOTE: In vitro resistance to nalidixic acid often predicts clinical failure of CIP (FQs) *(Ln 366:749, 2005)*	**CIP** 500 mg po bid times 10 (days) or **ceftriaxone** 2 gm IV q24h times 14 days). If associated shock, give **dexamethasone** a few minutes before antibiotic. In children, CIP superior to ceftriaxone	**Azithro** 1 gm po day 1, then 500 mg po times 6 days *(AAC 43:1441, 1999)* or 1 gm IV q24h times 5 days *(AAC 44:1855, 2000)* (See Comment) *(LnID 3:537, 2003)*	**Dexamethasone dose:** 3 mg per kg then 1 mg per kg q6h times 8 doses ↓ mortality *(NEJM 310:82, 1984)*. **Complications:** perforation of terminal ileum &/or cecum, osteo, septic arthritis, mycotic aneurysm (approx. 10% over age 50. AJM 110:62, 2001), meningitis. **Other rx options:** Controlled trial of CIP vs chloro. Efficacy equivalent. After 5 days, blood culture positive: CIP 18%, chloro 36% *(AAC 47:1727, 2003)*. **Ceftriaxone** 75 mg per kg per day and **azithro** (20 mg per kg per day or 1 gm max.) equal efficacy, More relapses with ceftriaxone *(CID 38:951, 2004)*
Sepsis: Following suggested empiric therapy assumes pt is bacteremic, mimicked by viral, fungal, rickettsial infections and pancreatitis				
Neonatal—early onset <1 week old	Group B strep, E. coli, kleb-siella, enterobacter, Staph. aureus (uncommon), listeria (rare in U.S.)	**AMP** 25 mg per kg IV q8h + **cefotaxime** 50 mg per kg q12h	(**AMP** + **APAG** or (**AMP** + **cefotaxime** 50 mg per kg IV/IM q12h) or (**AMP** + **ceftriaxone** 50 mg per kg q24h)	Blood cultures are key but only 5–10% +. Discontinue antibiotics after 72 hrs if cultures and course do not support diagnosis. In Spain, listeria predominates; in S. America, salmonella.
Neonatal—late onset 1–4 weeks old	As above + H. influenzae & S. epidermidis	(**AMP** 25 mg per kg IV q8h + **cefotaxime** 50 mg per kg q8h) or (**AMP** + **ceftriaxone** 75 mg per kg IV q24h)	(**AMP** + **APAG** 2.5 mg per kg per day IV or IM q8h IV/IM q(24h)	If MSSA/MRSA a concern, add vanco.

Abbreviations on page 2. NOTE: All dosage recommendations are for adults (unless otherwise indicated) and assume normal renal function.

TABLE 1 (52)

ANATOMIC SITE/DIAGNOSIS/ MODIFYING CIRCUMSTANCES	ETIOLOGIES (usual)	SUGGESTED REGIMENS*		ADJUNCT DIAGNOSTIC OR THERAPEUTIC MEASURES AND COMMENTS
		PRIMARY	ALTERNATIVE*	
SYSTEMIC FEBRILE SYNDROMES/Sepsis (continued)				
Child; not neutropenic	Strep. pneumoniae, meningococci, Staph. aureus (MSSA & MRSA), H. influenzae now rare	**Cefotaxime** 50 mg per kg IV q8h or **ceftriaxone** 100 mg per kg IV q24h) + **vanco** 15 mg per kg IV q6h	**Aztreonam** 7.5 mg per kg IV q6h + **linezolid** (see Table 16, page 168 for dose)	Major concerns are S. pneumoniae & community-acquired MRSA. Coverage for Gm-neg. bacilli included but H. influenzae infection now rare. Meningococcemia mortality remains high (Ln 356:961, 2000).
Adult; not neutropenic; NO HYPOTENSION but LIFE-THREATENING.—For Septic shock, see page 56				Systemic inflammatory response syndrome (SIRS): 2 or more of the following:
Source unclear—consider intra-abdominal as a source. **Life-threatening.**	Aerobic Gm-neg. bacilli; aureus; streptococci; others	**IMP or MER or ERTA** (**Dapto** 6 mg per kg IV q24h) or **vanco**	**(Dapto** 6 mg per kg IV q24h) or **PIP-TZ** or **TC-CL**	1. Temperature >38°C or <36°C 2. Heart rate >90 beats per min. 3. Respiratory rate >20 breaths per min. 4. WBC >12,000 per mL or >10% bands
		Could substitute linezolid for vanco or dapto; however, linezolid bacteriostatic vs S. aureus. Dosages in footnote[1]		Sepsis: SIRS + a documented infection (+ culture) Severe sepsis: Sepsis + organ dysfunction: hypotension or hypoperfusion abnormalities (lactic acidosis, oliguria, ↓ mental status) **Septic shock:** Sepsis-induced hypotension (systolic BP <90 mmHg) not responsive to 500 mL IV fluid challenge + peripheral hypoperfusion.
If suspect biliary source (see p.11)	Enterococci + aerobic Gm-neg. bacilli	**AM-SB, PIP-TZ** or **TC-CL**	**P Ceph 3 + metro; (CIP or Levo) + metro.** Dosages—footnote[1]	
If illicit use IV drugs	S. aureus	**Vanco** (if high prevalence of MRSA). Some empirically use vanco + oxacillin pending susceptibility results. Dosages—footnote[1]		
If suspect intra-abdominal source	Mixture aerobic & anaerobic Gm-neg. bacilli	See secondary peritonitis, page 42		
If petechial rash	Meningococcemia	**Ceftriaxone** 2 gm IV q12h (until sure no meningitis), consider Rocky Mountain spotted fever—see page 53		
If suspect urinary source	Aerobic Gm-neg. bacilli & enterococci	See pyelonephritis, page 30		
Neutropenic: Child or Adult (absolute PMN count <500 per mm3). Guideline: CID 34:730, 2002				
Prophylaxis—afebrile				
Post-chemotherapy—impending neutropenia	Aerobic Gm-neg. bacilli	**CIP** 750 mg po bid		Meta-analysis demonstrates substantive reduction in mortality with **CIP** 500 mg po bid. Similar results in observational study using **Levo** 500 mg po q24h (CID 40:1087 & 1094, 2005). Also NEJM 353:977, 988 & 1052, 2005.
Post-chemotherapy in AIDS ↑ risk pneumocystis	Pneumocystis (PCP)	**TMP-SMX-DS** po bid		Need TMP-SMX to prevent PCP. Hard to predict which leukemia/lymphoma/solid tumor pt at ↑ risk of PCP.
Allogeneic hematopoietic stem-cell transplant	↑ risk pneumocystis, herpes virus, candida	**TMP-SMX** as above + **fluconazole**	+ (either **acyclovir** or **ganciclovir**)	Combined regimen justified by combined effect of neutropenia and immunosuppression.
Empiric therapy—febrile neutropenia (≥38.3°C x1 or ≥38°C for ≥1 hr)				
Low-risk adults		**CIP** 500-750 mg po bid + **AM-CL** 875 mg po bid		**Treat as outpatients with 24/7 access to inpatient care if: no focal findings, no hypotension, no COPD, no fungal infection, age <60 & >16.** Neutropenic children with neg. blood cultures, safely switched to po ceftime 4 mg per kg q12h (CID 32:36, 2001).
Pads data pending (Def. low risk in Comment)	as above			

---

[1] **P Ceph 3** (**cefotaxime** 2 gm IV q8h, use q4h if life-threatening; **ceftizoxime** 2 gm IV q8h; **ceftriaxone** 2 gm IV q4h; **AP Pen** (**piperacillin** 3 gm IV q4h, **ticarcillin** 3 gm IV q4h), **TC-CL** 3.1 gm IV q4h, **PIP-TZ** 3.375 gm IV q4h, **AM-SB** 3 gm IV q4h; **APAG** (Table 10D, page 100), **AMP** 30 mg per kg IV q6h, **clinda** 900 mg IV q8h, **MER** IV q8h, **Nafcillin** or **oxacillin** 2 gm IV q4h; **aztreonam** 2 gm IV q8h; **metro** 1 gm IV q8h (loading dose then 0.5 gm q8h or 1 gm IV q12h; **vanco** 1 gm IV q12h; **vanco** 750 mg IV q12h; **P Ceph 3 AP** (**ceftazidime** 2 gm IV q8h), **P Ceph 4** [CFP 2 gm IV q12h (q8h if neutropenic), **cefpirome**]; CIP 400 mg IV q12h), **linezolid** 600 mg IV q12h.
Abbreviations on page 2.   NOTE: All dosage recommendations are for adults (unless otherwise indicated) and assume normal renal function.

56

TABLE 1 (53)

ANATOMIC SITE/DIAGNOSIS/ MODIFYING CIRCUMSTANCES	ETIOLOGIES (usual)	SUGGESTED REGIMENS* PRIMARY	ALTERNATIVE†	ADJUNCT DIAGNOSTIC OR THERAPEUTIC MEASURES AND COMMENTS
SYSTEMIC FEBRILE SYNDROMES/Sepsis/Neutropenia: Child or Adult/Empiric therapy—febrile neutropenia *(continued)*				
High-risk adults and children	Aerobic Gm-neg. bacilli; ceph-resistant viridans strep, MRSA	**Monotherapy:** **ceftaz or IMP or MER or CFP or PIP-TZ** *Dosages: Footnote 1 page 55 and Table 10.* Include empiric vanco if: suspect IV access infected; colonized with drug-resistant S. pneumo or MRSA; blood culture pos. for Gm-pos. cocci; pt hypotensive	**Combination therapy:** **(Gent or tobra) + (TC-CL or PIP-TZ or CIP)**	Increasing resistance of viridans streptococci to penicillins, cephalosporins & FQs (CID 34:1469 & 1524, 2002; CID 31:1126, 2000; JAC 47:87, 2001). **If severe β-lactam allergy?** No formal trials, but [APAG (or CIP) + aztreonam] ±vanco should work. In meta-analysis of monotherapies, **cefepime** (CFP) associated with higher 30 d all cause mortality; individual pt assessments pending (JAC 57:176, 2006). PIP-TZ & CFP: Equal efficacy (CID 43:447, 2006)
Persistent fever and neutropenia after 5 days of empiric antibacterial therapy—see CID 34:730, 2002—General guidelines				
	Candida species, aspergillus	Add either **caspofungin** 70 mg IV day 1, then 50 mg IV q24h **OR voriconazole** 6 mg per kg IV q12h times 2 doses, then 3 mg per kg IV q12h		Conventional ampho B more fever & nephrotoxicity & lower efficacy than liposomal ampho B (NEJM 340:764, 1999); both caspofungin & voriconazole bttr tolerated & perhaps more efficacious than liposomal ampho B (NEJM 346:225, 2002 & 351:1391 & 1445, 2005)
Shock syndromes				
Septic shock: Fever & hypotension Bacteremic shock, endotoxin shock. Overall review: Ln 365:63, 2005 Antimicrobial therapy: CCM 32(Suppl.):S495, 2004 Surviving sepsis campaign: CCM 32:858, 2004	Bacteremia with aerobic Gm-neg bacteria or Gm+ cocci	**Proven therapy: (1)** Replete intravascular volume, **(2)** correct, if possible, disease that allowed bloodstream invasion, **(3)** appropriate empiric antimicrobial rx, (see suggestions under organ system, page 54) **(4)** Decreased indication for **Comment**. **(5) Low-dose steroids** if document relative adrenal insufficiency (see Comment for criteria). Hydrocortisone 50 mg IV q6h + fludrocortisone (Florinef) 50 mcg po q24h) times 7 days. **(6) Low-dose vasopressin** reported effective for catecholamine-resistant septic shock (Sem Resp Crit Care Med 25:705, 2004). **(6) Blood glucose control:** 80–110 mg per dL		**Activ. Protein C: Drotrecogin (Xigris):** In a prospective randomized double-blind study (NEJM 344:699, 2001), 28-d. mortality ↓ from 31 to 25% in sickest pts. Study in less ill pts (APACHE II score <25) showed no benefit. Xigris not indicated in pts with single organ failure & recent surgery (NEJM 353:1332 & 1398, 2005). No evidence of increased mortality (NEJM 353:1332 & 1398, 2005). **Hemorrhage** (3.5% drotrecogin, 2% placebo) in initial NEJM trial. **Dose:** 24 mcg per kg per hr over 96 hrs by continuous IV infusion. Stop 2 hrs before & restart 12 hrs after surgery. Approx. **cost** of drug for 4-day course: $6,800. **Low-dose steroids** in controlled random double-blind trial, rx if low baseline cortisol & 9 mcg per dL response to 250 IV cosyntropin. 28-day mortality 63% (steroids) & 53% steroid group (JAMA 288:862 & 886, 2002). Results in question because "total" & not "free" plasma cortisol was measured (NEJM 350:1601 & 1629, 2004). Confirm. trial in process. **Low-dose vasopressin:** Dose should not exceed 0.04 units per min. **Targeted glucose levels:** Tight plasma glucose control appears to reduce mortality (NEJM 354:449, 2006) (NEJM 345:1359, 2001) (Mkt 164-2005, 2004)
Septic shock: post-splenectomy (asplenia)	S. pneumoniae, N. meningitidis, H. influenzae, Capnocytophaga (DF-2)	**Ceftriaxone** 2 gm IV q24h (1 to 2 gm q12h if meningitis) Other management as per Septic shock, above	**Levo** 750 mg IV or **Moxi** 400 mg IV/PO once IV q24h	Howell-Jolly bodies in peripheral blood smear confirm absence of functional spleen. Often results in symmetrical peripheral gangrene of digits due to severe DIC. For prophylaxis, see Table 15A, page 159
Toxic shock syndrome, Clostridium sordelli (CID 35:1441, 2002; NEJM 353:1449/vaforyinifepfex.htm)	S. pyogenes, S. aureus, Clostridium sordellii	**Fluids** and, **penicillin G** 18–20 million units per day div. q4-6h + **clindamycin** 900 mg IV q8h	Several deaths reported after use to abortifacient regimen of mifepristone (RU486) & misoprostol. Clinically: often afebrile, rapid progression (high Hct), neutrophilia.	

Abbreviations or page 2.   NOTE: All dosage recommendations are for adults (unless otherwise indicated) and assume normal renal function.

TABLE 1 (54)

ANATOMIC SITE/DIAGNOSIS/ MODIFYING CIRCUMSTANCES	ETIOLOGIES (usual)	SUGGESTED REGIMENS*		ADJUNCT DIAGNOSTIC OR THERAPEUTIC MEASURES AND COMMENTS
		PRIMARY	ALTERNATIVE¹	
SYSTEMIC FEBRILE SYNDROMES/Shock syndromes (continued)				
Toxic shock syndrome, staphylococcal. Superantigen review: LnID 2:156, 2002				
Colonization by toxin-producing Staph. aureus of: vagina (tampon-assoc.), surgical/traumatic-wounds, endometrium, burns	Staph. aureus (toxin-mediated)	**(Nafcillin** or **oxacillin** 2 gm IV q4h) or (if MRSA, **vanco** 1 gm q12h) OR **dapto** 6mg/kg IV + **IVIG**	**(Cefazolin** 1–2 gm IV q8h) or (if MRSA, **vanco** 1 gm q12h) OR **dapto** 6mg/kg IV q24h) + **IVIG**	**IVIG reasonable** (see Streptococcal TSS)—dose 1 gm per kg day 1, then 0.5 gm per kg days 2 & 3—once toxin antibodies present). "Turn off" toxin production with clinda; report of success with linezolid (CID 42:729, 2006).
Toxic shock syndrome, streptococcal (Ref.: JID 179(Suppl 2):S366–374, 1999). NOTE: Associated with invasive disease, i.e., erysipelas, necrotizing fasciitis, secondary strep infection of varicella. Secondary cases TSS reported (NEJM 335:547 & 590, 1996; CID 27:150, 1998).	Group A, B, C, & G Strep. pyogenes	**(Pen G** 24 million units per day IV in div. doses) + (**clinda** 900 mg IV q8h) **IVIG** associated with ↓ in sepsis-related organ failure (CID 37:333 & 341, 2003). IVIG dose: 1 gm per kg day 1, then 0.5 gm per kg days 2 & 3. IVIG preps vary in neutral. Antibody content (CID 43:743, 2006)	**Ceftriaxone** 2 gm IV q24h + **clinda** 900 mg IV q8h	**Definition:** Isolation of Group A strep, hypotension and ≥2 of: renal impairment, coagulopathy, liver involvement, ARDS, generalized rash, soft tissue necrosis (JAMA 269:390, 1993). Associated with invasive disease. **Surgery usually required.** Mortality with invasive disease: 30–50%; myositis 80% even with early rx (CID 14:2, 1992). Clinda ↓ toxin production. Use of NSAID may predispose to TSS. For discussion of pen G may fail in fulminant S. pyogenes infections, see JID 167:1401, 1993.
Other Toxin-Mediated Syndromes—no fever unless complicated				
Botulism (CID 41:1167, 2005. As biologic weapon: JAMA 285:1059, 2001; Table 1B, page 59; www.bt.cdc.gov)		For all types: Follow vital capacity; other supportive care if no ileus, purge GI tract		
Food-borne Dyspnea at presentation bad sign (CID 43:1247, 2006)	C. botulinum	Human botulinum immunoglobulin (BIG) IV, single dose. Call 510-540-2646. Do not use equine antitoxin.	Trivalent (types A, B, E) equine serum antitoxin from State Health Dept. or CDC (see Comment).	**Equine antitoxin:** Obtain from State Health Depts. or CDC (404-639-2206 M-F OR 404-639-2888 evenings/weekends). Skin test first & desensitize if necessary. One vial IV and one vial IM. **Antimicrobials:** May make infant botulism worse. Untested in wound botulism. When used, pen G 10-20 million units per day usual dose. If complications (pneumonia, UTI) occur, avoid antimicrobials with assoc. neuromuscular blockade, i.e., aminoglycosides, tetracycline.
Infant			No antibiotics; may lyse C. botulinum in gut and ↑ load of toxin	**Differential dx:** Guillain-Barré, myasthenia gravis, tick paralysis, organophosphate toxicity, West Nile virus.
Wound		Debridement & anaerobic cultures. No proven value of local antitoxin.	Trivalent equine antitoxin (see Comment)	Can result from spore contamination of far heroin.
Tetanus	C. tetani	**Pen G** 24 million units per day in div. doses or **doxy** 100 mg IV q12h times 7–10 days	**Metro** 500 mg po q6h or 1 gm q12h times 7–10 days (See Comment)	Multicosted treatment. Wound debridement. Tetanus immunoglobulin (250–500 units IM) antimicrobics, & tetanus toxoid (tetanus does not confer immunity). Options for control of muscle spasms: continuous infusion of midazolam, IV propofol, and/or intrathecal baclofen (CID 38:321, 2004).
VASCULAR Cavernous sinus thrombosis	Staph. aureus, Group A strep, H. influenzae, aspergillus/mucor/rhizopus	**Vanco** 1 gm IV q12h + **ceftriaxone** 2 gm IV q24h	**(Dapto** 6 mg per kg IV q24h^{NEW} or **linezolid** 600 mg IV q12h) + **ceftriaxone** 2 gm IV q24h	CT or MRI scan for diagnosis. Heparin indicated (Ln 338:597, 1991). If patient diabetic with ketoacidosis or post-desferrioxamine rx or nasal consider fungal etiology: aspergillus, mucor, rhizopus, see Table 11A, pages 94 & 103.

Abbreviations on page 2.   NOTE: All dosage recommendations are for adults (unless otherwise indicated) and assume normal renal function.

TABLE 1 (55)

ANATOMIC SITE/DIAGNOSIS/ MODIFYING CIRCUMSTANCES	ETIOLOGIES (usual)	SUGGESTED REGIMENS* PRIMARY	ALTERNATIVE†	ADJUNCT DIAGNOSTIC OR THERAPEUTIC MEASURES AND COMMENTS
VASCULAR (continued) **IV line infection** (see IDSA Guidelines: CID 32:1249, 2001): **Treatment:** (For Prevention, see below) Heparin lock, midline catheter, non-tunneled central venous catheter (subclavian, internal jugular), peripherally inserted central catheter (PICC) Avoid femoral vein if possible: ↑ risk of infection and/or thrombosis (JAMA 286:700, 2001)	Staph. epidermidis, Staph. aureus (MSSA/MRSA), Staph. aureus. Rarely; enterococci see BMC/Int.Dis 6:145, 2000.	**Vanco** 1 gm IV q12h. **Linezolid alternative—see Comment.** Other rx and duration: (1) **If S. aureus,** remove catheter. Can use TEE result to determine if 2 or 4 wks of rx. (2) **If S. epidermidis,** can try to "save" catheter. 80% cure after 7–10 days of rx. **Catheter-In-Situ: Infections may respond to "antibiotic lock" rx & allow salvage of catheter.** Drug **(vanco, gent, CIP)** at 1–5 mg per mL, mixed with 50–100 units heparin (or saline) in 2–5 mL volume; fill catheter when not in use. Continue 2 wks. **For S. aureus, need full course of parenteral therapy** (IJAC 48:597, 2001 & 55:90, 2005; 57:172, 2006). If candida, see *Hyperalimentation below and Table 11A, page 96.*		If no response to, or intolerant of, **vanco:** switch to **daptomycin** 6 mg per kg IV q24h. If intolerant of daptomycin or endocarditis or osteomyelitis, could use **linezolid** 600 mg IV/po bid. **Quinupristin-dalfopristin** an option: 7.5 mg per kg IV q8h via central line. **Dalbavancin** an option (if vanco cross-allergenicity is not an issue): 1000 mg IV day 1, then 500 mg IV 8 days later if needed. See *Table 6, page 73.* Culture removed catheter. With "roll" method, >15 colonies (NEJM 312:1142, 1985) suggests infection. Lines do not require "routine" changing when not infected. When infected, do not insert new catheter over a wire. Antimicrobial-impregnated catheters may ↓ infection risk; the debate is lively
Tunnel type indwelling venous catheters and ports (Broviac, Hickman, Groshong, Quinton), dual lumen hemodialysis catheters (Perma-cath)	Staph. epidermidis, Staph. aureus, (Candida sp.). Rarely; leuconostoc or lactobacillus—both resistant to vanco (see *Table 2, page 61*)	(**Vanco + P Ceph 3 AP**) or (**vanco + AP Pen**) or (**P Ceph 3 + APAG**). (*Dosage, see page 55*) If candida, see *Hyperalimentation below and Table 11A, page 96.*		**If S. epidermidis & catheter left in, vanco can cure 80%** of infections limited to exit site but only 25% cure if infection in subcutaneous tunnel between skin and subclavian vein. **If S. aureus & catheter left in, vanco cure rate 10% at exit site & 0% with tunnel infection** (AJM 89:137, 1990). Similar statistics for infected ports (CID 29:102, 1999). Infected hemodialysis access catheters should be removed (AnIM 127: 275, 1997).
Impaired host (burn, neutropenic)	As above + Pseudomonas sp., Enterobacteriaceae, Corynebacterium jeikeium, aspergillus, (Rhizopus)	(**Vanco + P Ceph 3 AP**) or (**P Ceph 3 + APAG**). (*Dosage, see page 55*)		Usually have associated septic thrombophlebitis. Biopsy of vein to rule out fungi. Surgical drainage, ligation or removal often indicated.
Hyperalimentation	As with tunnel + Candida (esp. *Candida albicans, C. tropicalis, C. krusei*) Staph. epidermidis, Malassezia furfur	If candida, **voriconazole** 3 mg per kg IV or **caspofungin** 70 mg IV q24h ... then 50 mg IV q24h		Remove venous catheter and discontinue antimicrobial agents if possible. Ophthalmology consultation recommended. **Rx all patients with + blood cultures.** See *Table 11A, Candidiasis, page 96.*
Intravenous lipid emulsion	Staph. epidermidis, Malassezia furfur	**Vanco** 1 gm IV q12h		Discontinue infusion (AJM 90:129, 1991)
IV line infection: Prevention (CID 35:1281, 2002 and 41:681, 2005; NEJM 348:1123, 2003)	To minimize risk of infection: 1. Maximal sterile barrier precautions during catheter insertion 2. Use 2% chlorhexidine for skin antisepsis 3. If infection rate high despite #1 & 2, use either chlorhexidine/silver sulfadiazine or minocycline/rifampin-impregnated catheters. 4. If possible, use subclavian vein			Small study, ↓ infection rate when catheter locked with gentamicin (5 mg per mL) + heparin 5000 units (per mL), p < 0.02 (Kidney Int 66:801, 2004).
Septic pelvic vein thrombophlebitis (with or without septic pulmonary emboli) Postpartum or postabortion or postpelvic surgery	Streptococci, bacteroides, Enterobacteriaceae	**Metro** → **P Ceph 3, cef-oxitin** or **TC-CL, PIP-TZ, AM-SB** ---- Dosages: *Table 10C, page 85*	**IMP** or **MER** or **ERTA** or (**clinda** + (**aztreonam** or [**clinda + APAG**])) Dosages: *Table 10C, page 85*	Use heparin during antibiotic regimen. Continued oral anticoagulation not recommended. Cefotetan less active than cefoxitin vs non-fragilis bacteroides. Cefotetan has methyltetrazole side-chain which is associated with hypoprothrombinemia (prevent with vitamin K).

Abbreviations on page 2.   NOTE: All dosage recommendations are for adults (unless otherwise indicated) and assume normal renal function.

TABLE 1B – PROPHYLAXIS AND TREATMENT OF ORGANISMS OF POTENTIAL USE AS BIOLOGICAL WEAPONS
(See page 2 for abbreviations)

DISEASE	ETIOLOGY	SUGGESTED EMPIRIC TREATMENT REGIMENS		SPECIFIC THERAPY AND COMMENTS
		PRIMARY	ALTERNATIVE	
Anthrax **Cutaneous, inhalational, gastrointestinal** Refs: Ln 364:393 & 449, 2004; MMWR 50:909, 2001; NEJM 345:1607 & 1621, 2001; CID 35:851, 2002; AnIM 144:270, 2006 or www.bt.cdc.gov Also see Table 1, pages 38 & 46	Bacillus anthracis Post-exposure prophylaxis Ref: Med Lett 43:91, 2001	**Adults (including pregnancy): Doxy** 100 mg po bid or **Levo** 500 mg po qd24hr) times 60 days **Children: CIP** 20–30 mg per kg per day div q12hr times 60 days	**Adults (including pregnancy): Doxy** 100 mg po bid times 60 days **Children** (see Comment): **Doxy** >8 y/o & >45 kg: 100 mg po bid; >8 y/o & <45 kg: 2.2 mg per kg po bid; <8 y/o: 2.2 mg per kg po bid. All for 60 days.	1. Once organism shows production, switch children to **amoxicillin** 80 mg per kg per day div q8h (max. 500 mg q8h); switch pregnant pt to **amoxicillin** 500 mg po tid 2. Do not use cephalosporins or TMP-SMX. 3. Other **FQs** (Gati, Moxi) & Clinitro should work but no clinical experience.
	Treatment—Cutaneous anthrax NEJM 345:1611, 2001 Skin lesions not painful	**Adults (including pregnancy): Doxy** 100 mg po bid or **Levo** 500 mg po q24hr times 60 days **Children: CIP** 20–30 mg per kg per day div q12hr times 60 days	**Adults (including pregnancy): Doxy** 100 mg po bid times 60 days **Children: Doxy** >8 y/o & >45 kg: 100 mg po bid; >8 y/o & <45 kg: 2.2 mg per kg po bid; <8 y/o: 2.2 mg per kg po bid. All for 60 days.	1. If penicillin susceptible, then: **Adults: Amox** 500 mg po q8h times 60 days **Children: Amox** 80 mg per kg per day div q8h (max. 500 mg q8h) 2. Usual treatment of cutaneous anthrax is 7–10 days; 60 days in setting of bioterrorism with presumed aerosol exposure 3. Other **FQs** (Gati, Levo, Moxi) should work based on in vitro susceptibility data.

To report bioterrorism event: 770-488-7100
Rationale for CID 39:303, 2004
	Treatment—Inhalational, gastrointestinal, or oropharyngeal
	Characteristic signs & symptoms—**Present**: Dyspnea, N/V; **Absent**: Rhinorrhea, sore throat.
	(AnIM 139:337, 2003)
		Adults (including pregnancy): CIP 400 mg IV q12hr) or **Levo** 500 mg IV q24hr) or **doxy** 100 mg IV q12hr) + **clinda** 900 mg IV q8h + **RIF** 300 mg IV q12hr. Switch to po when able &. **CIP** to 500 mg po bid; **clinda** to 450 mg po q8h; & **RIF** 300 mg po bid
		Treat times 60 days. See Table 2, page 6 for other alternatives.
			Children: CIP 10 mg per kg IV q12hr or 15 mg per kg po q12hr) or (**Doxy** >8 y/o & >45 kg: 100 mg IV q12hr; <8 y/o: 2.2 mg per kg IV q12hr) **plus clindamycin** 7.5 mg per kg IV q6h **plus RIF** 20 mg per kg IV qd. Treat times 60 days. See Table 16, page 168 for oral dosage.	1. Clinda may block toxin production.
				2. Rifampin penetrates CSF & intracellular sites.
				3. If isolate shown penicillin-susceptible
				  a. **Adult: Pen G** 4 million units IV q4h
				  b. **Child: Pen G** <12 y/o: 50,000 units per kg IV q6h; >12 y/o: 4 million units IV q4h
				4. Do not use cephalosporins or TMP-SMX.
				5. Constitutive & inducible β-lactamases—do not use pen or AMP alone.
				6. Erythro, azithro actively borderline, clarithro active.
				7. No person-to-person spread.

Botulism: CID 41:1167, 2005; JAMA 285:1059, 2001 **Food-borne** See Table 1, page 57	Clostridium botulinum	Purge GI tract if no ileus. **Trivalent antitoxin** (types A, B, & E): single 10 ml vial per pt, diluted in saline IV (slowly)	Antibiotics have no effect on toxin	Supportive care for all types. Follow vital capacity. Submit suspect food for toxin testing. Ref.: CID 39:357 & 363, 2004
Hemorrhagic fever viruses Ref. JAMA 287:2391, 2002 See Table 14, page 134	Ebola, Lassa, Hanta, yellow fever, & others	Fluid/electrolyte balance. Optimize circulatory volume.	For Lassa & Hanta. **Ribavirin** dose same as Adults. Pregnancy, Children: LD 30 mg per kg (max. 2 gm) IV times 1, then 16 mg per kg IV (max. 1 gm per dose) q6h times 4 days, then 8 mg per kg IV (max. 500 mg) q8h times 6 days	Ribavirin active in vitro; not FDA-approved for this indication. NOTE: Ribavirin contraindicated in pregnancy. However, in this setting, the benefits outweigh the risks.

TABLE 1B (2)

DISEASE	ETIOLOGY	SUGGESTED EMPIRIC TREATMENT REGIMENS		SPECIFIC THERAPY AND COMMENTS
		PRIMARY	ALTERNATIVE	
Plague Ref. *JAMA* 283:2281, 2000 **Inhalation pneumonic plague** See Table 1, page 52 *Both* **gentamicin** *and* **doxy** *alone efficacious (CID 42:614, 2006)*	Yersinia pestis **Treatment**	**Gentamicin** 5 mg per kg IV q24h *or* **streptomycin** 15 mg per kg IV b.id. Tobramycin should work.	(**Doxy** 200 mg IV times 1, & then 100 mg po or IV b/d) *or* (**CIP** 500 mg po bid or 400 mg IV q12h) *or* **gentamicin** plus **doxy** Ref. *CID* 38:663, 2004	1. **Chloro** also active: 25 mg per kg IV qid. 2. In mass casualty situation, may have to treat po 3. Pediatric doses: see Table 16, page 168 4. Pregnancy: as for non-pregnant adults 5. Isolate during first 48 hrs of treatment For community with pneumonic plague epidemic: Pediatric doses: see Table 16, page 133. Pregnancy: As for non-pregnant adults
	Post-exposure prophylaxis	**Doxy** 100 mg po bid times 7 days	**CIP** 500 mg po bid times 7 days	
Smallpox Ref. *NEJM* 346:1300, 2002 See Table 14, page 140	Variola virus	Smallpox vaccine up to 4 days after exposure; isolation; gloves, gown, & N&S respirator	**Cidofovir** protected mice against aerosol cowpox (*JID* 181:10, 2000)	**Immediately notify State Health Dept.** & State notifies CDC (770-488-7100). Vaccinia immune globulin of no benefit. For vaccination complications, see *JAMA* 288:1901, 2002.
Tularemia **Inhalational tularemia** Ref. *JAMA* 285:2763, 2001 See Table 1, page 53	Francisella tularemia **Treatment**	(**Streptomycin** 15 mg per kg IV b/d) *or* (**gentamicin** 5 mg per kg IV qd) times 10 days.	**Doxy** 100 mg IV or po bid times 14–21 days *or* **CIP** 400 mg IV (or 750 mg po) bid times 14–21 days	For pediatric doses, see Table 16, page 168. Pregnancy: As for non-pregnant adults. **Tobramycin** should work.
	Post-exposure prophylaxis	**Doxy** 100 mg po bid times 14 days	**CIP** 500 mg po bid times 14 days	For pediatric doses, see Table 16, page 168. Pregnancy: As for non-pregnant adults

TABLE 2 – RECOMMENDED ANTIMICROBIAL AGENTS AGAINST SELECTED BACTERIA

BACTERIAL SPECIES	ANTIMICROBIAL AGENT (See page 2 for abbreviations)		
	RECOMMENDED	ALTERNATIVE	ALSO EFFECTIVE[1] (COMMENTS)
Alcaligenes xylosoxidans (Achromobacter xylosoxidans)	IMP, MER, AP Pen	TMP-SMX. Some strains susc. to ceftaz (AAC 40:772, 1996)	Resistant to APAG; P Ceph 1, 2, 3, 4; aztreonam; FQ (AAC 40:772, 1996)
Acinetobacter calcoaceticus—baumannii complex	IMP or MER or [FQ + (amikacin or ceftaz)]	AM-SB (CID 24:932, 1997; CID 34:1425, 2002). Sulbactam[NUS] also effective (JAC 42:793, 1998); colistin (CID 36:1111, 2003)	Up to 10% isolates resistant to IMP; resistance to FQs, amikacin increasing. Doxy + amikacin effective in animal model (JAC 45: 493, 2000). (See Table 5, pg 72)
Actinomyces israelii	AMP or Pen G	Doxy, ceftriaxone	Clindamycin, erythro
Aeromonas hydrophila	FQ	TMP-SMX or (P Ceph 3, 4)	APAG; ERTA; IMP; MER; tetracycline (some resistant to carbapenems)
Arcanobacterium (C.) haemolyticum	Erythro	Benzathine Pen G	Sensitive to most drugs, resistant to TMP-SMX (AAC 38:142, 1994)
Bacillus anthracis (anthrax): inhalation	See Table 1B, page 59		
Bacillus cereus, B. subtilis	Vancomycin, clinda	FQ, IMP	
Bacteroides fragilis (ssp. fragilis)	Metronidazole	Cefoxitin, ERTA, IMP, MER, TC-CL, PIP-TZ, AM-SB, cefotetan, AM-CL	Resist to clindamycin limits utility against B.frag. (JAC 53(Suppl2):ii29, 2004)
"DOT" group of bacteroides			(not cefotetan)
Bartonella (Rochalimaea) henselae, quintana See Table 1, pg 40, 46, 51	Azithro, clarithro, CIP (bacillary angiomatosis), azithro (catscratch) (PIDJ 17:447, 1998; AAC 48:1921, 2004)	Erythro or doxy	Other drugs: TMP-SMX (IDC N.Amer 12: 137, 1998). Consider doxy + RIF for severe bacillary angiomatosis (IDC N.Amer 12: 137, 1998); doxy + gentamicin optimal for endocarditis (AAC 47:2204, 2003)
Bordetella pertussis	Erythro	TMP-SMX	An erythro-resistant strain reported in Arizona (MMWR 31:807, 1994)
Borrelia burgdorferi, B. afzelii, B. garinii	Ceftriaxone, cefuroxime axetil, doxy, amox (See Comments)	Penicillin G (HD), cefotaxime	Clarithro. Choice depends on stage of disease, Table 1, pg 52
Borrelia sp.	Doxy	Erythro	Penicillin G
Brucella sp.	Doxy + either gent or SM(IDCP 7, 2004; CID 42:1075, 2006)	(Doxy + RIF) or (TMP-SMX + gentamicin)	FQ + RIF (AAC 41:80,1997; EID 3: 213, 1997; CID 21:283,1995). Mino + FQ (J Chemother 15:248, 2003).
Burkholderia (Pseudomonas) cepacia	TMP-SMX or MER or CIP	Minocycline or chloramphenicol	(Usually resist to APAG, AG, polymyxins) (AAC 37: 123, 1993 & 43:213, 1999; Int Med 18:49, 2001) (Some resist to carbapenems). May need combo rx (AJRCCM 161:1206, 2000).
Burkholderia (Pseudomonas) pseudomallei See Table 1, pg 36, & Ln 361:1715, 2005)	Initially, IV ceftaz or IMP (CID 29:381, 1999; CID 41:1105, 2005)	Then po TMP-SMX + doxy x 3 mo ± chloro (AAC 49:4020, 2005)	(Thai, 12–80% strains resist to TMP-SMX). FQ active in vitro. Combo chloro, TMP-SMX, doxy ↑ effective than doxy alone for maintenance (pg 29:375, 1999). MER also effective (AAC 48: 1763, 2004)
Campylobacter jejuni	Erythro	FQ (↑ resistance, NEJM 340:1525,1999)	Clindamycin, doxy, azithro, clarithro (see Table 5, pg 72)
Campylobacter fetus	Gentamicin	P Ceph 3	AMP, chloramphenicol, erythro
Capnocytophaga ochracea (DF-1) and canimorsus (DF-2)	Clinda or AM-CL	CIP, Pen G	P Ceph 3, INP, cefoxitin, FQ, (resist to APAG, TMP-SMX). C. haemolytica & C. granulosa often resist to β-lactams & aminoglycosides (CID 35 (Suppl.1): S17, 2002].
	AM-CL		
Chlamydophila pneumoniae	Doxy	Erythro, FQ	Azithro, clarithro
Chlamydia trachomatis	Doxy or azithro	Erythro or oflox	Levofloxacin
Chryseobacterium (Flavobacterium) meningosepticum	Vancomycin ± RIF (CID 26:1169, 1998)	CIP, levofloxacin	In vitro susceptibilities may not correlate with clinical efficacy (AAC 41:1301, 1997; CID 26:1169, 1998)
Citrobacter diversus (koseri), C. freundii	AP Pen	FQ	APAG
Clostridium difficile	Metronidazole (po)	Vancomycin (po)	Bacitracin (po); nitazoxanide (CID 43:421, 2006)
Clostridium perfringens	Pen G ± clindamycin	Doxy	Erythro, chloramphenicol, cefazolin, cefoxitin, AP Pen, CARB
Clostridium tetani	Metronidazole or Pen G	Doxy	AP Pen
Corynebacterium jeikeium	Vancomycin	Pen G + APAG	
C. diphtheriae	Erythro	Clindamycin	RIF. Penicillin reported effective (CID 27:845, 1998)
Coxiella burnetii (Q fever) acute disease	Doxy (see Table 1, page 27)	Erythro	In meningitis consider FQ (CID 20: 489, 1995). Endocarditis: doxy + hydroxychloroquine (JID 188:1322, 2003; LnID 3:709, 2003).
chronic disease	(CIP or doxy) + RIF	FQ + doxy x 3 yrs (CID 20:489, 1995)]	CQ + doxy (AAC 37:1773, 1993). ? gamma interferon (Ln 20:546, 2001)

TABLE 2 (2)

BACTERIAL SPECIES	ANTIMICROBIAL AGENT (See page 2 for abbreviations)		
	RECOMMENDED	**ALTERNATIVE**	**ALSO EFFECTIVE[1] (COMMENTS)**
Ehrlichia chaffeensis, Ehrlichia ewubguum Anaplasma (Ehrlichia) phagocytophilium	Doxy	Tetracycline, RIF (CID 27:213, 1998)	CIP, oflox, chloramphenicol also active in vitro. Resist to clinda, TMP-SMX, IMP, AMP, erythro, & azithro (AAC 41:76, 1997).
Eikenella corrodens	Penicillin G or AMP or AM-CL	TMP-SMX, FQ	Doxy, cefoxitin, cefotaxime, IMP (Resistant to clinda, cephalexin, erythro, & metro)
Enterobacter species	Recommended agents vary with clinical setting. See Table 1 & Table 4		
Enterococcus faecalis	See Table 5, pg 71		
Enterococcus faecium, β-lactamase +, high-level aminoglycoside resist., vancomycin resist.: See Table 5, pg 71			
Erysipelothrix rhusiopathiae	Penicillin G or AMP	P Ceph 3, FQ	IMP, AP Pen (vancomycin, APAG, TMP-SMX resistant)
Escherichia coli	Recommended agents vary with clinical setting. See Table 1 & Table 4		
Francisella tularensis (tularemia) See Table 1B, pg 60	Gentamicin, tobramycin, or streptomycin	Doxy or CIP	Chloramphenicol, RIF. Doxy/chloro bacteriostatic → relapses
Gardnerella vaginalis (bacterial vaginosis)	Metronidazole	Clindamycin	See Table 1, pg 23 for dosage
Hafnia alvei	Same as Enterobacter spp.		
Helicobacter pylori	See Table 1, pg 18		Drugs effective in vitro often fail in vivo.
Hemophilus aphrophilus	[(Penicillin or AMP) ± gentamicin] or [AM-SB ± gentamicin]	P Ceph 2, 3 ± gentamicin	(Resistant to vancomycin, clindamycin, methicillin)
Hemophilus ducreyi (chancroid)	Azithro or ceftriaxone	Erythro, CIP	Most strains resistant to tetracycline, amox, TMP-SMX
Hemophilus influenzae Meningitis, epiglottitis & other life-threatening illness	Cefotaxime, ceftriaxone	TMP-SMX, AP Pen, FQs (AMP if ß-lactamase neg) (US 25–30% AMP resist, Japan 35%)	Chloramphenicol (downgrade from 1st choice due to hematotoxicity). 9% US strains resist to TMP-SMX (AAC 41:292, 1997).
non-life threatening illness	AM-CL, O Ceph 2/3, TMP-SMX, AM-SB		Azithro, clarithro, telithro
Klebsiella ozaenae/ rhinoscleromatis	FQ	RIF + TMP-SMX	(Ln 342:122, 1993)
Klebsiella species	Recommended agents vary with clinical setting. See Table 1 & Table 4		
Lactobacillus species	(Pen G or AMP) ± gentamicin	Clindamycin, erythro	**May be resistant to vancomycin**
Legionella sp. (42 species & 60 serotypes recognized) (Sem Resp Inf 13:90, 1998)	FQ, or azithro, or (erythro + RIF)	Clarithro	TMP-SMX, doxy. Most active FQs in vitro: Gemi, Levo, Moxi. See AnIM 129:328, 1998. Telithro active in vitro.
Leptospira interrogans	Penicillin G	Doxy	Ceftriaxone (CID 36:1507, 2003), cefotaxime (CID 39:1417, 2004)
Leuconostoc	Pen G or AMP	Clinda, erythro, minocycline	APAG **NOTE: Resistant to vancomycin**
Listeria monocytogenes	AMP	TMP-SMX	Erythro, penicillin G (high dose), APAG may be synergistic with β-lactams. **Cephalosporin-resistant!**
Moraxella (Branhamella) catarrhalis	AM-CL or O Ceph 2/3, TMP-SMX	Azithro, clarithro, dirithromycin, telithro	Erythro, doxy, FQs
Morganella species	Recommended agents vary with clinical setting. See Table 1 & Table 4		
Mycoplasma pneumoniae	Erythro, azithro, clarithro, dirithro, FQ	Doxy	(Clindamycin & ß lactams NOT effective)
Neisseria gonorrhoeae (gonococcus)	Ceftriaxone, cefixime, cefpodoxime	Ofloxacin & other FQs (Table 1, pg 19–20), spectinomycin, azith	Kanamycin (used in Asia). FQ resistance in Asia, rare in U.S., but ↑ (MMWR 47:405, 1998)
Neisseria meningitidis (meningococcus)	Penicillin G	Ceftriaxone, cefuroxime, cefotaxime	Sulfonamide (some strains), chloramphenicol. Chloro-resist strains in SE Asia (NEJM 339:868, 1998) (Prophylaxis: pg9)
Nocardia asteroides	TMP-SMX, sulfonamides (high dose),	Minocycline	Amikacin + (IMP or ceftriaxone or cefuroxime) for brain abscess
Nocardia brasiliensis	TMP-SMX, sulfonamides (high dose)	AM-CL	Amikacin + ceftriaxone
Pasteurella multocida	Pen G, AMP, amox	Doxy, AM-CL, P Ceph 2, TMP-SMX	Ceftriaxone, cefpodoxime, FQ (active in vitro), azithro (active in vitro) (DMID 30:99, 1998; AAC 43:1475, 1999)
Plesiomonas shigelloides	CIP	TMP-SMX	AM-CL, P Ceph 1,2,3,4, FQ, tetracycline, aztreonam
Proteus mirabilis (indole−)	AMP	TMP-SMX	Most agents except nafcillin/oxacillin. β-lactamase (including ESBL) production now being described in P. mirabilis (J Clin Micro 40:1549, 2002)
vulgaris (indole +)	P Ceph 3 or FQ	APAG	Aztreonam, BL/BLI, AP-Pen
Providencia sp.	Amikacin, P Ceph 3, FQ	TMP-SMX	AP-Pen + amikacin, IMP

TABLE 2 (3)

BACTERIAL SPECIES	ANTIMICROBIAL AGENT (See page 2 for abbreviations)		
	RECOMMENDED	**ALTERNATIVE**	**ALSO EFFECTIVE[1] (COMMENTS)**
Pseudomonas aeruginosa	AP Pen, AP Ceph 3, IMP, MER, tobramycin, CIP, aztreonam. For serious inf., use AP β-lactam + tobramycin or CIP (*LnID 4:519, 2004*)	For UTI, single drugs usually effective: AP Pen, AP Ceph 3, cefepime, IMP, MER, APAG, CIP, aztreonam	Resistance to β-lactams (IMP, ceftaz) may emerge during rx. β-lactam inhibitor adds nothing to activity of TC or PIP against P. aeruginosa. Clavulanic acid antag TC in vitro (*AAC 43:882, 1999*). (*See also Table 5*). Recommend combination therapy for serious infections, but value of combos controversial (*LnID 5:192, 2005*).
Rhodococcus (C. equi)	IMP, APAG, erythro, vanco, or RIF (Consider 2 agents)	CIP (variable) [resistant strains in SE Asia (*CID 27:370, 1998*)], TMP-SMX, tetra, or clinda	Vancomycin active in vitro but intracellular location of R. equi may impair efficacy (*Sem Resp Inf 12:57, 1997; CID 34:1379, 2002*)
Rickettsiae species	Doxy	Chloramphenicol	FQ; clari, azithro effective for Mediterranean spotted fever in children (*CID 34:154, 2002*).
Salmonella typhi	FQ, ceftriaxone	Chloramphenicol, amox, TMP-SMX, azithro (for uncomplicated disease: *AAC 43:1441, 1999*)	Multi drug strains (chloramphenicol, AMP, TMP-SMX) common in many developing countries, seen in immigrants. FQ resistance now being reported (*AJTMH 61:163, 1999*).
Serratia marcescens	P Ceph 3, ERTA, IMP, MER, FQ	Aztreonam, gentamicin	TC-CL, PIP-TZ
Shigella sp.	FQ or azithro	TMP-SMX and AMP (resistance common in Middle East, Latin America). Azithro ref.: *AnIM 126:697, 1997*	
Staph. aureus, methicillin-susceptible	Oxacillin/nafcillin	P Ceph 1, vanco, teicoplanin[NUS], clinda, dalbavancin	ERTA, IMP, MER, BL/BLI, FQ, erythro, clarithro, dirithromycin, azithro, telithro, quinu-dalfo, linezolid, dapto
Staph. aureus, methicillin-resistant (health-care associated)	Vancomycin	Teicoplanin[NUS], TMP-SMX (some strains resistant), quinu-dalfo, linezolid, daptomycin, dalbavancin	Fusidic acid[NUS], >60% CIP-resistant in U.S. (Fosfomycin + RIF), novobiocin. Partially vancomycin-resistant strains (GISA, VISA) & highly resistant strains now described—*see Table 6, pg 73.*
Staph. aureus, methicillin-resistant [community-acquired (CA-MRSA)]			CA-MRSA usually not multiply-resistant (*Ln 359: 1819, 2002; JAMA 286: 1201, 2001*). Oft resist. to erythro & variably to FQ. Vanco, teico[NUS], daptomycin or dalbavancin can be used in pts requiring hospitalization (*see Table 6, pg 73*).
Mild-moderate infection	(TMP-SMX or doxy or mino) ± RIF (*CID 40: 1429, 2005*)	Clinda (if D-test neg—see Table 5)	
Severe infection	Vanco or teico[NUS]	Linezolid or daptomycin or dalbavancin	
Staph. epidermidis	Vancomycin + RIF	RIF + (TMP-SMX or FQ), dalbavancin, FQs. (See Table 5)	Cephalothin or nafcillin/oxacillin if sensitive to nafcillin/oxacillin but 75% are resistant.
Staph. haemolyticus	TMP-SMX, FQ, nitrofurantoin	Oral cephalosporin	Recommendations apply to UTI only.
Staph. lugdunensis	Oxacillin/nafcillin or penicillin G (if β-lactamase neg.) (*Inf Dis Alert 22:193, 2003*)	P Ceph 1 or vancomycin or teico[NUS]	Approx. 75% are penicillin-susceptible. Usually susceptible to gentamicin, RIF (*AAC 32:2434, 1990*).
Staph. saprophyticus (UTI)	Oral cephalosporin or AM-CL	FQ	Suscept to most agents used for UTI; occ. failure of sulfonamides, nitrofurantoin reported (*JID 155:170, 1987*). Resist to fosfomycin.
Stenotrophomonas (Xanthomonas, Pseudomonas) maltophilia	TMP-SMX	TC-CL (aztreonam + TC-CL) (*AAC 41:2612, 1997*)	Minocycline, doxy, ceftaz. [In vitro synergy (TC-CL + TMP-SMX) & (TC-CL + CIP), *AAC 39:2220, 1995; CMR 11:57, 1998*]
Streptobacillus moniliformis	Penicillin G or doxy	Erythro, clindamycin	
Streptococcus, anaerobic (Peptostreptococcus)	Penicillin G	Clindamycin	Erythro, doxy, vancomycin
Streptococcus pneumoniae penicillin-susceptible	Penicillin G	Multiple agents effective, e.g., amox	*See footnote 2 pg 10*
penicillin-resistant (MIC ≥2.0)	(Vancomycin ± RIF) or Moxi) See footnote 1 pg 7 and Table 5, pg 72)	(Gemi, Gati, Levo, or	For non-meningeal infec: P Ceph 3/4, AP Pen, quinu-dalfo, linezolid, telithro
Streptococcus pyogenes, Groups A, B, C, G, F, **Strep. milleri** (constellatus, intermedius, anginosus)	Penicillin G or V (some add genta for serious Group B infec & some add clinda for severe invasive Group A) (*SMJ 96:968, 2003*)	β all lactams, erythro, azithro, dirithromycin, clarithro, telithro	Macrolide resistance increasing.
Vibrio cholerae	Doxy, FQ	TMP-SMX	Strain 0139 is resistant to TMP-SMX
Vibrio parahaemolyticus	Antibiotic rx does not ↓ course		Sensitive in vitro to FQ, doxy
Vibrio vulnificus, alginolyticus, damsela	Doxy + ceftaz	Cefotaxime, FQ (eg, levo, *AAC 46:3580, 2002*)	APAG often used in combo with ceftaz
Yersinia enterocolitica	TMP-SMX or FQ	P Ceph 3 or APAG	*CID 19:655, 1994*
Yersinia pestis (plague)	*See Table 1B, pg 59*		

[1] Agents are more variable in effectiveness than "Recommended" or "Alternative". Selection of "Alternative" or "Also Effective" based on in vitro susceptibility testing, pharmacokinetics, host factors such as auditory, renal, hepatic function, & cost.

TABLE 3 – SUGGESTED DURATION OF ANTIBIOTIC THERAPY IN IMMUNOCOMPETENT PATIENTS[1,2]

SITE	CLINICAL SITUATION / CLINICAL DIAGNOSIS	DURATION OF THERAPY (Days)
Bacteremia	Bacteremia with removable focus (no endocarditis)	10–14 (*CID 14:75, 1992*) (*See Table 1*)
Bone	Osteomyelitis, adult; acute	42
	adult; chronic	Until ESR normal (often > 3 months)
	child; acute; staph. and enterobacteriaceae[3]	21
	child; acute; strep, meningococci, hemophilus[3]	14
Ear	Otitis media with effusion	<2 yr: 10 (or 1 dose ceftriaxone); >2yr: 5-7
	Recent meta-analysis suggests 3 days of azithro (*JAC 52:469, 2003*) or 5 days of "short-acting" antibiotics effective for uncomplicated otitis media (*JAMA 279:1736, 1998*), but may be inadequate for severe disease (*NEJM 347:1169, 2002*).	
Endocardium	Infective endocarditis, native valve	
	Viridans strep	14 or 28 (*See Table 1, page 24*)
	Enterococci	28 or 42 (*See Table 1, page 25*)
	Staph. aureus	14 (R-sided only) or 28 (*See Table 1, page 26*)
Gastrointestinal *Also see Table 1*	Bacillary dysentery (shigellosis)/traveler's diarrhea	3
	Typhoid fever (S. typhi): Azithro	5 (children/adolescents)
	Ceftriaxone	14*
	FQ	5-7
	Chloramphenicol	14
		*[Short course ↓ effective (*AAC 44:450, 2000*)]
	Helicobacter pylori	10–14
	Pseudomembranous enterocolitis (C. difficile)	10
Genital	Non-gonococcal urethritis or mucopurulent cervicitis	7 days doxy or single dose azithro
	Pelvic inflammatory disease	14
Heart	Pericarditis (purulent)	28
Joint	Septic arthritis (non-gonococcal) Adult	14–28 (*Ln 351:197, 1998*)
	Infant/child	Rx as osteomyelitis above
	Gonococcal arthritis/disseminated GC infection	7 (*See Table 1, page 20*)
Kidney	Cystitis (bladder bacteriuria)	3 (Single dose extended-release cipro also effective) (*AAC 49:4137, 2005*)
	Pyelonephritis	14 (7 days if CIP used)
	Recurrent (failure after 14 days rx)	42
Lung	Pneumonia, pneumococcal	Until afebrile 3–5 days (minimum 5 days)
	Pneumonia, enterobacteriaceae or pseudomonal	21, often up to 42
	Pneumonia, staphylococcal	21–28
	Pneumocystis carinii in AIDS,	21
	other immunocompromised	14
	Legionella, mycoplasma, chlamydia	7–14
	Lung abscess	Usually 28–42[4]
Meninges[5] (*CID 39:1267, 2004*)	N. meningitidis	7
	H. influenzae	7
	S. pneumoniae	10–14
	Listeria meningoencephalitis, gp B strep, coliforms	21 (longer in immunocompromised)
Multiple systems	Brucellosis (*See Table 1, page 19*)	42 (add SM or gent for 1st 7–14 days)
	Tularemia (*See Table 1, pages 40, 53*)	7–14
Muscle	Gas gangrene (clostridial)	
Pharynx *Also see Pharyn- gitis,Table 1, page 43*	Group A strep pharyngitis	O Ceph 2/3, azithromycin effective at 5 days (*JAC 45, Topic TI 23, 2000*). 3 days less effective (*Int Med 18:515, 2001*)
	Diphtheria (membranous)	7–14
	Carrier	7
Prostate	Chronic prostatitis (TMP/SMX)	30–90
	(FQ)	28–42
Sinuses	Acute sinusitis	5–14[6]
Skin	Cellulitis	Until 3 days after acute inflamm disappears
Systemic	Lyme disease	See Table 1, page 52
	Rocky Mountain spotted fever (*See Table 1, page 53*)	Until afebrile 2 days

---

[1] It has been shown that early change from parenteral to oral regimens (about 72 hours) is cost-effective with many infections, i.e., intra-abdominal (*AJM 91:462, 1991*)

[2] The recommended duration is a minimum or average time and should not be construed as absolute

[3] These times are with proviso: sx & signs resolve within 7 days and ESR is normalized (*J.D. Nelson, APID 6:59, 1991*)

[4] After patient afebrile 4-5 days, change to oral therapy

[5] In children relapses seldom occur until 3 days or more after termination of rx. Practice of observing in hospital for 1 or 2 days after rx is expensive and non-productive. For meningitis in children, *see Table 1, page 8*

[6] Duration of therapy dependent upon agent used and severity of infection. Longer duration (10-14 days) optimal for beta-lactams and patients with severe disease. For sinusitis of mild-moderate severity shorter courses of therapy (5-7 days) effective with "respiratory FQ's" (including gemifloxacin, levofloxacin 750mg), azithromycin and telithromycin. Courses as short as 3 days reportedly effective for TMP-SMX and azithro and one study reports effectiveness of single dose extended-release azithro. Authors feel such "super-short" courses should be restricted to patients with mild-mod disease (*JAMA 273:1015, 1995; AAC 47:2770, 2003; Otolaryngol-Head Neck Surg 133:194, 2005; Otolaryngol-Head Neck Surg 127:1, 2002; Otolaryngol-Head Neck Surg 134:10, 2006*).

TABLE 4 – COMPARISON OF ANTIMICROBIAL SPECTRA

(These are generalizations; major differences exist between countries/areas/hospitals depending on antibiotic usage—verify for individual location. See Table 5 for resistant bacteria)

Organisms	Penicillin G	Penicillin V	Methicillin	Nafcillin/Oxacillin	Cloxacillin^NUS/Diclox.	AMP/Amox	Amox/Clav	AMP-Sulb	Ticarcillin	Ticar-Clav	Pip-Tazo	Piperacillin	Ertapenem	Imipenem	Meropenem	Aztreonam	Ciprofloxacin	Ofloxacin	Lomefloxacin	Pefloxacin^NUS	Levofloxacin	Moxifloxacin	Gemifloxacin	Gatifloxacin
	Penicillins		Antistaphylococcal Penicillins			Amino-Penicillins			Anti-Pseudomonal Penicillins				Carbapenems				Fluoroquinolones							
GRAM-POSITIVE:																								
Strep. Group A,B,C,G	+	+	+	+	+	+	+	+	+	+	+	+	+	+	+	0	±	±		0	+	+	+	+
Strep. pneumoniae	+	+	+	+	+	+	+	+	+	+	+	+	+	+	+	0	±	±		0	+	+	+	+
Viridans strep	±	±	±	±	±	±	±	±	±	±	±	±	+	+	+	0	0	0		0	0	+	+	±
Strep. milleri	+	+	+	+	+	+	+	+	+	+	+	+	+	+	+	0	0	0		0	±	+	+	+
Enterococcus faecalis	+	+	0	0	0	+	+	+	±	+	+	+	0	+	+	0	±	±		±	±	±		±
Enterococcus faecium	0	0	0	0	0	0	0	0	0	0	0	0	0	0	0	0	0	0		0	0	±		0
Staph. aureus (MSSA)	0	0	+	+	+	0	+	+	0	+	+	0	+	+	+	0	+	+	+	+	+	+	+	+
Staph. aureus (MRSA)	0	0	0	0	0	0	0	0	0	0	0	0	0	0	0	0	0	0	0	0	0	±	±	±
Staph. aureus (CA-MRSA)	0	0	0	0	0	0	0	0	0	0	0	0	0	0	0	0	+	+	+	0	+	+	+	+
Staph. epidermidis	0	0	0	0	0	0	0	0	0	0	0	0	0	0	0	0	0	0	0	0	0	±	±	±
C. jeikeium	0	0	0	0	0	0	0	0	0	0	0	0	0	±	±	0	+	+		+	+	+		+
L. monocytogenes	+	+	0	0	0	+	+	+	±	+	+	+	0	+	+	0	0	0		0	±	+		+
GRAM-NEGATIVE:																								
N. gonorrhoeae	0	0	0	0	0	0	+	+	+	+	+	+	+	+	+	+	+	+	+	+	+	+	+	+
N. meningitidis	+	+	0	0	0	+	+	+	+	+	+	+	+	+	+	+	+	+	+	+	+	+	+	+
M. catarrhalis	0	0	0	0	0	0	+	+	±	+	+	±	+	+	+	+	+	+	+	+	+	+	+	+
H. influenzae	0	0	0	0	0	±	+	+	±	+	+	±	+	+	+	+	+	+	+	+	+	+	+	+
E. coli	0	0	0	0	0	±	+	+	±	+	+	±	+	+	+	+	+	+	+	+	+	+	+	+
E. coli/Klebs sp ESBL+	0	0	0	0	0	0	0	0	0	0	±	0	+	+	+	0	±	±			±	±		+
Enterobacter sp.	0	0	0	0	0	0	0	0	±	±	+	±	+	+	+	+	+	+	+	+	+	+		+
Serratia sp.	0	0	0	0	0	0	0	0	+	+	+	+	+	+	+	+	+	+	+	+	+	+		+
Salmonella sp.	0	0	0	0	0	±	+	+	±	+	+	±	+	+	+	+	+	+	+	+	+	+		+
Shigella sp.	0	0	0	0	0	±	+	+	±	+	+	±	+	+	+	+	+	+	+	+	+	+		+
Proteus mirabilis	0	0	0	0	0	+	+	+	+	+	+	+	+	±	+	+	+	+	+	+	+	+	+	+
Proteus vulgaris	0	0	0	0	0	0	+	+	+	+	+	+	+	±	+	+	+	+	+	+	+	+		+
Providencia sp.	0	0	0	0	0	0	0	0	+	+	+	+	+	±	+	+	+	+	+	+	+	+		+

+ = usually effective clinically or >60% susceptible; ± = clinical trials lacking or 30–60% susceptible; 0 = not effective clinically or <30% susceptible; blank = data not available

** Most strains ±; can be used in UTI, not in systemic infection

TABLE 4 (2)

Organisms	Penicillin G	Penicillin V	Methicillin	Nafcillin/Oxacillin	Cloxacillin^NUS/Diclox.	AMP/Amox	Amox/Clav	AMP-Sulb	Ticarcillin	Ticar-Clav	Pip-Tazo	Piperacillin	Ertapenem	Imipenem	Meropenem	Aztreonam	Ciprofloxacin	Ofloxacin	Lomefloxacin	Pefloxacin^NUS	Levofloxacin	Moxifloxacin	Gemifloxacin	Gatifloxacin
Morganella sp.	0	0	0	0	0	0	±	+	+	+	+	+	+	+	+	+	+	+	+	+	+	+		+
Citrobacter sp.	0	0	0	0	0	0	0	0	+	+	+	+	+	+	+	+	+	+	+	+	+	+		+
Aeromonas sp.	0	0	0	0	0	0	0	+	0	+	+	+	+	+	+	+	+	+	+		+	+		+
Acinetobacter sp.	0	0	0	0	0	0	±	+	±	±	+	+	0	+	+	0	+	±	±		±	±	±	±
Ps. aeruginosa	0	0	0	0	0	0	0	0	+	+	+	+	0	+	+	+	+	±	±	±	±	0	0	±
B. (Ps.) cepacia	0	0	0	0	0	0	0	0	+	+	+	+	0	0	+	0	0	0	0	0	+	0		0
S. (X.) maltophilia	0	0	0	0	0	0	0	0	+	+	0	0	0	0	0	0	0	0	0	0	+	+		+
Y. enterocolitica	0	0	0	0	0	0	+	+	+	+	+	+	+	+	+	+	+	+	+	+	+	+		+
Legionella sp.	0	0	0	0	0	0	0	0	0	0	0	0	0	±	+	0	+	+	±	+	+	+	+	+
P. multocida	+	+	0	0	0	+	+	+	+	+	+	+	+	+	+	+	+	+	+	+	+	+	+	+
H. ducreyi		0	0	0	0	0	+	+	±	+	+	±	+	+	+	+	+	+	+	+	+	+		+
MISC.:																								
Chlamydia sp.	0	0	0	0	0	0	0	0	0	0	0	0	0	0	0	0	±	+	0	±	+	+	+	+
M. pneumoniae	0	0	0	0	0	0	0	0	0	0	0	0	0	0	0	0	+	+	0	+	+	+	+	+
ANAEROBES:																								
Actinomyces	+	+	0	0	0	+	+	+	+	+	+	+	+	+	+	0	0	±	0	0	±	+		+
Bacteroides fragilis	+†	0	0	0	0	0	+	+	+	+	+	+	+	+	+	0	0	±	0	0	±	+		±
P. melaninogenica	+	±	0	0	0	±	+	+	+	+	+	+	+	+	+	0	±	±	0	0	+	+		+
Clostridium difficile	+†		0	0	0		+	+	+	+	+	+	+	+	+	0	0	0	0	0	0	0		0
Clostridium (not difficile)	+	+	0	0	0	+	+	+	+	+	+	+	+	+	+	0	±	±	0	0	±	+		+
Peptostreptococcus sp.	+	+	+	+	+	+	+	+	+	+	+	+	+	+	+	0	±	±	0	0	±	+		+

+ = usually effective clinically or >60% susceptible; ± = clinical trials lacking or 30–60% susceptible; 0 = not effective clinically or <30% susceptible; blank = data not available

† No clinical evidence that penicillins or fluoroquinolones are effective for C. difficile enterocolitis (but they may cover this organism in mixed intra-abdominal and pelvic infections)

TABLE 4 (3)

Organisms	1st Generation	2nd Generation			3rd/4th Generation					Oral Agents 1st Generation		Oral Agents 2nd Generation			Oral Agents 3rd Generation		
	Cefazolin	Cefotetan	Cefoxitin	Cefuroxime	Cefotaxime	Ceftizoxime	Ceftriaxone	Ceftazidime	Cefepime	Cefadroxil	Cephalexin	Cefaclor/Loracarbef*	Cefprozil	Cefuroxime axetil	Cefixime	Ceftibuten	Cefpodox/Cefdinir/Cefditoren
GRAM-POSITIVE:																	
Strep. Group A,B,C,G	+	+	+	+	+	+	+	±	+	+	+	+	+	+	+	+	+
Strep. pneumoniae	+	+	+	+	+	+	+	±[1]	+	+	+	+	+	+	+	±	+
Viridans strep	+	+	+	+	+	+	+	+	+	+	+	+	±	+	+	0	+
Enterococcus faecalis	0	0	0	0	0	0	0	0	0	0	0	0	0	0	0	0	0
Staph. aureus (MSSA)	+	+	+	+	+	+	+	±	+	+	+	+	+	+	0	0	+
Staph. aureus (MRSA)	0	0	0	0	0	0	0	0	0	0	0	0	0	0	0	0	0
Staph. aureus (CA-MRSA)	0	0	0	0	0	0	0	0	0	0	0	0	0	0	0	0	0
Staph. epidermidis	±	±	±	±	±	±	±	±	±	±	±	±	±	±	0	0	±
C. jeikeium	0	0	0	0	0	0	0	0	0	0	0	0	0	0	0	0	0
L. monocytogenes	0	0	0	0	0	0	0	0	0	0	0	0	0	0	0	0	0
GRAM-NEGATIVE																	
N. gonorrhoeae	±	+	+	+	+	+	+	+	+	0	0	±	±	+	+	±	+
N. meningitidis	0	±	±	±	+	+	+	+	+	0	0	±	±	±	±	±	+
M. catarrhalis	+	+	+	+	+	+	+	+	+	0	0	+	+	+	+	+	+
H. influenzae	+	+	+	+	+	+	+	+	+	0	0	+	+	+	+	+	+
E. coli	+	+	+	+	+	+	+	+	+	+	+	+	+	+	+	+	0
Klebsiella sp.	+	+	+	+	+	+	+	+	+	0	0	0	0	+	+	+	0
E. coli/Klebs sp ESBL+	0	0	0	0	0	0	0	0	0	0	0	0	0	0	0	0	0
Enterobacter sp.	0	0	0	0	±	±	±	+	+	0	0	0	0	0	0	+	+
Serratia sp.	0	+	0	0	±	±	±	+	+	0	0	0	0	0	±	±	+
Salmonella sp.	+	+	+	+	+	+	+	+	+	0	0				±	±	+
Shigella sp.	+	+	+	+	+	+	+	+	+	0	0				+	+	+
Proteus mirabilis	+	+	+	+	+	+	+	+	+	+	+	+	+	+	+	+	±
Proteus vulgaris	0	+	+	+	+	+	+	+	+	0	0	0	0	0	+	+	0
Providencia sp.	0	+	0	0	+	+	+	+	+	0	0	0	0	0	0	0	
Morganella sp.	0	+	±	±	+	+	+	+	+	0	0	0	0	±	0	0	0

+ = **usually effective clinically or >60% susceptible**; ± = **clinical trials lacking or 30-60% susceptible**; 0 = **not effective clinically or <30% susceptible**; blank = **data not available**

* A 1-carbacephem best classified as a cephalosporin

[1] Ceftaz 8-16 times less active than cefotax/ceftriax, effective only vs Pen-sens. strains (AAC 39:2193, 1995). Oral cefuroxime, cefprozil, cefpodoxime most active in vitro vs resistant S. pneumo (PIDJ 14:1037, 1995).

TABLE 4 (4)

CEPHALOSPORINS

Organisms	1st Generation — Cefazolin	2nd Generation — Cefotetan	2nd Generation — Cefoxitin	2nd Generation — Cefuroxime	3rd/4th Generation — Cefotaxime	3rd/4th Generation — Ceftizoxime	3rd/4th Generation — Ceftriaxone	3rd/4th Generation — Ceftazidime	3rd/4th Generation — Cefepime	Oral 1st Gen — Cefadroxil	Oral 1st Gen — Cephalexin	Oral 2nd Gen — Cefaclor/Loracarbef*	Oral 2nd Gen — Cefprozil	Oral 2nd Gen — Cefuroxime axetil	Oral 3rd Gen — Cefixime	Oral 3rd Gen — Ceftibuten	Oral 3rd Gen — Cefpodox/Cefdinir/Cefditoren
C. freundii	0	0	0	0	0	0	0	0	+	0	0	0	0	0		0	0
C. diversus	0	±	±	±	+	+	+	+	+	0	0	±	0	±	+	+	+
Citrobacter sp.	0	±	±	±	+	+	+	+	+	0	0	0	0	0	+	+	
Aeromonas sp.	0	±	±	±	0	0	0	±	+	0	0	0	0	0	0	+	0
Acinetobacter sp.	0	0	0	0	±	±	0	+	±	0	0	0	0	0	0	0	0
Pa. aeruginosa (Ps.)	0	0	0	0	±	±	±	+	+	0	0	0	0	0	0	0	
B. (Ps.) cepacia	0	0	0	0	±	±	0	±	0	0	0	0	0	0	0	+	
S. (X.) maltophilia	0	0	0	0	0	0	0	0	0	0	0	0	0	0	0	0	
Y. enterocolitica	0	0	0	0	±	±	+	±	+	0	0	0	0	0	+	+	0
Legionella sp.	0	0	0	0	0	0	0	0	0	0	0	0	0	0	+		+
P. multocida		+	0	0	+	+	+	0	+						0		
H. ducreyi					+	+	+	+	+						+	0	+
ANAEROBES:																	
Actinomyces	0	±¹ +			0	±	0	0	0	0						0	
Bacteroides fragilis		+	+	0	+	±	0	+	+						+		
P. melaninogenica		+	+	0	+	0	+								0		
Clostridium difficile																	
Clostridium (not difficile)	0	+	0	+	+	+	+	+	+	0	0	0	+	+	0	+	0
Peptostreptococcus sp.		+	+	+	+	+	+	0	+	+	+	+	+	+	+	+	+

+ = **usually effective clinically or >60% susceptible**; ± = clinical trials lacking or 30-60% susceptible; 0 = not effective clinically or <30% susceptible; blank = data not available

* A 1-carbacephem best classified as a cephalosporin

¹ Cefotetan is less active against B. ovatus, B. distasonis, B. thetaiotamicron

TABLE 4 (5)

Class	Drug	Strep Group A,B,C,G	Strep. pneumoniae	Enterococcus faecalis	Enterococcus faecium	Staph. aureus (MSSA)	Staph. aureus (MRSA)	Staph. aureus (CA-MRSA)	Staph. epidermidis	C. jeikeum	L. monocytogenes	N. gonorrhoeae	N. meningitidis	M. catarrhalis	H. influenzae	Aeromonas	E. coli	Klebsiella sp.	E. coli/Klebs. sp ESBL+	Enterobacter sp.	Salmonella sp.	Shigella sp.	Serratia marcescens
MISCELLANEOUS	Colistimethate (Colistin)	o	o	o	o	o	o	o	o		o				o	o	+	+	+	+			
	Daptomycin	+	+	±[2]	+	+	+	+	+	+	±	o	o	o	o	o	o	o	o	o	o	o	o
	Linezolid	+	+	+	+	+	+	+	+	+	+	o		±			o	o	o	o	o	o	o
	Quinupristin-dalfopristin	+	+	o	+	o	+	+	+	+	+	o		±			o	o	o	o	o	o	o
	Metronidazole	o	o	o	o	o	o	o	o	o	o	o	o	o	o	o	o	o	o	o	o	o	o
	Rifampin	+	+	±	o	+	+	+	+	+		+	+	+	o	o	o	o		o	o	o	o
URINARY TRACT AGENTS	Fosfomycin			+	±												+		±	±			±
	Nitrofurantoin	+	+	+	+	+	+	+		o							+	o	±	±		o	o
	TMP-SMX	+[1]	+	+[1]	o	+	+	+	±	o	+	±	+	±	+	±	±	±		±	±	±	±
	Trimethoprim	+	+	±	o	±	±	±	+	o	+	o	±		±		+	+	±	±	±	±	o
	Fusidic Acid[NUS]	±	±			+	+	+	+	+		+	+				o	o	o	o	o	o	o
GLYCOPEPTIDES	Dalbavancin	+	+	+	±	+	+	+	+	+	+	o	o				o	o	o	o	o	o	o
	Teicoplanin	+	+	+	±	+	+	+	±	+	±	o	o				o	o	o	o	o	o	o
	Vancomycin	+	+	+	±	+	+	+	+	+	±	o	o				o	o	o	o	o	o	o
GLYCYLCYCLINE	Tigecycline	+	+	+	+	+	+	+	+	+	+	+		+	+	+	+	+	o	+	+	+	+
TETRACYCLINES	Minocycline	+	+	o	o	+	+	+	+	±	+	+	+	+	+	±	+	+	±	+	±	+	o
	Doxycycline	±	+	o	o	±	±	o	+	+	+	+	+	+	+	±	±	+	o	+	±	+	o
KETOLIDE	Telithromycin	+	+	+	+	o	o	o	+	+	+												
MACROLIDES	Clarithromycin	±	+	o	o	+	o	+	o	+	+		+	+	+	o	o	o	o	o	o	o	o
	Azithromycin	±	+	o	o	+	o	+	o	+	+	+	+	+	+	o	o	o	o	o	±	o	o
	Erythro/Dirithro	±	+	o	o	±	o	±	o	+	+	±	+	+	±	o	o	o	o	o	o	±	o
	Clindamycin	+	+	o	o	+	o	±	o	±	o	o	o	o	o								
	Chloramphenicol	+	+	±	±	±	o		o	o	+	+	+	+	+	+	+	±		+	o	+	o
AMINOGLYCOSIDES	Netilmicin[NUS]	o	o	S	S	o	+	o		±	o	o	+		+	+	+	+		+	+	+	+
	Amikacin	o	o	S	S	o	+	o		±	o	o	+		+	+	+	+		+	+	+	+
	Tobramycin	o	o	S	S	o	+	o		±	o	o	+		+	+	+	+		+	+	+	+
	Gentamicin	o	o	S	S	o	+	o		±	S	o	+		+	+	+	+		+	+	+	+

+ = usually effective clinically or >60% susceptible; ± = clinical trials lacking or 30–60% susceptible; o = not effective clinically or <30% susceptible; blank = data not available. Antimicrobials such as azithromycin have high tissue penetration and hence in vivo activity may exceed in vitro activity.

(ampicillin); S = synergistic with penicillins; o = not effective clinically or <30% susceptible; blank = data not available. Antimicrobials such as clarithromycin are metabolized to more active compounds, and some such as clarithromycin have high tissue penetration.

[1] Although active in vitro, TMP-SMX is not clinically effective for Group A strep pharyngitis or for infections due to E. faecalis.

[2] Although active in vitro, daptomycin is not chemically effective for pneumonia caused by strep pneumonia.

TABLE 4 (6)

Organisms	Colistimethate (Colistin)	Daptomycin	Linezolid	Quinupristin-dalfopristin	Metronidazole	Rifampin	Fosfomycin	Nitrofurantoin	TMP-SMX	Trimethoprim	Fusidic Acid[NUS]	Dalbavancin	Teicoplanin	Vancomycin	Tigecycline	Minocycline	Doxycycline	Telithromycin	Clarithromycin	Azithromycin	Erythro/Dirithro	Clindamycin	Chloramphenicol	Netilmicin[NUS]	Amikacin	Tobramycin	Gentamicin
	MISCELLANEOUS						URINARY TRACT AGENTS					GLYCOPEPTIDES			GLYCYLCYCLINE	TETRACYCLINES		KETOLIDE	MACROLIDES					AMINOGLYCOSIDES			
Proteus vulgaris	o	o	o	o	o	o	±	o	o	o	o	o	o	o	±	o	o	o	o	o	o	o	±	+	+	+	+
Acinetobacter sp.	+	o	o	o	o	o			±	o	o	o	o	o	+	o	o	o	o	o	o	o	o	o	±	o	o
Pa. aeruginosa	+	o	o	o	o	o			o	o	o	o	o	o	+	o	o	o	o	o	o	o	+	+	o	o	o
B. (Ps.) cepacia	o	o	o	o	o				+	+	o	o	o	o	±	o	o	o	o	o	o	o	+	o	o	o	+
S. (X.) maltophilia	o	o	o	o	o				+	+	o	o	o	o	+	o	o	o	o	o	o	o	+	o	o	+	+
Y. enterocolitica		o			o	+		o	+	+					+	+	+	+	o	o	o	+	+	+			+
F. tularensis		o			o	+			+	+						+	+		+	+	+		+	+			+
Brucella sp.									+	+	±				+	+	+	+	+	+	±	±	+	±	±		±
Legionella sp.			+	o		+			±		o			o	o	+	+	+	+	+	+	±	+				
H. ducreyi			o						+		o			o	o	±	±		+	+	o	o	+				
V. vulnificus			o			+					o				+	+	+	+	+	+	±	+	+	o			
MISC.:																											
Chlamydophilia sp.									o	o	o			o	o	+	+	+	+	+	+	+	+	o	o	o	o
M. pneumoniae			o	+							o			o	o	±	±	+	+	+	+	±	+	o	o	o	o
Rickettsia sp.			o								o				o	+	+	+	o	o	o	o	+	o	o	o	o
Mycobacterium avium			o			+			o		o				o	+	+	+	+	+	±	+	±	o	+	o	o
ANAEROBES:																											
Actinomyces			±	+	o						+	+	+	+	+	+	+	+	+	+	+	+	+	o	o	o	o
Bacteroides fragilis			±	+	+				o		+	o	o	o	+	±	±		o	o	o	±	±	o	o	o	o
P. melaninogenica			+	+	+						+	o	o	o	o	±	±		+	+	o	±	+	o	o	o	o
Clostridium difficile			+	+	+	+			o		+	+	+	+	±	±	±		+	+	±	±	±	o	o	o	o
Clostridium (not difficile) **			±	±	+	+					+	+	+	+	+	+	+	+	+	+	±	+	+	o	o	o	o
Peptostreptococcus sp.			+	+	+						+	+	+	+	+	+	+	+	+	+	+	+	+	o	o	o	o

+ = usually effective clinically or >60% susceptible; ± = clinical trials lacking or 30–60% susceptible; 0 = not effective clinically or <30% susceptible; blank = data not available.

Antimicrobials such as azithromycin have high tissue penetration & some such as clarithromycin are metabolized to more active compounds, hence in vivo activity may exceed in vitro activity.

** Vancomycin, metronidazole given po active vs C. difficile; IV vancomycin not effective

TABLE 5 – TREATMENT OPTIONS FOR SELECTED HIGHLY RESISTANT BACTERIA
(See page 2 for abbreviations)

ORGANISM/RESISTANCE	THERAPEUTIC OPTIONS	COMMENT[1]
E. faecalis. Resistant to:		
Vanco + strep/gentamicin (MIC >500 mcg per mL), β-lactamase neg. (JAC 40:161, 1997).	Penicillin G or AMP (systemic infections); Nitrofurantoin, fosfomycin (UTI only). Usually resistant to Synercid.	Non-BL+ strains of E. faecalis resistant to penicillin and AMP described in Spain, but unknown for strains) in U.S. and elsewhere (AAC 40:2420, 1996). Linezolid effective in 60-70% of cases (AnIM 138:135, 2003). Daptomycin, tigecycline active in vitro (JAC 52:123, 2003).
Penicillin (β-lactamase producers)	Vanco, AM-SB	Appear resistant to AMP and penicillin by standard in vitro methods. Must use direct test for β-lactamase with chromogenic cephalosporin (nitrocefin) to identify. Rare since early 1990s.
E. faecium. Resistant to:		
Vanco and high levels (MIC >500 mcg per mL) of streptomycin and gentamicin	Penicillin G or AMP (systemic infections); fosfomycin, nitrofurantoin (UTI only)	For strains with pen/AMP MIC or >8 ≤64 mcg per mL, anecdotal evidence that high-dose (300 mg per kg per day) AMP ± may be effective. Daptomycin, tigecycline active in vitro (JAC 52:123, 2003).
Penicillin, AMP, vanco, & high-level resist to streptomycin and gentamicin (NEJM 342:710, 2000)	Linezolid 600 mg po or IV q12h and quinu-dalfo 7.5 mg per kg q8h are bacteriostatic against most strains of E. faecium. Can try combinations of cell wall-active antibiotics with other agents (including FQ, chloramphenicol, RIF, or doxy). Chloramphenicol alone effective in some cases of bacteremia (Clin Micro Inf 7:17, 2001). Nitrofurantoin or fosfomycin may work for UTI.	For strains with Van B phenotype (vanco R, teico S), teicoplanin[a,e], preferably in combination with streptomycin or gentamicin (if not highly AG resistant), may be effective. Synercid roughly 70% effective in clinical trials (CID 30:790, 2000; & 33:1816, 2001). Linezolid shows similar efficacy. (AAC 45, CID) response rates to linezolid ~85%. (AAC 48) Emergence of resistance with therapeutic failure has occurred during monotherapy with either quinu-dalfo or linezolid (CID 30:790, 2000; Ln 357:1179, 2001). Nosocomial spread of linezolid-resistant E. faecium possible (Clin Micro Inf 346:867, 2002). Daptomycin active in vitro against most strains (JAC 52:123, 2003). Tigecycline also active in vitro (Circulation 111:e384, 2005). **Infectious disease consultation imperative**
S. aureus. Resistant to:		
Methicillin (health-care associated) (CID 32:108, 2001)	Vanco [For persistent bacteremia (≥7 days) on vanco or teicoplanin[a,e], see Table 6]	Alternatives[A,s]: daptomycin (AAC 49:770, 2005; NEJM 355:653, 2006), linezolid (Chest 124:1789, 2003), dalbavancin (EMID 48:137, 2004), TMP-SMX (test susceptibility first), minocycline & doxy (some strains), tigecycline (CID 41(Suppl 5):S303, 2005), or quinu-dalfo (CID 34:1481, 2002). Fusidic acid[NUS], fosfomycin.
For community-acquired MRSA infections, see Table 6		mycin, RIF may be active; use only in combination to prevent in vitro emergence of resistance. Staphylococci (incl. CA-MRSA) with inducible MLSB resistance may appear susceptible to clindamycin in vitro. Clinda therapy may result in therapeutic failure (CID 37:1257, 2003). Test for inducible resistance [double-disk ("D test")] before treating with clinda (Ln 358:207, 2004). Investigational drugs with activity against MRSA include oritavancin (LY333328), telavancin, ceftobiprole.
Vanco, methicillin (VRMRSA) (NEJM 339:520, 1998; CID 32:108, 2001; MMWR 51:902, 2002; NEJM 348:1342, 2003)	Unknown, but even high-dose vanco may fail. Linezolid, quinu-dalfo, daptomycin active in vitro.	Most clinical isolates of VRMRSA have had only low levels (MIC 516 mcg per mL) of vanco resistance (MMWR 51:565, 1997; JAC 40:135, 1997). Some call these strains VISA or GISA. Only anecdotal data on therapeutic regimens. Most susceptible to TMP-SMX, minocycline, doxycycline, RIF and AGs (CID 32:108, 2001). RIF should always be combined with a 2nd therapeutic agent to prevent emergence of RIF resistance during therapy. 6 clinical isolates of truly vancomycin-resistant (MIC >64) MRSA described. Organisms still susceptible to TMP-SMX, chloro, linezolid, minocycline, quinu-dalfo (MMWR 51:902, 2002; NEJM 348:1342, 2003).
S. epidermidis. Resistant to:		
Methicillin	Vanco (+ RIF and gentamicin for prosthetic valve endocarditis).	Vanco more active than teicoplanin[As] (Clin Micro Rev 8:585, 1995).
Methicillin, glycopeptides (AAC 48: 770, 2005)	Quinu-dalfo (see comments on E. faecium generally active in vitro as are linezolid, daptomycin, & dalbavancin).	New FQs (levofloxacin, gatifloxacin, moxifloxacin active in vitro, but development of resistance is a potential problem.

---

[1] Guideline on prevention of resistance: CID 24:584, 1997

TABLE 5 (2)

ORGANISM/RESISTANCE	THERAPEUTIC OPTIONS	COMMENT
S. pneumoniae. Resistant to: Penicillin G (MIC >0.1 ≤1.0)	Ceftriaxone or cefotaxime. High-dose penicillin (≥10 million units per day) or AMP (amox) likely effective for nonmeningeal sites of infection (e.g. pneumonia), telithro	IMP, ERTA, cefepime, cefpodoxime, cefuroxime also active (IDCP 3:75, 1994). MER less active than IMP (AAC 38:898, 1994). Gemi, moxi, gati, levo also have good activity (AAC 38:898, 1994; DMID 31:45, 1998; Exp Opin Invest Drugs 8:123, 1999).
Penicillin G (MIC ≥2.0)	High-dose cefotaxime (300 mg per kg per day, max. 24 gm per day) with cefotaxime MICs as high as 2 mcg per mL (AAC 40:218, 1996). Review: IDCP 6(Suppl 2):S21, 1997.	
Penicillin erythro, tetracycline, chloramphenicol, TMP-SMX.	Vanco ± RIF. (Gemi, moxi, gati, or levo), telithro (non-meningeal infections)	66-80% of strains susceptible to clindamycin (DMID 25:201, 1996).
Acinetobacter baumannii. Resistant to: IMP, P Ceph 3 AP, AP Pen, APAG, FQ (see page 2 for abbreviations)	AM-SB (CID 34:1425, 2002). Subactam alone is active against some A. baumannii (JAC 42:793, 1998)	6/8 patients with A. baumannii meningitis (7 organisms resistant to IMP) cured with AM-SB (CID 24: 932, 1997). Various combinations of FQs and AGs, IMP and AGs or RIF, AP Pens or P Ceph 3 APs with AGs may show activity against **some** multiresistant strains (CID 36:1268, 2003). IV colistin also effective (CID 36:111, 2003; JAC 54:1085, 2004). MER + subactam active in vitro & in vivo (AAC 53:393, 2004). Active in vitro: triple drug combinations of polymyxin B, IMP, & RIF (AAC 48:753, 2004) & tigecycline (CID 41:S315, 2005).
Campylobacter jejuni. Resistant to: FQs	Erythro, azithro, clarithro, doxy, clindamycin	Resistance to **both** FQs & macrolides reported (CID 22:868, 1996; EID 7:24, 2002; AAC 47:2358, 2003).
Klebsiella pneumoniae (producing ESBL). Resistant to: Ceftazidime & other 3rd generation cephalosporins (see Table 10C), aztreonam	IMP, MER, (CID 39:31, 2004) (See Comment)	P Ceph 4, TC-CL, PIP-TZ show in vitro activity, but not proven entirely effective in animal models (LJAA 8:37, 1997); some strains w/hyperproduce ESBLs are primarily resistant to TC-CL and PIP-TZ (J Clin Micro 34:358, 1996). Note: there are strains of ESBL-producing klebsiella sensitive in vitro to P Ceph 2, 3 but resistant to ceftazidime, infections with such strains do not respond to P Ceph 2 or 3 (J Clin Micro 39:2206, 2001). FQ may be effective if susceptible but many strains resistant. Note Klebsiella sp. with carbapenem resistance due to class A carbapenemase. Some of these organisms resistant to all antimicrobials except colistin (CID 39:55, 2004).
Pseudomonas aeruginosa. Resistant to: IMP, MER	CIP (check susceptibility), APAG (check susceptibility)	Many strains remain susceptible to aztreonam & ceftazidime or (AP Pen & APAG) or (AP Ceph 3 + APAG) may show in vitro activity (AAC 39:2411, 1995). IV colistin may have some utility (CID 28:1008, 1999).

TABLE 6 – SUGGESTED MANAGEMENT OF SUSPECTED OR CULTURE-POSITIVE COMMUNITY-ACQUIRED PHENOTYPE OF METHICILLIN-RESISTANT S. AUREUS (CA-MRSA) INFECTIONS

In the absence of definitive comparative efficacy studies, the Editors have generated the following guidelines. With the magnitude of the clinical problem and a number of new drugs, it is likely new data will require frequent revisions of the regimens suggested. Ref: CID 40:562, 2005. (See page 2 for abbreviations)

CLINICAL ILLNESS	ABSCESS, AFEBRILE, & IMMUNO-COMPETENT: OUTPATIENT CARE	ABSCESS(ES) WITH FEVER, OUTPATIENT CARE	VENTILATOR-ASSOCIATED[3][4] PNEUMONIA	BACTEREMIA OR POSSIBLE ENDOCARDITIS OR BACTEREMIC SHOCK	BLOOD CULTURES DRAWN ON DAY 7 OF VANCO ARE POSITIVE (See footnote[3])
Management (for drug doses, see footnote)	TMP-SMX-DS or doxycycline or minocycline (CID 40:1429, 2005) **NOTE:** for abscesses <5 cm diameter, I&D only sufficient (PED 123:123, 2004) Culture abscess. I&D. Hot packs.	(TMP-SMX-DS + rifampin) or linezolid or 1 dose of dalbavancin IV. ┄┄┄┄┄┄┄┄┄┄┄ Culture abscess & maybe blood. I&D. Hot packs.	Vanco[ars] IV or linezolid IV Ref. Chest 124:1632, 2003 ┄┄┄┄┄┄┄┄┄┄┄ Need quant. cultures for diagnosis: e.g., protected specimen brush	Vanco or teico[ars] IV or dapto IV. Could start with **nafcillin (or oxacillin) + vanco;** DC inactive drug when suscept. data available ┄┄┄┄┄┄┄┄┄┄┄ Blood cultures. Target trough level of vanco 15 (range 10-20) mcg per mL.	**Dapto** (or vanco or vice versa). **Quinupristin–dalfopristin** (Q-D) 2nd choice ± with **vanco.** Linezolid –70% effective in compassionate use (JAC 50:1017, 2002). No strong data that adding **rifampin** helps. Adding **gentamicin** to **vanco** ↑ risk of nephrotoxicity with little evidence of enhanced efficacy. Could try **Levo,** or **Moxi** if isolate susceptible. In retrospective evaluation, linezolid & vanco equivalent efficacy–roughly 30% microbiologic failure with both drugs (JAC 56:923, 2005).
Comments	Close followup. Fever should resolve quickly post I&D. Rarely S. pyogenes MRSA: **TMP-SMX** not active vs S. pyogenes: **rifampin** active or add **Pen V-K**	Linezolid superior to vanco in retrospective subset analysis; prospective study in progress.	Can't rely on **clinda** without in vitro documentation of absence of inducible resistance (CID 40:280, 2005). **TMP-SMX** IV of limited efficacy vs bacteremic S. aureus (AnIM 117:390, 1992).	If MRSA resistant to **erythro**, likely that Q-D will have bacteriostatic & not bactericidal activity. Interest in Q-D + vanco, but no data. Do not add **linezolid** to **vanco**: no benefit & may be antagonistic. Linezolid successful in compassionate use (JAC 50:1017, 2002) & in pts with reduced vanco suscept. (CID 38:521, 2004). To date, no data for **dalbavancin** in vanco failures.	

Dalbavancin: 1000 mg IV, then 500 mg IV 8 days later. **Daptomycin:** 6 mg per kg IV q24h. **Doxycycline or minocycline:** 100 mg po bid. **Linezolid:** 600 mg po/IV bid. **Nafcillin or oxacillin:** 2 gm IV q4h. **Quinupristin-dalfopristin (Q-D):** 7.5 mg per kg IV q8h via central line. **Rifampin:** Long serum half-life justifies dosing 600 mg po q24h; however, frequency of nausea less with 300 mg po bid. **TMP-SMX-DS:** Standard dose 8-10 mg per kg per day. For 70 kg person = 750 mg TMP component per day. TMP-SMX-DS contains 160 mg TMP. Hence, suggest **2** TMP-SMX-DS po bid. 50% failure rate with one TMP-SMX-DS bid (J Am Acad Derm 50:854, 2004). **Vancomycin:** 1 gm IV q12h

---

[2] Bacteremia may persist 7 days after starting vanco (AnIM 115:674, 1991). Longer duration of bacteremia, greater likelihood of endocarditis (JID 190:1140, 2004).

[3] Before switching, look for undrained abscess(es) &/or infected foreign body. Recheck vanco and dapto MICs to exclude intermediate or high-level vanco resistance that may develop during therapy.

TABLE 7 – METHODS FOR PENICILLIN DESENSITIZATION (CID 35:26, 2002)
(See Table 10C, page 91, for TMP/SMX desensitization)

Perform in ICU setting. Discontinue all β-adrenergic antagonists. Have IV line, ECG and spirometer (CCTD 13:131, 1993). A history of allergic reactions ↑. Once desensitized, rx must not lapse or risk of allergic reactions ↑.
Stevens-Johnson syndrome, exfoliative dermatitis, erythroderma are nearly absolute contraindications to desensitization (use only as a last resort, and only if pt has hypersensitivity).

Oral Route: If oral prep. available and pt has functional GI tract, oral route is preferred. [13 pts will develop transient reaction during desensitization or treatment, usually mild.]

Step	1	2	3	4	5	6	7	8	9	10	11	12	13	14
Drug (mg per mL)	0.5	0.5	0.5	0.5	0.5	0.5	5.0	5.0	5.0	5.0	50	50	50	50
Amount (mL)	0.1	0.2	0.4	0.8	1.6	3.2	0.64	1.2	2.4	4.8	1.0	2.0	4.0	8.0

** Interval between doses: 15 min. After Step 14, observe for 30 minutes, then 1.0 gm IV

Parenteral Route:

Step **	1	2	3	4	5	6	7	8	9	10	11	12	13	14	15	16	17
Drug (mg per mL)	0.1	0.1	0.1	0.1	1.0	1.0	1.0	10	10	10	100	100	100	1000	1000	1000	1000
Amount (mL)	0.1	0.2	0.4	0.8	0.16	0.32	0.64	0.12	0.24	0.48	0.1	0.2	0.4	0.8	0.16	0.32	0.64

** Interval between doses: 15 min. After Step 17, observe for 30 minutes, then 1.0 gm IV. [Adapted from Sullivan, T.J., in Allergy: Principles and Practice, C.V. Mosby, 1993, p. 1726, with permission.]

TABLE 8 – RISK CATEGORIES OF ANTIMICROBICS IN PREGNANCY

DRUG	FDA CATEGORIES*
Antibacterial Agents	
Aminoglycosides:	
Amikacin, gentamicin, isepamicin^NUS, netilmicin^NUS, streptomycin & tobramycin	D
Beta Lactams	
Penicillins, pens + BLI; cephalosporins; aztreonam	B
Imipenem/cilastatin	C
Meropenem, ertapenem	B
Chloramphenicol	C
Clindamycin	B
Dalbavancin	C
Daptomycin	B
Fosfomycin	B
Fusidic acid	see Footnote ‡
Linezolid	C
Macrolides:	
Erythromycins/azithromycin	B
Clarithromycin	C
Metronidazole	B
Nitrofurantoin	B
Rifaximin	C
Sulfonamides/trimethoprim	C
Telithromycin	C
Tetracyclines, tigecycline	D
Tinidazole	C
Vancomycin	C
Antifungal Agents: (CID 27:1151, 1998)	
Amphotericin B preparations	B
Anidulafungin	C
Caspofungin	C
Fluconazole, itraconazole, ketoconazole, flucytosine	C

DRUG	FDA CATEGORIES*
Antifungal Agents: (continued)	
Micafungin	C
Posaconazole	C
Terbinafine	B
Voriconazole	D
Antiparasitic Agents:	
Albendazole/mebendazole	C
Atovaquone/proguanil; atovaquone alone	C
Chloroquine, eflornithine	C
Ivermectin	C
Mefloquine	C
Miltefosine	X
Nitazoxanide	B
Pentamidine	C
Praziquantel	B
Pyrimethamine/pyrisulfadoxine	C
Quinine	X
Antimycobacterial Agents:	
Clofazimine/cycloserine	C
Dapsone	C
Ethambutol	"avoid"
Ethionamide	C
INH, pyrazinamide	"safe"
Rifabutin	"do not use"
Rifampin	C
Thalidomide	X
Antiviral Agents:	
Abacavir	C
Acyclovir	B
Adefovir	C
Amantadine	C

DRUG	FDA CATEGORIES*
Antiviral Agents: (continued)	
Atazanavir	B
Cidofovir	C
Darunavir	B
Delavirdine	D
Didanosine (ddI)	B
Efavirenz	D
Emtricitabine	B
Entecavir	C
Etravirine	B
Famciclovir	B
Foscarnet	C
Fosamprenavir	C
Ganciclovir	C
Indinavir	C
Interferons	C
Lamivudine	C
Lopinavir/ritonavir	C
Maraviroc	B
Nelfinavir	B
Nevirapine	B
Oseltamivir	C
Ribavirin	X
Rimantadine	C
Ritonavir	B
Saquinavir	B
Stavudine	C
Telbivudine	B
Tenofovir	B
Tipranavir	C
Valacyclovir	B
Valganciclovir	C
Zalcitabine	C
Zanamivir	C
Zidovudine	C

* **FDA Pregnancy Categories:** A—studies in pregnant women, no risk; B—animal studies no risk, but human studies not adequate or animal toxicity but human studies no risk; C—animal studies show toxicity, human studies inadequate but benefit of use may exceed risk; D—evidence of human risk, but benefits may outweigh; X—fetal abnormalities in humans, risk > benefit.

‡Fusidic acid: no problems reported

TABLE 9A – SELECTED PHARMACOLOGIC FEATURES OF ANTIMICROBIAL AGENTS

DRUG	DOSE, ROUTE OF ADMINISTRATION	FOR PO DOSING—Take Drug WITH FOOD	WITHOUT FOOD³	WITH OR WITHOUT FOOD³	% AB¹	PEAK SERUM LEVEL mcg per mL¹	PROTEIN BINDING, %	SERUM T½² HOURS	BILIARY EXCRETION, %³	CSF⁴/BLOOD, %	CSF LEVEL POTENTIALLY THERAPEUTIC⁵
PENICILLINS: Natural											
Benzathine Pen G	1.2 million units IM					0.15					
Penicillin G	2 million units IV					20	65	0.5	500	5-10	Yes for Pen-sens. S. pneumo
Penicillin V	500 mg po		X		60-73	5-6	65	0.5			
PEN'ASE-RESISTANT PENICILLINS											
Dicloxacillin	500 mg po		X		50	10-15	95-98	0.5			
Nafcillin/Oxacillin	500 mg po		X		Erratic	10-15	90-94	0.5	>100/25	9-20	Yes-high-dose IV therapy
AMINOPENICILLINS											
Amoxicillin	250 mg po			X	75	4-5	17	1.2	100-3000	13-14	Yes
AM-CL	875/125 mg po			X		11.6/2.2	20/30	1.4/1.1	100-3000		
AM-CL-ER		X				17/2.1	18/25	1.3/1.0			
Ampicillin	2 gm IV					47	18-22	1.2	100-3000	13-14	Yes
AM-SB	3 gm IV					109-150	28/38	1.2			
ANTIPSEUDOMONAL PENICILLINS											
Carbenicillin indanyl	382 mg po			X	35	6.5	50	1.0			
Piperacillin	4 gm IV					400	16-48	1.0	3000-6000	30	Not for P. aeruginosa; marginal for coliforms
PIP-TZ	3/3.375 gm IV					209	16-48	1.0	>100		
Ticarcillin	3 gm IV					260	45	1.2		40	Not for P. aeruginosa; marginal for coliforms
TC-CL	3.1 gm IV					330	45/25	1.1			
CEPHALOSPORINS—1st Generation											
Cefadroxil	500 mg po			X	90	16	20	1.5	22		
Cefazolin	1 gm IV					188	73-87	1.9	29-300	1-4	No
Cephalexin	500 mg po		X		90	18-38	5-15	1.0	216		
CEPHALOSPORINS—2nd Generation											
Cefaclor	500 mg po		X		93	9.3	22-25	0.8	≥60		
Cefaclor-CD	500 mg po		X			8.4	22-25	0.8	≥60		
Cefotetan	1 gm IV					124	78-91	4.2	2-21	3	±
Cefoxitin	1 gm IV					110	65-79	0.8	280		
Cefprozil	500 mg po			X	95	10.5	36	1.5			
Cefuroxime	1.5 gm IV					100	50	1.5	35-80	17-88	Yes
Cefuroxime axetil	250 mg po	X			52	4.1	50	1.5			
Loracarbef				X	90	8	25	1.2			
CEPHALOSPORINS—3rd Generation											
Cefdinir	300 mg po			X	25	1.6	60-70	1.7			
Cefditoren pivoxil	400 mg po	X			16	4	88	1.6			
Cefixime	400 mg po			X	50	3-5	65	3.1	800		
Cefotaxime	1 gm IV					100	30-51	1.5	15-75	10	Yes
Cefpodoxime proxetil	200 mg po	X			46	2.9	40	2.3	115		

See page 79 for all footnotes; see page 2 for abbreviations

TABLE 9A (2)

DRUG	DOSE, ROUTE OF ADMINISTRATION	WITH FOOD	WITHOUT FOOD[1]	WITH OR WITHOUT FOOD[1]	% AB[1]	PEAK SERUM LEVEL mcg per mL[1]	PROTEIN BINDING, %	SERUM T½[2], HOURS[2]	BILIARY EXCRETION, %[3]	CSF[4]/BLOOD, %	CSF LEVEL POTENTIALLY THERAPEUTIC[5]
CEPHALOSPORINS—3rd Generation (continued)											
Ceftazidime	1 gm IV					60	<10	1.9	13-54	20-40	Yes
Ceftibuten	400 mg po		X		80	15	65	2.4			
Ceftizoxime	1 gm IV					132	30	1.7	34-82	8-16	Yes
Ceftriaxone	1 gm IV					150	85-95	8	200-500	10	Yes
CEPHALOSPORIN—4th Generation											
Cefepime	2 gm IV					193	20	2.0	∞ 5	10	Yes
CARBAPENEMS											
Ertapenem	1 gm IV					154	95	4	10	8.5	+[b]
Imipenem	500 mg IV					40	15-25	1	minimal	Approx. 2	+
Meropenem	1 gm IV					49	2	1	3-300	3-52	
MONOBACTAM											
Aztreonam	1 gm IV					125	56	2	115-405		±
AMINOGLYCOSIDES											
Amikacin, gentamicin, kanamycin, tobramycin—see Table 10D, page 93, for dose & serum levels										< 3	
Neomycin	po					0			10-60	0-30	No; intrathecal: 5-10 mg
FLUOROQUINOLONES	po										
Ciprofloxacin	750 mg po / 1000 mg ER po / 400 mg IV			X	70	1.8-2.8 / 4.6	20-40 / 20-40	4 / 4	2800-4500 / 2600-4500	26	1 mcg per mL [inadequate] for Strep. species (CID 31:1131, 2000)
Gatifloxacin	400 mg po/IV			X	96	4.2-4.6	20	7-8		36	
Gemifloxacin	320 mg po			X	71	1.6	55-73	7			
Levofloxacin	500 mg po/IV / 750 mg po/IV			X	99	5.7 / 5.6	24-38 / 24-38	6.6 / 6.3		30-50	
Moxifloxacin	400 mg po / 400 mg IV			X	89	4.5	30-50	10-14			
Ofloxacin	400 mg po/IV			X	98	4.6 / 6.2	32	9			
MACROLIDES, AZALIDES, LINCOSAMIDES, KETOLIDES											
Azithromycin	500 mg po / 500 mg IV			X	37	0.4 / 3.6	7-51 / 7-51	68 / 12/68	High		
Azithromycin-ER	2 gm po			X	30	0.8	7-50	59	High		
Clarithromycin	500 mg po			X	50	3-4	65-70	5-7	7000		
Clarithromycin-ER	500-1000 mg po	X				2-3	65-70	5-7			
Dirithromycin	500 mg po	X			10	0.4	15-30	8			
Erythromycin — Oral (various)	500 mg po				18-45	0.1-2	70-74	2-4			
Lactobionate	500 mg po					3-4	70-74	2-4			
Telithromycin	800 mg po				57	2.3	60-70	10	7	2-13	No
Clindamycin	150 mg po / 600 mg IV			X	90	2.5 / 10	85-94 / 85-94	2.4 / 2.4	250-300 / 250-300		No / No

See page 79 for all footnotes; see page 2 for abbreviations

TABLE 9A (3)

DRUG	DOSE, ROUTE OF ADMINISTRATION	FOR PO DOSING—Take Drug WITH FOOD	FOR PO DOSING—Take Drug WITHOUT FOOD	FOR PO DOSING—Take Drug WITH OR WITHOUT FOOD	% AB[1]	PEAK SERUM LEVEL mcg per mL[2]	PROTEIN BINDING, %	SERUM T½, HOURS[3]	BILIARY EXCRETION, %[4]	CSF[5]/BLOOD, %	CSF LEVEL POTENTIALLY THERAPEUTIC[6]
MISCELLANEOUS ANTIBACTERIALS											
Chloramphenicol	1 gm po			X	High	11-18	25-50	4.1		45-89	Yes
Colistin	150 mg IV					5-7.5		2-3			No
Dalbavancin	1 gm, then 0.5 gm IV on day 8					240	93	168	0		No (26%)
Daptomycin	4-6 mg per kg IV					58-99	92	8-9			
Doxycycline	100 mg po			X		1.5-2.1	93	18	200-3200		
Fosfomycin	3 gm po		X			26	<10	5.7			
Fusidic acid	500 mg p.o.	X			91	30	95-99	5-15			
Linezolid	600 mg po/IV			X	100	15-20	31	5	60-70		
Metronidazole	500 mg po/IV			X		20-25	20	6-14	100	45-89	
Minocycline	200 mg po			X		2.0-3.5	76	16	200-3200		
Polymyxin B	20,000 units per kg IV					1-8		4.3-6			
Quinu-Dalfo	7.5 mg per kg IV					5		1.5			No
Rifampin	600 mg po		X			4-32	80	2-5	10,000		
Rifaximin	200 mg po				<0.4	0.004-0.01		7-12			
Sulfamethoxazole (SMX)	2 gm po				70-90	50-120	71-89	8-15			
Trimethoprim (TMP)	100 mg po				80	1	<10-55			50/40	
TMP-SMX-DS	160/800 mg po; 160/800 mg IV			X	85	1-2/40-60; 9/105			100-200; 40-70		Most meningococci resistant. Static vs coliforms
Tetracycline	250 mg po				58 ± 21	1.5-2.2		6-12	200-3200		No (7%)
Tigecycline	50 mg IV q12h					0.63		42	138	22-100	Need high doses. See *Meningitis, Table 1, page 6*
Vancomycin	1 gm IV					20-50	<10-55	4-6	50	7-14	
ANTIFUNGALS											
Amphotericin B											
Standard: 0.4-0.7 mg per kg IV						0.5-3.5	90	24		0	
Ampho B lipid complex (ABLC): 5 mg per kg IV						1.2		24			
Ampho B cholesteryl complex: 4 mg per kg IV						2.5		39			
Liposomal ampho B: 5 mg per kg IV						2.9		7-10/100			
Azoles											
Fluconazole	400 mg po/IV	X		X	90	6.7		20-50		50-94	Yes
Itraconazole	Oral soln 200 mg po; 200 mg po	X	X		55 LOW	0.4-0.6/Itracox 1.4	99.8	20-50		0	No
Posaconazole	200 mg po	X			98	0.3-1.0	98-99	20-66			No
Voriconazole	200 mg po/IV		X		96	3	58	6		22-100	Yes UAC 56:745, 2605; Yes CID 37:728, 2003
Anidulafungin	200 mg IV x1, then 100 mg IV q24h					7.2	84	26.5			No
Caspofungin	70 mg IV x1, then 50 mg IV qd					9.9	97	9-11		0	No
Flucytosine	2.5 gm po			X	78-90	30-40		3-6		60-100	Yes
Micafungin	150 mg IV					5-16	>99	15-17			No

See page 79 for all footnotes; see page 2 for abbreviations

TABLE 9A (4)

DRUG	DOSE, ROUTE OF ADMINISTRATION	FOR PO DOSING—Take Drug WITH FOOD	WITHOUT FOOD[4]	WITH OR WITHOUT FOOD	% AB[1]	PEAK SERUM LEVEL mcg per mL[6]	PROTEIN BINDING, %	SERUM T½, HOURS[1]	BILIARY EXCRETION, %[3]	CSF/BLOOD, %	CSF LEVEL POTENTIALLY THERAPEUTIC[5]
ANTIMYCOBACTERIALS											
Ethambutol	25 mg per kg po	X			80	2-6	10-30	4		25-50	No
Isoniazid	300 mg po		X		100	3-5		0.7-4		90	Yes
Pyrazinamide	20-25 mg per kg po		X		95	30-50	5-10	10-16		100	Yes
Rifampin	600 mg po		X		70-90	4-32	80	1.5-5	10,000	7-56	Yes
Streptomycin	1 gm IV (see Table 10D, page 93)					25-50	0-10	2.5	10-60	0-30	No. Intrathecal 5-10 mg
ANTIPARASITICS											
Albendazole	400 mg po	X				0.5-1.6	70			<1	No
Atovaquone suspension	750 mg po			X	47	15	99.9	67			
Dapsone	100 mg po				100	1.1		10-50			
Ivermectin	12 mg po		X			0.05-0.08		13-24 days			
Mefloquine	1.25 gm po	X				0.5-1.2	98				
Nitazoxanide	200 mg po	X				3	99				
Proguanil[13]											
Pyrimethamine	25 mg po	X			"High"	0.1-0.3	75	96			
Praziquantel	20 mg per kg po	X			80	0.2-2.0	87	0.8-1.5			
Tinidazole	2 gm po	X			48	13	12	13	Chemically similar to metronidazole		
ANTIVIRAL DRUGS—NOT HIV											
Acyclovir	400 mg po	X		X	10-20	1.21	9-33	2.5-3.5			
Adefovir	10 mg po			X	59	0.02	≤4	7.5			
Entecavir	0.5 mg po		X		100	4.2 ng/mL	13	128-149			
Famciclovir	500 mg po			X	77	3-4	<20	2-3			
Foscarnet	60 mg per kg IV					155		4		<1	No
Ganciclovir	5 mg per kg IV			X		8.3	1-2	3.5			
Oseltamivir	75 mg po			X	75	0.065/3.5[14]	3	1-3			
Ribavirin	600 mg po			X	64	0.8		44			
Rimantadine	100 mg po			X		0.1-0.4		25			
Valacyclovir	1000 mg po			X	55	5.6	13-18				
Valganciclovir	900 mg po			X	59	5.6	1-2	4			

DRUG	DOSE, ROUTE OF ADMINISTRATION	FOR PO DOSING—Take Drug WITH FOOD	WITHOUT FOOD[4]	WITH OR WITHOUT FOOD	% AB[1]	PEAK SERUM LEVEL mcg per mL	PROTEIN BINDING, %	SERUM T½, HOURS[2]	INTRACELLULAR T½, HOURS[6]	CYTOCHROME P450
ANTI-HIV VIRAL DRUGS										
Abacavir	600 mg po			X	83	3.0	50	1.5	12-26	
Amprenavir	1200 mg po			X	No data	6-9	90	7-11		Inhibitor
Atazanavir	400 mg po	X			"Good"	2.3	86	7		
Darunavir	600 mg with 100 mg ritonavir	X			82		95	15		
Delavirdine	400 mg po			X	85	19 ± 11	98	5.8		Inhibitor
Didanosine	400 mg EC* po		X		30-40		<5	1.4	25-40	
Efavirenz	600 mg po		X		42	13 mcM[14]	99	52-76		Inducer/inhibitor
Emtricitabine	200 mg po			X	93	1.8	<4	10	39	

See page 79 for all footnotes; see page 2 for abbreviations

TABLE 9A (6)

DRUG	DOSE, ROUTE OF ADMINISTRATION	FOR PO DOSING—Take Drug/			% AB[1]	SERUM LEVEL mcg per mL[6]	PROTEIN BINDING, %	INTRACELLULAR T½, HOURS[5]	SERUM T½, HOURS[2,3]	CYTOCHROME P450
		WITH FOOD	WITHOUT FOOD[7]	WITH OR WITHOUT FOOD						
ANTI-HIV VIRAL DRUGS *(continued)*										
Enfuvirtide	90 mg sc				84	5	92		4	
Fosamprenavir	1400 mg po			X	No data	5	90	No data	7.7	Inducer/inhibitor
Indinavir	800 mg po		X		65	12.6 mcM[14]	60		1.2-2	Inhibitor
Lamivudine	300 mg po			X	86	2.6	<36	18-22	5-7	
Lopinavir	400 mg po	X			No data	9.6	98-99		5-6	Inhibitor
Nelfinavir	1250 mg po	X			20-80	3-4	98		3.5-5	Inhibitor
Nevirapine	200 mg po			X	>90	2	60		25-30	Inducer
Ritonavir	300 mg po	X			65	7.8	98-99		3-5	Potent inhibitor
Saquinavir	1000 mg po (with 100 mg ritonavir)	X			4	3.1	97		1-2	Inhibitor
Stavudine	40 mg po			X	86	1.4	<5	7.5	1	
Tenofovir	300 mg po	X			39	0.12	<1-7	>60	17	
Tipranavir	500 mg + 200 mg ritonavir	X				78-95 mcM[6]	99.9		5.5-6	
Zalcitabine	0.75 mg po			X	85	0.03	<4	Unknown	1.2	
Zidovudine	300 mg po			X	60	1-2	<38	>	0.5-3	

FOOTNOTES:

1. % absorbed under optimal conditions
2. Assumes CrCl >80 mL per min.
3. Peak concentration in bile/peak concentration in serum x 100. If blank, no data.
4. CSF levels with inflammation
5. Judgment based on drug dose & organ susceptibility. CSF concentration ideally ≥10 above MIC.
6. Total drug; adjust for protein binding to determine free drug concentration.
7. For adult oral preps; not applicable for peds suspensions.
8. Food decreases rate and/or extent of absorption.
9. Concern over seizure potential; see *Table 10*

10. Take all po FQs 2–4 hours before sucralfate or any multivalent cations: Ca^{++}, Fe^{++}, Zn^{++}.
11. Given with atovaquone as Malarone for malaria prophylaxis.
12. Oseltamivir/oseltamivir carboxylate
13. EC = enteric coated
14. mcM=micromolar

TABLE 9B – PHARMACODYNAMICS OF ANTIBACTERIALS*

BACTERIAL KILLING/PERSISTENT EFFECT	DRUGS	THERAPY GOAL	PK/PD MEASUREMENT
Concentration-dependent/Prolonged persistent effect	Aminoglycosides; daptomycin; ketolides; quinolones	High peak serum concentration	24-hr AUC/MIC
Time-dependent/No persistent effect	Penicillins; cephalosporins; carbapenems	Long duration of exposure	Time above MIC
Time-dependent/Moderate to long persistent effect	Clindamycin; erythromycin/clarithro; linezolid; tetracyclines; vancomycin	Enhanced amount of drug	24-hr AUC/MIC

1 **AUC** = area under drug concentration curve

* Adapted from Craig, WA. IDC No. Amer 17:479, 2003

See page 79 for all footnotes; see page 2 for abbreviations

TABLE 10A – SELECTED ANTIBACTERIAL AGENTS—ADVERSE REACTIONS—OVERVIEW

Adverse reactions in individual patients represent all-or-none occurrences, even if rare. After selection of an agent, the physician should read the manufacturer's package insert [statements in the product labeling (package insert) must be approved by the FDA].

Numbers = frequency of occurrence (%); + = occurs, incidence not available; ++ = significant adverse reaction; 0 = not reported; R = rare, defined as <1%. NOTE: Important reactions in bold print. A blank means no data found.

Column groups: **PENICILLINS, CARBAPENEMS, MONOBACTAMS, AMINOGLYCOSIDES** | **MISC.**
- Penicillinase-Resistant Anti-Staph Penicillins: Penicillin G,V; Dicloxacillin; Nafcillin; Oxacillin
- Aminopenicillins: Amoxicillin; Amox-Clav; Ampicillin; Amp-Sulb
- AP Pens: Piperacillin; Pip-Taz; Ticarcillin; Ticar-Clav
- Carbapenems: Ertapenem; Imipenem; Meropenem
- Monobactam: Aztreonam
- Aminoglycosides: Amikacin, Gentamicin, Kanamycin, Netilmicin[NUS], Tobramycin
- Misc.: Linezolid; Telithromycin

ADVERSE REACTIONS	Penicillin G,V	Dicloxacillin	Nafcillin	Oxacillin	Amoxicillin	Amox-Clav	Ampicillin	Amp-Sulb	Piperacillin	Pip-Taz	Ticarcillin	Ticar-Clav	Ertapenem	Imipenem	Meropenem	Aztreonam	Aminoglycosides	Linezolid	Telithromycin
Rx stopped due to AE					2–4.4			3	3.2	3.2	3		4	4	1.2	<1		3/1	7/2
Local, phlebitis	+		++										4	3	1	4			
Hypersensitivity																			
Fever	+		+	+	+	+	+	+	+		+		+	+	+	+			+
Rash	**3**		**4**	**4**	**5**	**3**	**5**	**2**	**1**	**4**	**3**	**2**	+	+	+	**2**	+	+	+
Photosensitivity	0		0	0	0	R	0	0	0	0	0	0							
Anaphylaxis	R		R	R	R	R	R	R	+	+	+	+	+	+	+	R	R		
Serum sickness	4					R													
Hematologic																			
+ Coombs	3		R	R	2	+	+		6		+		+	2	+	R			
Neutropenia	R	0	+	+	+	+	+	+	+	+	+	+	+	+	+	+			
Eosinophilia	R	+	**22**	**22**	2	+	2	**22**	**7**	**11**	**3**	+	+	+	8	8		1.1	
Thrombocytopenia	R	+	**22**	**22**	R	+	R	R	+	+	R	R	+	+	+	+			
↑ PT/PTT	R	0	R	0	0	0	R	0	+	+	+	+		R		R			
GI																			
Nausea/vomiting	3	+	0	0	**2**	**3**	**2**	**2**	**2**	**7**	+	**1**	**3**	**2**	**4**	+	+	**4**	**2**
Diarrhea	4	+	+	+	**5**	**9**	**5**	**10**	**2**	**11**	**3**	**1**	**6**	**2**	**5**	+	+		**10**
C. difficile colitis	R	0	0	0	R	R	R	R	0	0	0	0	+	+	4	2			+
Hepatic																			
Hepatic, LFTs	R	R	R	R	R	+	R	6	+	0	+	0	6	4	4	2		1.3	3–10 (see IOC)
Hepatic failure	0	0	0	0	0	0	0	0	0	0	0	0	+	+	+	0			+
Renal: ↑ BUN, Cr	R	R	R	R	R	R	R	R	R	R	R	R	R	R	R	R	**5–25**[1]		
CNS																			
Headache	R	R	R	R	0	0	R	R	+	8	R	R	2	+	+	3	+	2	2
Confusion	R	R	R	R	0	0	R	R	R	R	R	R	+	+	+			+	+
Seizures	R	R	R	R	0	0	R	R	R	R	R	R	See footnote[2]			+		+	

[1] Varies with criteria used

[2] **All β-lactams in high concentration can cause seizures** (JAC 45:5, 2000). In rabbit, IMP 10x more neurotoxic than benzylpenicillin (JAC 22:687, 1988). In clinical trial of IMP for ped meningitis, trial stopped due to seizures in 7/25 IMP recipients; hard to interpret as purulent meningitis causes seizures (PIDJ 10:122, 1991). Risk with IMP with careful attention to dosage (Epilepsia 42:1590, 2001).
Postulated mechanism: Drug binding to GABA₍A₎ receptor; IMP binds with greater affinity than MER.
Package insert, percent seizures: ERTA 0.5; IMP 0.4; MER 0.7. However, in 3 clinical trials of MER for bacterial meningitis, no drug-related seizures (Scand J Inf Dis 31:3, 1999; Drug Safety 22:191, 2000). In clinical trials of ERTA, seizures reported at 2% (CID 32:381, 2001; Peds Hem Onc 17:585, 2000). In febrile neutropenic cancer pts, IMP-related seizures reported at 2% (Peds Hem Onc 17:585, 2000).

TABLE 1:0A (2)

PENICILLINS, CARBAPENEMS, MONOBACTAMS, AMINOGLYCOSIDES

ADVERSE REACTIONS	Penicillin G,V	Dicloxacillin	Nafcillin	Oxacillin	Amoxicillin	Amox-Clav	Ampicillin	Amp-Sulb	Piperacillin	Pip-Taz	Ticarcillin	Ticar-Clav	Ertapenem	Imipenem	Meropenem	Aztreonam	Aminoglycosides (Amikacin, Gentamicin, Kanamycin, Netilmicin[NUS], Tobramycin)	Linezolid	Telithromycin
Special Senses																			
Ototoxicity	O	O	O	O	O	O	O	O	O	O	O	O		R		O	3-14[1]		
Vestibular	O	O	O	O	O	O	O	O	O	O	O	O		O		O	4-6[2]		
Cardiac																			
Dysrhythmias	R	O	O	O	O	O	O	O	O	O	O	O		O		O		+	+
Miscellaneous, Unique (table 10C)	+	+	+	+	+	+	+	+	O	O	O	O	+	+		+	+	+	++
Drug/drug interactions, common (table 22)	O	O	O	O	O	O	O	O	O	O	O	O	O	O		O	+	+	+

CEPHALOSPORINS/CEPHAMYCINS

ADVERSE REACTIONS	Cefazolin	Cefotetan	Cefoxitin	Cefuroxime	Cefotaxime	Ceftazidime	Ceftizoxime	Ceftriaxone	Cefepime	Cefpirome[NUS]	Cefaclor/Cef.ER[1]/Loracarb	Cefadroxil	Cefdinir	Cefixime	Cefpodoxime	Cefprozil	Ceftibuten	Cefditoren pivoxil	Cefuroxime axetil	Cephalexin
Rx stopped due to AE	3								1.5	1	1		3		2.7				2.2	
Local, phlebitis	3	R	R	2	5	1	2	2	1	3	2			2		2	2	2		
Hypersensitivity																				
Fever	5	1	+	2	+	R	4	2	+	+	1	+	R	1	R	+	1	1	R	
Rash	+	2	2	R	2	R	2	2	2	+	1	+	R	1	R	+	R	1	R	1
Photosensitivity	O	O	O		O	O	O	O												
Anaphylaxis	R	+	+	R	R	R	O	O			R									+
Serum sickness											<0.5* +									
Hematologic																				
+ Coombs	3	2	2	R	6	4	1	2	14	3	R		R	R	R	R	R	R	R	3
Neutropenia	+	2	+	R	+	+	+	2	1	1	+		R	R	R	R	R	R	R	3

[1] Cefaclor extended release tablets

[2] Serum sickness requires biotransformation of parent drug plus inherited defect in metabolism of reactive intermediates (Ped Pharm & Therap 125:805, 1994)

* See note at head of table, page 80

TABLE 10A (3)
CEPHALOSPORINS/CEPHAMYCINS

ADVERSE REACTIONS	Cefazolin	Cefotetan	Cefoxitin	Cefuroxime	Cefotaxime	Ceftazidime	Ceftizoxime	Ceftriaxone	Cefepime	Cefpirome[NUS]	Cefaclor/Cef.ER[1]/Loracarb	Cefadroxil	Cefdinir	Cefixime	Cefpodoxime	Cefprozil	Ceftibuten	Cefditoren pivoxil	Cefuroxime axetil	Cephalexin
Eosinophilia	+	+	3	7	1	8	4	6	1	1			R	R	3	3	5	R	1	9
Thrombocytopenia				R							2			R	R	2	2			
↑ PT/PTT	+	+ +	2		+	+	+	+	+	+										
GI																				
Nausea/vomiting			+	R	R	R	+	R			3	+	3	13	R	+	R	6/1	3	2
Diarrhea	+	4	3	4	1	1		3	1	+	1–4		15	7/16	4/7	4	6/2	1.4	4	+
C. difficile colitis	+	+	+		+	6		+	+	+	3	+	+			3	3		+	+
Hepatic. ↑ LFTs	0	1	3		1	4	0	3	+	+	+		1	+	+	+	+	R	2	+
Renal ↑ BUN, Cr	+	0	3	0	0	R	0	1	0	0		0	R	R	4	2	R	R		+
CNS																				
Headache	0					1		R	2		3		2	+	1	R	R	2	R	+
Confusion	0										+			4		R	R			+
Seizures	0																			
Special Senses																				
Ototoxicity	0	0	0		0	0	0	0			0	0	0	0	0	0	0	0	0	0
Vestibular	0	0	0		0	0	0	0			0	0	0	0	0	0	0	0	0	0
Cardiac																				
Dysrhythmias	0	0	0		0	0	0	0			0	0	0	0	0	0	0	+	0	0
Miscellaneous, Unique (Table 10C)							+	+			+[R]							+		
Drug/drug interactions, common (Table 22)	0	0	0		0	0	0	0			0	0	0	0	0	0	0	0	0	0

[1] Cefaclor extended release tablets
[2] Serum sickness requires biotransformation of parent drug plus inherited defect in metabolism of reactive intermediates (Ped Pharm & Therap. 125;805, 1994)
* See note at head of table, page 80

TABLE 10A (4)

ADVERSE REACTIONS (AE)	MACROLIDES			QUINOLONES						OTHER AGENTS											
	Azithromycin, Reg. & ER[1]	Clarithromycin, Reg. & ER[1]	Erythromycin	Ciprofloxacin/Cipro XR	Gatifloxacin^NUS	Gemifloxacin	Levofloxacin	Moxifloxacin	Ofloxacin	Chloramphenicol	Clindamycin	Colistimethate (Colistin)	Dalbavancin	Daptomycin	Metronidazole	Quinupristin-dalfopristin	Rifampin	Tetracycline/Doxy/Mino	Tigecycline	TMP-SMX	Vancomycin
Rx stopped due to AE	1	3		3.5	2.9	2.2	4	3.8	4					2.8					5	2	
Local phlebitis			++		5									6		++					13
Hypersensitivity																					
Fever										+	+						1	+			
Rash	R		+	R	R	1-22[a]	R	R	2	+	+		1.8	2		R	+	+	7	++	8
Photosensitivity	R		+	R	R	R	1.7	R	R	+	+		1.8	4			+	R	2.4	+	1
Anaphylaxis				R	R	R	R	R	R							R	+	+	+	+	3
Serum sickness										+	+										0
Hematologic																					
Neutropenia	R	1		R					1	+								R		+	R
Eosinophilia				R						+	+							+		+	
Thrombocytopenia	R	R								+	+				+			+		+	2
↑ PT/PTT	R					1.5													4		
GI																					
Nausea/vomiting	3	3[3]	25	5	8/<3	2.7	7/2	7/2	7	+	7		3/2	6.3	12		+		30/20	3	
Diarrhea	5	3-6	8	2	4	3.6	1.2	5	4		++		2.5	5	R	R	R	+	13	+	+
C. difficile colitis				R	R	1.5	+	2	2		+			+				+			+
Hepatic, LFTs	R	R	+	2	R	+	2.5	3	R	+	++		+	+		2	R	+	4	+	
Hepatic failure	0	0	+							+							+				0
Renal																					
↑ BUN, Cr				1							0	R		R							R
CNS																					
Dizziness, light headedness	+	4		R	3	0.8	2	3	3				2		++		+		2	+	5
Headache	R	2		1	4	5.4	+	2			+		5		+		+	+	3.5		
Confusion									R	+					+					+	
Seizures				+	2	+	+	R	2						+					+	

[1] Regular and extended-release formulations
[2] **Highest frequency**: females <40 years of age after 14 days of rx, with 5 days or less of Gemi; incidence of rash <1.5%
[3] Less GI upset/abnormal taste with ER formulation

* See note at head of table, page 80

TABLE 10A (5)

ADVERSE REACTIONS (AE)	MACROLIDES			QUINOLONES						OTHER AGENTS											
	Azithromycin, Reg. & ER[1]	Clarithromycin, Reg. & ER[1]	Erythromycin	Ciprofloxacin/Cipro XR	Gatifloxacin[NUS]	Gemifloxacin	Levofloxacin	Moxifloxacin	Ofloxacin	Chloramphenicol	Clindamycin	Colistimethate (Colistin)	Dalbavancin	Daptomycin	Metronidazole	Quinupristin-dalfopristin	Rifampin	Tetracycline/Doxy/Mino	Tigecycline	TMP-SMX	Vancomycin
Special senses Ototoxicity	+			O					O												R
Vestibular	+																	21[3]			
Cardiac Dysrhythmias	+	+	+	R	+[4]	+	+	+[4]	+[4]		R										O
Miscellaneous, Unique (*Table 10C*)	+		+	+	+	+	+	+	+	+	+	+	+	+	+	++	+	+	+	+	+
Drug/drug interactions, common (*Table 22*)	+	+	+	+	+	+	+	+	+						+	++	+	+	+	+	+

[3] Minocycline has 21% vestibular toxicity

[4] Fluoroquinolones as class assoc. **with QT₄ prolongation.** Ref.: *CID* 34:861, 2002.

TABLE 10B – ANTIMICROBIAL AGENTS ASSOCIATED WITH PHOTOSENSITIVITY

The following drugs are known to cause photosensitivity in some individuals. There is no intent to indicate relative frequency or severity of reactions.

Source: 2006 Drug Topics Red Book, Medical Economics, Montvale, NJ. Listed in alphabetical order:

Azithromycin, benznidazole, ciprofloxacin, dapsone, doxycycline, erythromycin ethyl succinate, flucytosine, ganciclovir, gatifloxacin, gemifloxacin, griseofulvin, interferons, lomefloxacin, ofloxacin, pyrazinamide, saquinavir, sulfonamides, tetracyclines, tigecycline, tretinoins, voriconazole

* See note at head of table, page 80

TABLE 10C – SUMMARY OF CURRENT ANTIBIOTIC DOSAGE*, SIDE-EFFECTS, AND COST

CLASS, AGENT, GENERIC NAME (TRADE NAME)	USUAL ADULT DOSAGE* (Cost†)	ADVERSE REACTIONS, COMMENTS (See Table 10A for Summary)
NATURAL PENICILLINS		
Benzathine penicillin G (Bicillin L-A)	600,000–1.2 million units IM q2–4 wks Cost: 600,000 units $26	**Most common adverse reactions are hypersensitivity.** Anaphylaxis in up to 0.05%, 5–10% fatal. Commercially available skin test antigen (penicilloyl polylysine) does not predict anaphylactic reactions. Rare anaphylactic
Penicillin G	Low: 600,000–1.2 million units IM per day High: >20 million units IV q24h(=12gm) Cost: 5 million units $42	(seizures) reactions usually seen with high dose (>20 million per day) and renal failure. With procaine pen G and benzathine pen G, an immediate but transient (<30min. after injection) toxic reactions can occur with bizarre behavior & neurologic
Penicillin V	0.25–0.5gm po bid, tid, qid before meals & at bedtime. Cost: 500 mg po $0.39	reactions can occur (Hoignes syndrome). Coombs test positive hemolytic anemias are rare but typically severe; in contrast, the Coombs test is often + with cephalosporin therapy, but clinically significant hemolysis is rare. Penicillin allergy ref.: *JAMA 278:1895, 1997*
PENICILLINASE-RESISTANT PENICILLINS		
Dicloxacillin (Dynapen)	0.125–0.5gm po q6h ac. Cost: 500mg G $0.20	Blood levels ~2 times greater than cloxacillin. Acute hemorrhagic cystitis reported. Acute abdominal pain with GI bleeding without antibiotic-associated colitis also reported.
Flucloxacillin^NUS^ (Floxapen, Lutropin, Staphcil)	0.25–0.5gm po q6h	In Australia, cholestatic hepatitis (women predominate, age >65, rx mean 2 weeks, onset 3 weeks from starting rx) (*Ln 339:679, 1992*), 16 deaths since 1980; recommendation use only in severe infection (*Ln 344:676, 1994*).
Nafcillin (Unipen, Nallpen)	1–2gm IV q4h. Cost: 2 gm IV $16.75	Extravasation can result in tissue necrosis. With dosages of 200–300 mg per day hypokalemia may occur.
Oxacillin (Prostaphlin)	1–2gm IV/IM q4h. Cost: 2 gm IV $20.11	**Reversible neutropenia (over 10% with ≥21-day rx, occasionally WBC <1000 per mm³).** **Hepatic dysfunction with ≥2 gm per day.** LFTs usually ↑ 2–24 days after start of rx, reversible. In children, more rash and liver toxicity with oxacillin as compared to nafcillin (*CID 34:50, 2002*)
AMINOPENICILLINS		
Amoxicillin (Amoxil, Polymox)	250mg–1gm po tid. Cost: 500 mg G $0.13, NB $0.55	IV available in UK, Europe. IV amoxicillin rapidly converted to ampicillin. Rash with infectious mono—see *Ampicillin*.
Amoxicillin-clavulanate (Augmentin)	See Comment (c: adult products/cost)	500–875 mg po bid listed in past, may be inadequate due to ↑ resistance. With bid regimen, less clavulanate & less diarrhea. Clavulanate assoc. with rare reversible cholestatic hepatitis, esp.
AM-CL extra-strength peds suspension (ES-600)	Peds ES susp.: 600/42.9 per 5mL. Dose: 90/6.4mg/kg/div bid. Cost: 100 mL $82	men >60 yrs, on rx >2 weeks (*AJM 156:1327, 1996*). 2 cases anaphylactoid to clavulanic acid (*J All Clin Immun 96:748, 1995*). **Comparison adult Augmentin product dosage regimens:**
AM-CL-ER—extended release adult tabs	For adult formulations, see Comments	Cost for 10 days rx: Augmentin 500/125 1 tab po tid $145 NB $97 G Augmentin 875/125 1 tab po bid $129 NB $137 G Augmentin-XR 1000/62.5 2 tabs po bid $132
Ampicillin (Principen)	0.25–0.5gm po q6h. Cost: 500mg po G $0.30 150–200mg/kg IV/day. Cost: 1gm IV G $7.38	A maculopapular rash occurs (not urticarial), **not true penicillin allergy**, in 65–100% pts with infectious mono, 90% with chronic lymphocytic leukemia, and 15–20% with allopurinol therapy.
Ampicillin-subbactam (Unasyn)	1.5–3gm IV q6h. Cost: 3gm NB $16.40 (see Comment)	Supplied in vials: ampicillin 1 gm, subbactam 0.5 gm or amp 2 gm, subbactam 1 gm. Antibiotic is not active vs pseudomonas. Total daily dose subbactam ≤4 gm.
ANTIPSEUDOMONAL PENICILLINS		
	NOTE: Platelet dysfunction may occur with any of the antipseudomonal penicillins, esp. in renal failure patients.	
Piperacillin (Pipracil) (Canada only)	IV: 3gm IV q4–6h (200–300 mg per kg per day up to 24gm per day). **For urinary tract infection: 2 gm IV q6h.** Cost: 3 gm NB $12.52	1.85 mEq Na⁺ per gm
ANTIPSEUDOMONAL PENICILLINS		
Piperacillin-tazobactam (Zosyn)	3.375gm IV q6h. Cost: 3.375gm NB $18 4.5gm q8h available For P. aeruginosa: 4.5gm IV q6h + tobra	Supplied as: piperacillin 3 gm + tazobactam 0.375 gm. TZ similar to clavulanate, more active than subbactam as β-lactamase inhibitor. Has ↑ activity over pip alone vs gram-negatives and anaerobes. PIP-TZ 3.375 gm q6h monotherapy **not adequate for serious pseudomonas infections. For empiric or specific treatment of P. aeruginosa use 4.5gm IV q6h + tobramycin.** Rx longer than 10 d. may ↑ risk of neutropenia (*CID 37:1568, 2003*). Piperacillin can cause false-pos. test for galactomannan—α test for invasive aspergillosis.

* NOTE: all dosage recommendations are for adults (unless otherwise indicated) & assume normal renal function.

* Cost = average wholesale price from 2006 DRUG TOPICS RED BOOK, Medical Economics
† (See page 2 for abbreviations)

TABLE 10C (2)

CLASS, AGENT, GENERIC NAME (TRADE NAME)	USUAL ADULT DOSAGE* (Cost†)	ADVERSE REACTIONS, COMMENTS (See Table 10A for Summary)
ANTIPSEUDOMONAL PENICILLINS (continued)		
Ticarcillin disodium (Ticar)	3gm IV q4-6h. Cost: 3.0 gm NB $12.38	Coagulation abnormalities common with large doses, interferes with platelet function, ↑ bleeding times; may be clinically significant in pts with renal failure. (4.5 mEq Na⁺ per gm).
Ticarcillin-clavulanate (Timentin)	3.1gm IV q4-6h. Cost: 3.1 gm NB $16	Supplied as 3gm ticarcillin + 0.1 gm clavulanate (0.1 gm/vial. 4.5-5 mEq Na⁺ per gm. Diarrhea due to clavulanate. Rare reversible cholestatic hepatitis secondary to clavulanate (AnIM 156:1327, 1986).
CARBAPENEMS. NOTE: In pts with pen allergy, 11% had allergic reaction after imipenem or meropenem (CID 38:1102, 2004); 9% in a 2nd study (JAC 54:1155, 2004); and 0% in a 3rd study (NEJM 354:23835, 2006).		
Ertapenem (Invanz)	1gm IV/IM q24h. Cost: 1gm $56.50	Lidocaine diluent for IM use; ask about lidocaine allergy. Standard dosage may be inadequate in obesity (BMI >40) (AAC 50:1222, 2006).
imipenem + cilastatin (Primaxin)	0.5gm IV q6h. for P. aeruginosa. 1gm q6-8h (see Comment). Cost: 500mg NB $33	For moderate or severe infection due to P. aeruginosa, dosage can be increased to 3 or 4 gm per day div. q6h or q8h. Pharmacokinetic studies suggest that continuous infusion of carbapenems may be more efficacious & safer (J Clin Pharm 43:1116, 2003; AAC 49:1881, 2005). For seizure comment, see footnote, Table 10A, page 80.
Meropenem (Merrem)	0.5-1gm IV q8h. Up to 2gm IV q8h for meningitis. Cost: 1gm NB $65.52	For seizure incidence comment, see Table 10A, page 80. Comments. Does not require a dehydropeptidase inhibitor (cilastatin). Activity vs aerobic gm-neg., slightly ↑ over IMP, activity vs staph & strep slightly ↓, anaerobes → to meropenem. B. distasonis more resistant to meropenem.
MONOBACTAMS		
Aztreonam (Azactam)	1gm q8h-2gm IV q6h. Cost: 1gm NB $27	Can be used in pts with allergy to penicillins/cephalosporins. Animal data and a letter raise concern about cross-reactivity with ceftazidime (Rev Inf Dis 7:613, 1985); side-chains of aztreonam and ceftazidime are identical
CEPHALOSPORINS (1st parenteral, then oral drugs).	NOTE: Prospective data demonstrate correlation between use of cephalosporins (esp. 3rd generation) and ↑ risk of C. difficile toxin-induced diarrhea. May also ↑ risk of colonization with vancomycin-resistant enterococci. For cross-allergenicity, see Oral, on page 87.	
1st Generation, Parenteral		
Cefazolin (Ancef, Kefzol)	0.25gm q8h-1.5gm IV/IM q6h. Cost: 1gm G $1.74	Do not give into lateral ventricles—seizures!
2nd Generation Parenteral		
Cefotetan (Cefotan)	1-3gm IV/IM q12h. (Max. dose not >6gm q24h). Cost: 1gm NB $16.72	Increasing resistance of B. fragilis, Prevotella bivivus, Prevotella disiens (most common in pelvic infections). Ref.: CID 35 (Suppl 1):S126, 2002. Methyltetrazole (MTT) side-chain can inhibit vitamin K activation.
Cefoxitin (Mefoxin)	1gm q6h-2gm IV/IM q4h. Cost: 1gm G $11.23, NB $15.29	In vitro may induce β-lactamase, esp. in Enterobacter sp.
Cefuroxime (Kefurox, Ceftin, Zinacef)	0.75-1.5gm IV/IM q8h. Cost: 1.5gm IV G $13.46	More stable vs staphylococcal β-lactamase than cefazolin.
3rd Generation, Parenteral		
Cefoperazone-sulbactam (Sulperazon)	Usual dose 1-2gm IV q12h; if severe infection should use 2-3gm IV q6h	Use of P Ceph 3 drugs correlates with incidence of C. difficile toxin diarrhea, perhaps due to no cephalosporin resistance of C. difficile (CID 38:646, 2004). Cefoperazone used to treat intra-abdominal, biliary, & gyn. infections. Other uses due to broad spectrum of activity. Possible clotting problem due to side-chain. For dose logic: JAC 15:156, 1985
Cefotaxime (Claforan)	1gm q8-12h to 2gm IV q4h. Cost: 2gm G $18, NB $25.38	Maximum daily dose: 12 gm.
Ceftazidime (Fortaz, Tazicef)	1gm q8-12h. Cost: 2gm NB $21-28.93	Excessive use may result in ↑ incidence of cephalosporin resistance and/or selection of vancomycin-resistant E. faecium. Ceftaz is susceptible to extended-spectrum cephalosporinases (CID 27:76 & 81, 1998). Maximum daily dose: 12 gm.
Ceftizoxime (Cefizox)	1-2gm IV/IM q8-12h. Cost: 2gm NB $24.64	Maximum daily dose: 12 gm.

---

* NOTE: all dosage recommendations are for adults (unless otherwise indicated) & assume normal renal function.
† Cost = average wholesale price from 2006 Drug Topics Red Book, Medical Economics
(See page 2 for abbreviations)

TABLE 10C (3)

CLASS, AGENT, GENERIC NAME (TRADE NAME)	USUAL ADULT DOSAGE* (Cost†)	ADVERSE REACTIONS, COMMENTS (See Table 10A for Summary)
CEPHALOSPORINS/3rd Generation, Parenteral *(continued)*		
Ceftriaxone (Rocephin)	Commonly used IV dosage in adults: < Age 65: 2gm once daily > Age 65: 1gm once daily Purulent meningitis: 2gm q12h. Can give IM in 1% lidocaine. Cost: 1gm NB $51.16, G $21	Dosage: 2 gm IV q12h gives higher tissue levels than 1 gm q12h (overcomes protein binding) (see footnote†) "Pseudocholelithiasis"² to sludge in gallbladder by ultrasound (50%), symptomatic (9%) (NEJM 322:1821, 1990). More likely with 2 gm per day with pt on total parenteral nutrition and not eating (AnIM 115:712, 1991). Clinical significance still unclear but has led to cholecystectomy (JID 17:356, 1995) and gallstone pancreatitis (Ln 17:662, 1998).
4th Generation, Parenteral		
Cefepime (Maxipime)	1-2gm IV q12h. Cost: 2gm NB $36.59	Active vs P. aeruginosa and many strains of Enterobacter, serratia. C. freundii resistant to ceftazidime, cefotaxime, aztreonam (CID 20:56, 1995). More active vs S. aureus than 3rd generation cephalosporins.
Cefpirome^ab,^FnR^810	1-2gm IV q12h	Similar to cefepime; ³⁄₄ activity vs enterobacteriaceae, P. aeruginosa, Gn + organisms. Anaerobes: less active than cefoxitin, more active than cefotax or ceftaz.
		Cross-Allergenicity: Patients with a history of IgE-mediated allergic reactions to a penicillin (e.g., anaphylaxis, angioneurotic edema, immediate urticaria) should not receive a cephalosporin. If the history is a 'measles-like' rash to a penicillin, available data suggest a 5–10% risk of rash in such patients; there is no enhanced risk of anaphylaxis. Cephalosporin skin tests, if available, predictive of reaction (AnIM 141:16, 2004). Any of the cephalosporins can result in **C. difficile toxin-mediated diarrhea/enterocolitis.** The reported frequency of nausea/vomiting and non-C. difficile toxin diarrhea is summarized in Table 10A. **Cefaclor:** Serum sickness-like reaction 0.1–0.5%—arthralgia, rash, erythema multiforme but no adenopathy, proteinuria or demonstrable immune complexes. Anecdotal reports of similar reaction to loracarbef. Appear due to mixture of drug biotransformation and genetic susceptibility (Ped Pharm & Thera 125:805, 1994). **Cefdinir:** Drug-iron complex causes red stools in roughly 1% of pts. **Cefditoren pivoxil:** Hydrolysis yields pivalate. Pivalate absorbed (70%) & becomes pivaloylcarnitine which is renally excreted; 39–63% ↓ in serum carnitine concentrations. Carnitine involved in fatty acid (FA) metabolism & FA transport into mitochondria. Effect transient & reversible. No clinical events documented to date (Med Lett 44:5, 2002). Also contains caseinate (milk protein); **avoid if milk allergy** (not same as lactose intolerance). Need gastric acid for optimal absorption. **Cefpodoxime:** There are rare reports of acute liver injury, bloody diarrhea, pulmonary infiltrates with eosinophilia. **Cefdinir:** Now available from Lupin Pharmaceuticals. **Cephalexin:** Can cause false-neg urine dipstick test for leukocytes.
Oral Cephalosporins **1st Generation, Oral**		
Cefadroxil (Duricef)	0.5-1gm po q12h. Cost: 0.5gm G $2.48, NB $5.38	
Cephalexin (Keflex, Keftab, generic)	0.25-0.5gm pc q6h. Cost: 0.5gm G $0.44, NB $3.45	
2nd Generation, Oral		
Cefaclor (Ceclor)	0.25-0.5 gm po q8h. Cost: 0.25 gm G $1.08, NB $2.40	
Cefaclor-ER (Ceclor)	0.375-0.5 gm po q12h. Cost: 0.5 gm $3.50	
Cefprozil (Cefzil)	0.25-0.5 gm po q12h. Cost: 0.5 gm NB $9.64	
Cefuroxime axetil po (Ceftin)	0.125-0.5 gm po q12h. Cost: 0.5 gm NB $12.85	
3rd Generation, Oral		
Loracarbef [Lorabid]	0.4 gm po q12h. Cost: 0.4 gm NB $6.37	
Cefdinir (Omnicef)	300 mg po q 2h or 600 mg q24h. Cost: 300 mg $4.75	
Cefditoren pivoxil (Spectracef)	200–400 mg po bid. Cost: 200 mg $2.08	
Cefixime [Suprax]	0.4 gm po q12-24h. Cost: 0.4 gm NB $10.26	
Cefpodoxime proxetil (Vantin)	0.1-0.2 gm po q12h. Cost: 0.2 gm G $4.44, NB $1.22	
Ceftibuten (Cedax)	0.4 gm po q24h. Cost: 0.4 gm NB $9.10	

¹ The age-related dosing of ceftriaxone is based on unpublished pharmacokinetic data that show an age-related reduction in hepatic clearance of ceftriaxone; hence, there is possible underdosing in younger pts, therefore the suggested 2 gm per day dose.

* NOTE: all dosage recommendations are for adults (unless otherwise indicated) & assume normal renal function.

§ Cost = average wholesale price from 2006 Drug Topics Red Book, Medical Economics
(See page 2 for abbreviations)

TABLE 10C (4)

CLASS, AGENT, GENERIC NAME (TRADE NAME)	USUAL ADULT DOSAGE* (Cost†)	ADVERSE REACTIONS, COMMENTS (See Table 10A for Summary)
AMINOGLYCOSIDES and RELATED ANTIBIOTICS—See Table 10D, page 93, and Table 17A, page 169		
GLYCOPEPTIDES		
Dalbavancin (Zeven)	1gm IV, then 0.5gm IV on day 8. No cost data.	Semi-synthetic lipoglycopeptide with very long serum half-life. So far, 2 published clinical trials (CID 40:374, 2005 & 37:1298, 2003). No serious AEs.
Teicoplanin† (Targocid)	**For septic arthritis—maintenance dose** 12mg/kg per day; S. aureus endocarditis— trough serum levels >20mcg/mL required (12mg/kg) iq12h times 3 loading dose, then 12mg/kg q24h)	Hypersensitivity: fever (at 3mg/kg 2.2%, at 24 mg per kg 8.2%), skin reactions 2.4%. Marked ↓ platelets (high dose ≥15 mg per kg per day). Red neck syndrome less common than with vancomycin.
Vancomycin (Vancocin)	**Normal weight pt:** 15mg/kg IV q12h (if critically ill load with 25mg/kg) at 500 mg/hr IV. **Morbidly obese (90% over ideal body weight):** 30mg/kg per day divided q8h (Eur J Clin Pharm 54:621, 1998). **For intrathecal—see comment P.O. for C. diff colitis:** 125mg po q6h Cost: 1gm IV iq6 $6.70, NB $34.50; 125mg po $16.15	Measure serum levels if: planned dose ≥2gm per day, rapidly changing renal function, or on hemodialysis Target levels: peak 20-50mcg/mL, trough 5-10mcg/mL. Rapid infusion (over <1hr) can cause non-specific histamine release manifest as angioneurotic edema, flushed skin ("red neck syndrome"), or hypotension. Can continue vanco but ↓ rate of infusion over 1-2hrs. **Ototoxicity & nephrotoxicity now rare** unless vanco given with an aminoglycoside; aminoglycoside amplifies the risk of nephrotoxicity. Neutropenia, rash occur. Rarely assoc with linear IgA bullous dermatosis (CID 38:442, 2004). **Intrathecal vanco:** not used for meningitis &/or ventriculitis/shunt infections. **Initial** dosing ranges from 5-10mcg/day (infants) to 10-20mcg/day (children/adults) adjusted to achieve trough CSF conc: of 10-20mcg/mL (AnPharmacotherapy 27:912, 1993)
CHLORAMPHENICOL, CLINDAMYCIN(S), ERYTHROMYCIN GROUP, KETOLIDES, OXAZOLIDINONES, QUINUPRISTIN-DALFOPRISTIN (SYNERCID)		
Chloramphenicol (Chloromycetin)	0.25–1 gm po/IV q6h. Max. of 4 gm per day Cost: 1 gm IV $22.75; po $6.60	No oral drug distrib in U.S. Hematologic: (↓ RBC, aplastic anemia 1:21,600 courses). Gray baby syndrome in premature infants, anaphylactoid reactions, optic atrophy or neuropathy (very rare), digital paresthesias, minor disulfiram-like reactions.
Clindamycin (Cleocin)	0.15–0.45 gm po q6h. 600–900 mg IV/IM q8h Cost: 300 mg po NB $5.71, G ⎍ (Lincomycin) $4.64 600 mg IV NB $11.15, G $4.13	Based on number of exposed pts, these drugs are the most frequent cause of C. difficile toxin-mediated diarrhea. In most severe form can cause pseudomembranous colitis/toxic megacolon.
Lincomycin (Lincocin)	0.6 gm IV/IM q8h. Cost: 600 mg IV $10.51	
Erythromycin Group (Review drug interactions before use)		Motilin is gastric hormone that activates duodenal/jejunal receptors to initiate peristalsis. Erythro (E) and E esters, both po and IV, activate motilin receptors and cause uncoordinated peristalsis with resultant anorexia, nausea or vomiting (Gut 38:397, 1992). Less binding and GI distress with azithromycin/clarithromycin. Systemic erythro in 1st 2 wks of life associated with infantile hypertrophic pyloric stenosis (J Ped 139:380, 2001). **Frequent drug/drug interactions**, see Table 22, page 164. Major concern is prolonged QT interval on EKG. **Prolonged QTc/**QT: Mutations in 6 genes (LQT 1-6) produce abnormal cardiac K+/Na+ channels. Variable penetrance: no symptoms, repeated syncope, to sudden death. **↑ risk if female & QTc >500 msec! Risk amplified by drugs** (macrolides, antiarrhythmics, & drug-drug interactions (see FQs page 90 for list)). Can result in torsades de pointes (ventricular tachycardia) and/or cardiac arrest. Refs: NEJM 348:1837 & 1866, 2003; 351:1053 & 1089, 2004; www.qtdrugs.org. Cholestatic hepatitis in approx 1:1000 adults (children) given E estolate. Transient reversible tinnitus or deafness with 24 gm per day of E or erythro IV in pts with renal or hepatic impairment. Reported with ≥600 mg per day of azithro (AJM 89:76, 1997). Dosages of oral erythro preparations expressed as base equivalents. With differences in absorption/biotransformation, variable amounts of erythro esters required to achieve same free erythro serum level, e.g., 400 mg E ethyl succinate = 250 mg E base. Dirithromycin available as 1/day macrolide. **Very low serum levels; do not use if potential for bacteremic disease.**
Azithromycin (Zithromax) Azithromycin ER (ZMax)	0.5 gm po q24h times 3 Tabs: 250 & 600mg. Peds suspension: 100 & 200mg per 5mL. Adult ER suspension: 2gm Dose varies with indication, see Table 1. Acute otitis media (page 10), acute exac. chronic bronchitis (page 32). Comm.-acq. pneumonia (pages 34–36) & sinusitis (page 44). Cost: 250 mg IV: 0.5gm per day. Cost: $32	
Base and esters (Erythro, Ilosone) V name: E. lactobionate	0.25gm q6h–0.5 gm po/IV q6h: 15–20mg/kg up to 4gm q24h. Infuse over 30+ min. Cost: po 250mg base G $0.18, stearate $0.19, estolate $0.31, ESS 400 $0.23, IV/gm NB $15.29	
Clarithromycin (Biaxin) or clarithromycin extended release (Biaxin XL)	Extended release: Two 0.5 gm tabs po per day Cost: 500 mg ER $3.34; 500mg G $4.50	
Dirithromycin (Dynabac)	0.5 gm po q24h Cost: 250 mg $4.25	

* NOTE: all dosage recommendations are for adults (unless otherwise indicated) & assume normal renal function.
† Cost = average wholesale price from 2006 Drug Topics Red Book, Medical Economics
(See page 2 for abbreviations)

TABLE 10C (5)

CLASS, AGENT, GENERIC NAME (TRADE NAME)	USUAL ADULT DOSAGE* (Cost)	ADVERSE REACTIONS, COMMENTS (See Table 10A for Summary)
CHLORAMPHENICOL, CLINDAMYCIN), ERYTHROMYCIN GROUP, KETOLIDES, OXAZOLIDINONES, QUINUPRISTIN-DALFOPRISTIN (continued)		
Ketolide		
Telithromycin (Ketek) (Med Lett 46:66, 2004)	**Two 400 mg tabs po q24h.** Cost: 400 mg $5.76 300 mg tabs available	As of 9/06, 2 cases acute liver failure & 23 cases serious liver injury reported, or 23 cases per 10 million prescriptions. Occurred during or immediately after treatment. (AnIM 144:415, 447, 2006). **Uncommon: blurred vision 2°** slow accommodation, may cause exacerbation of **myasthenia gravis (Black Box Warning)**. Potential QT_c prolongation. Several **drug-drug interactions** (Table 22, pages 184–188) (NEJM 355:2260, 2006).
Oxazolidinones		
Linezolid (Zyvox)	**PO or IV dose: 600 mg q12h all indications except 400 mg q12h for uncomplicated skin infections.** Available as 400 & 600 mg tabs, oral suspension (100 mg per 5 mL), & IV solution. 600 mg po $65; 600 mg IV $82.	**Reversible myelosuppression:** thrombocytopenia, anemia, & neutropenia reported. Most often after ≥2 wks of therapy. Incidence of thrombocytopenia after 2 wks of rx: 7/20 osteomyelitic pts; 5/7 pts treated with vanco & then linezolid. Refs. CID 37:1609, 2003 & 38:1058 & 1065, 2004. 6-fold increased risk in pts with ESRD (CID 42:66, 2006). **Lactic acidosis:** inhibition of intramitochondrial protein synthesis (CID 42:1111, 2006; AAC 50:2042, 2006) and dose-dependent inhibition of mitochondrial function. Risk of severe hypertension if taken with foods rich in tyramine. Avoid concomitant **Inhibitor of monoamine oxidase**: risk of severe hypertension if taken with foods rich in tyramine. Avoid concomitant pseudoephedrine, phenylpropanolamine, and caution with SSRIs. **Serotonin syndrome** (fever, agitation, mental status changes, tremors, etc.) none with central venous line. **Serotonin syndrome** with concomitant SSRIs: (CID 42:1578 and 43:180, 2006)
Quinupristin + dalfopristin (Synercid) (CID 36:473, 2003)	**7.5 mg per kg IV q8h via central line** Cost: 350 mg–150 mg $138	Venous irritation (5%); none with central venous line. Asymptomatic ↑ in unconjugated bilirubin. **Arthralgia** 2%–50% arthralgias, many more—see Table 22. **Drug-drug interactions:** Cyclosporine, nifedipine, midazolam, many more—see Table 22. (CID 36:476, 2003)
TETRACYCLINES (Mayo Clin Proc 74:727, 1999)		
Doxycycline (Vibramycin, Doryx, Monodox, Adoxa)	**0.1 gm po/IV q12h.** Cost: 100 mg po G $0.08–0.11, NB $5.40; 100 mg IV NB $14.75	Similar to other tetracyclines. ↑ nausea on empty stomach. Erosive esophagitis, esp. if taken at bedtime. Phototoxicity + but less than with tetracycline. Deposition in teeth less. Can be used in patients with renal failure. **Comments:** Effective in treatment and prophylaxis for malaria, leptospirosis, typhus fevers.
Minocycline (Minocin, Dynacin)	**0.1 gm po q12h.** Cost: 100 mg po G $2.73, NB $4.02	Similar to other tetracyclines. **Vestibular symptoms** (30–90% in some groups, none in others): vertigo 33%, ataxia 43%, nausea 50%, vomiting 3%, women more frequently than men. Hypersensitivity pneumonitis, reversible, −34 cases reported (BMJ 310:1520, 1995).
Tetracycline, Oxytetracycline (Sumycin) (CID 36:462, 2003)	**0.25–0.5 gm po q6h, 0.5–1 gm IV q12h.** Cost: 250 mg po $0.06	Similar to other tetracyclines vs staph and in prophylaxis of meningococcal disease. P. acnes: many resistant to other tetracyclines, not to minocycline. Active vs some M. chelonei, M. marinum. **GI** (nausea, vomiting, diarrhea). Allergic reactions (rare), deposition in teeth, negative N balance, hepatotoxicity, enamel hypoplasia, pseudotumor cerebri/encephalopathy. Outdated drug: Fanconi syndrome. **Contraindicated in pregnancy, hepatotoxicity in mother, transplacental to fetus.** Comments: IV dosage over 2.0 gm per day may be associated with fatal hepatotoxicity. False-neg, urine dipstick for leukocytes.
Tigecycline (Tygacil)	**100 mg IV initially, then 50 mg IV q12h** If severe liver dis. (Child Pugh C): 100 mg IV initially, then 25 mg IV q12h. Cost: 50 mg $54.28	Derivative of tetracycline. High incidence of nausea (25%) & vomiting (20%) but only 1% of pts discontinued therapy due to an adverse event. Pregnancy Category D. Do not use in children under age 18. Like other tetracyclines, may cause photosensitivity, pseudotumor cerebri, pancreatitis, & a catabolic state (elevated BUN).

SSRI = selective serotonin reuptake inhibitors, e.g. fluoxetine (Prozac).

* **NOTE:** all dosage recommendations are for adults unless otherwise indicated) & assume normal renal function.

‡ Cost = average wholesale price from 2006 Drug Topics Red Book, Medical Economics

(See page 2 for abbreviations)

TABLE 10C (6)

CLASS, AGENT, GENERIC NAME (TRADE NAME)	USUAL ADULT DOSAGE* (Cost*)	ADVERSE REACTIONS, COMMENTS (See Table 10A for Summary)
FLUOROQUINOLONES (FQs)	All can cause false-positive urine drug screen	for opiates (Pharmacother 26:435, 2006)
Ciprofloxacin (Cipro) and **Ciprofloxacin-extended release** (Cipro XR, Proquin XR)	**500-750 mg po bid. Urinary tract infection: 250 mg bid po or Cipro XR 500 mg q24h Parenteral** rx 200–400 mg q12h. Cost: 500 mg po G $15, NB $6.00, Cipro XR 500 mg XR 500 mg $8.32; Proquin XR 500 mg $10.30. **Cipro 400 mg IV** $30.00. **Ophthalmic solution** $47.30 for 5 ml	**All can cause false-positive urine drug screen for opiates** (Pharmacother 26:435, 2006) **Children:** No FQ approved for use under age 16 based on joint cartilage injury in immature animals. Articular SEs in children are at 2–3% (IJID 3:537, 2003). **CNS toxicity:** Poorly understood. Varies from mild (lightheadedness) to moderate (confusion) to severe (seizures). May be aggravated by NSAIDs. **Gemi skin rash:** Macular rash after 8–10 d. of rx. Incidence of rash with ≤5 d of therapy only 1.5%. Frequency highest in females: < age 40, treated 14 d. frequency 14.2%. In men, < age 40, frequency 7.7%. Mechanism unclear. Inclination to DC therapy.
Gatifloxacin (Tequin)⁵⁵ See comments	**200–400 mg IV/po q24h**. (See comment) [Ophthalmic solution (Zymar) $58 for 5 ml	**Hypoglycemia/hyperglycemia** Due to documented hypo and hyperglycemic reactions (NEJM 354:1352, 2006), US distribution of Gati in US ceased in 6/2006. Gati ophthalmic solution remains available.
Gemifloxacin (Factive)	**320 mg po q24h** Cost: 320 mg $19.80	**Opiate screen false-positive** FQs can cause false-positive urine assay for opiates (JAMA 286:3115, 2001; AnPharmacother 38:1525, 2004). **Photosensitivity:** See Table 10B, page 84
Levofloxacin (Levaquin)	**250–750 mg po/IV q24h** Cost: 750 mg po $22; 750 mg IV $58; ophthal solution (Quinix) $52 for 5 ml	**QT (corrected QT) interval prolongation:** ↑ QT, (>500msec or >60msec from baseline) is considered possible with any FQ. ↑ QT can lead to torsades de pointes and ventricular fibrillation. Risk low with current marketed drugs). Risk ↑ in women, ↓ K⁺, ↓ Mg⁺⁺, bradycardia. (Refs.: NEJM 348: 1837 & 1866, 2003). Major problem is ↑ risk with concomitant drugs.
Moxifloxacin (Avelox)	**400 mg po/IV q24h** Cost: 400 mg po $11, IV $42 Ophthalmic solution (Vigamox) $58 for 3 ml	**Avoid concomitant drugs with potential to prolong QTc:**
Ofloxacin (Floxin)	**200–400 mg po bid.** Cost: 400 mg po $120 200–400 mg IV bid. Ophthalmic solution (Ocuflox) $51 for 5 ml	

Avoid concomitant drugs with potential to prolong QTc:

Antiarrhythmics:	Anti-Infectives:	CNS Drugs	Misc.
Amiodarone	Clarithro	Fluoxetine	Salmeterol
Disopyramide	Erythro	Sertraline	Naratriptan
Dofetilide	Foscarnet	Tricyclics	Sumatriptan
Flecainide	Halofantrine	Venlafaxine	Dolasetron
Ibutilide	Pentamidine	Haloperidol	Droperidol
Mefloquine	**Anti-Hypertensives:**	Phenothiazines	Fosphenytoin
Procainamide	Bepridil	Pimozide	Indapamide
Quinidine	Isradipine	Quetiapine	Tamoxifen
Sotalol	Nicardipine	Ziprasidone	Tizanidine
		Risperidone	

Updates online: www.qtdrugs.org; www.torsades.org. ↑ risk with concomitant steroid or renal disease (CID 36:1404, 2003).

CLASS, AGENT, GENERIC NAME (TRADE NAME)	USUAL ADULT DOSAGE* (Cost*)	ADVERSE REACTIONS, COMMENTS
POLYMYXINS		
Polymyxin B (Poly-Rx)	15,000–25,000 units/kg/day divided q12h Cost:50mg/$11	Also used as/for: bladder irrigation, intrathecal, ophthalmic preps. Source: Bedford Labs, Bedford, OH. Differs from colistin by one amino acid. **Intrathecal** 10 mg/day and **intraventricular** 1.6 mg/day reported successful.
Colistin (=Polymyxin E) (IJID 6:589 2006) Don't confuse dose calc for the "base" vs the "salt"! 10,000 units = 1mg base 2.4 mg colistathimate sodium salt. In US, label refers to mgs of base. See AAC 50:2274 & 401, 2006	**Parenterals:** **In US: Colymycin-M** 2.5-5 mg/kg per day divided into 2-4 doses = 6.7-13.3 mg/kg per day (max 800 mg/day). Cost: colistimethate sodium (Coly-Mycin) [50mg] $17. **Enteral:** Colomycin ≤60 kg 50,000-75,000 IU/kg per day IV in 3 divided doses (=4-6mg/kg per day or ≥60kg: 1.2 mill IU IV tid	**Inhalation:** Colistimethate 80 mg bid with cystic fibrosis and other ± (CID 41:1754, 2005) **Combination therapy:** Few studies – 1) some reports of efficacy of colistin & rifampin vs A. baumannii and P. aeruginosa combining p.o cipro + nebulized aerosolized colistin for P. aeruginosa in cystic fibrosis pts, attempts at eradication of P. aeruginosa. **Topical & oral:** Colistin sulfate used. **Nephrotoxicity:** Reversible tubular necrosis. Exact frequency unclear **Neurotoxicity:** Reversible Paresthesias. Vertigo, facial paresthesia, abnormal vision, confusion, ataxia, & neuromuscular blockade → respiratory failure. Dose-dependent. In cystic fibrosis pts, 29% experienced paresthesia, ataxia or both.

NOTE: all dosage recommendations are for adults (unless otherwise indicated) & assume normal renal function.
* Cost = average wholesale price from 2006 Drug Topics Red Book, Medical Economics
(See page 2 for abbreviations)

TABLE 10C (7)

CLASS, AGENT, GENERIC NAME (TRADE NAME)	USUAL ADULT DOSAGE* (Cost)	ADVERSE REACTIONS, COMMENTS (See Table 10A for Summary)
MISCELLANEOUS AGENTS		
Daptomycin (Cubicin) (CID 38/994, 2004; NEJM 355:653 & 727, 2006)	**Skin/soft tissue:** 4 mg per kg IV q24h **Bacteremia/right-sided endocarditis:** 6 mg per kg IV q24h **Morbid obesity:** base dose on total body weight (J Clin Pharm 45:48, 2005) Cost: 500 mg $182.	**Potential muscle toxicity:** At 4 mg per kg per day, ↑ CPK in 2.8% dapto pts & 1.8% comparator-treated pts. Suggest weekly CPK. DC dapto if CPK exceeds 10x normal level or if symptoms of myopathy and CPK > 1000. Manufacturer suggests stopping statins during dapto tx). With selected reagents, can falsely prolong PT & INR (4/12/06 Dear Doctor letter). **NOTE:** Dapto well-tolerated in healthy volunteers at doses up to 12 mg/kg q24h x 14d (AAC 50:3245, 2006).
Fosfomycin (Monurol)	3 gm with water po times 1 dose. Cost $39.50	Diarrhea in 9% compared to 6% of pts given nitrofurantoin and 2.3% given TMP-SMX.
Fusidic acid[NUS] (Fucidin) (CID 42:394, 2006) available in Canada)	500 mg po/IV tid (Leo Laboratories, Denmark)	Mild GI; occ. skin rash, jaundice (17% with IV & po). (None in CSF; <1% in urine) CID 42:394, 2006)
Immune globulin IV therapy	Dosage, frequency vary with the indication At least 7 manufacturers. Cost for 10–12 gm ranges from $600–$1100.	Reported adverse effects range from 1–15%. Fever, headache, myalgia, N/V relate to rate of infusion, mild, & self-limited. **More serious:** anaphylactoid reactions, thromboemboli, aseptic meningitis, & renal injury in 6.7% (QJM 93:751, 2000).
Methenamine hippurate (Hiprex, Urex)	**1 gm po/h** Cost: 1 gm $1.23 1 gm = 480 mg methenamine	Nausea and vomiting, skin rash or dysuria. Overall ~3%. Methenamine requires (pH <5.5) urine to liberate formaldehyde. Useful in suppressive therapy after infecting organisms cleared; do not use for pyelonephritis. *Comment:* Do not force fluids; may dilute formaldehyde. Of no value in pts with chronic Foley. If urine pH >5.0, co-administer ascorbic acid (1–2 gm q4h) to acidify the urine; cranberry juice (1200–4000 mL per day) has been used, results ±.
Methenamine mandelate (Mandelamine)	1 gm po q6h (480 mg methenamine) Cost: 1 gm NB $0.29	
Metronidazole (Flagyl) Roe, Mayo Clin Proc 74:825, 1999	**Anaerobic infections:** usually IV, 7.5 mg per kg (500 mg) q6h (do not exceed 4 gm q24h). **With food/po, 7.5 mg per kg (500 mg q12h. If life-threatening, can use loading dose of IV 15 mg per kg.** Oral Cost: 500 mg Cost: 500 mg tab G $0.21, NB $4.56; 500 mg IV G $2.80, NB $2.75; 70 gm vaginal gel $78.54. Ext. release 750 mg po q24h	Can be given rectally (enema or suppository). In pts with **decompensated liver disease** (manifest by ↓↓ of ascites, encephalopathy, ↑ prothrombin time, ↓ serum albumin) ↑½ ordinary dose + by approx. ¾. **side-effects:** nausea, vomiting and serum trans-vaginal gel. **Neurol.:** headache, rare paresthesias or peripheral neuropathy, ataxia, seizures, aseptic meningitis; report of reversible metro-induced cerebellar lesions (NEJM 346:68, 2002). **Avoid alcohol during & 48 hrs after (disulfiram-like reaction).** Very dark urine (common but harmless). Skin: urticaria. Mutagenic in Ames test. Tumorigenic in animals (high dose over lifetime). No evidence of risk in man. No teratogenicity.
Mupirocin (Bactroban)	**5 gm crush or ointment 2%: Apply tid times 10 days.** 15 gm $31.48. **Nasal ointment 2%: apply bid times 5 days.** 22 gm NB $53.39; G $41.45	Skin cream: itch, burning, stinging 1–1.5%. Nasal: headache 9%, rhinitis 6%, respiratory congestion 5%.
Nitrofurantoin macrocrystals (Macrodantin, Furadantin)	**100 mg po q6h** Cost: 100 mg G $1.21, NB $2.44 Dose for long-term UTI suppression: 50–100 mg at bedtime	Absorption ↑ with meals. Increased activity in acid urine, much reduced at pH 8 or over. Not effective in endstage renal disease (JAC 33[Suppl. A]:121, 1994). Nausea and vomiting, hypersensitivity, peripheral neuropathy. Pulmonary reactions (with chronic rx) acute ARDS type, **chronic desquamative interstitial pneumonia with fibrosis**. Intrahepatic cholestasis & **hepatitis**. Hemolytic anemia in G6PD deficiency.
monohydrate/macrocrystals (Macrobid)	**100 mg po bid** Cost: 100 mg $2.44	**Contraindicated in renal failure.** Should not be used in infants <1 month of age.
Rifaximin (Xifaxan)	**200 mg tab po tid** times 3 days. Cost: 200 mg $3.78	Efficacy of Macrobid 100 mg bid = Macrodantin 50 mg qid. Adverse effects 5.6%, less nausea than with Macrodantin. For traveler's diarrhea. In general, adverse events equal to or less than placebo.

* NOTE: all dosage recommendations are for adults (unless otherwise indicated) & assume normal renal function.

* Cost = average wholesale price from 2006 Drug Topics Red Book, Medical Economics (See page 2 for abbreviations)

TABLE 10C (8)

CLASS, AGENT, GENERIC NAME (TRADE NAME)	USUAL ADULT DOSAGE* (Cost†)	ADVERSE REACTIONS, COMMENTS (See Table 10A for Summary)
Sulfonamides [e.g. sulfisoxazole (Gantrisin), sulfamethoxazole (Gantanol), (Truxazole)]	Dose varies with indications. Cost 500 mg: $0.09	**Short-acting are best:** high urine concentration and good solubility at acid pH. More active in alkaline urine. **Allergic reactions:** skin rash, drug fever, pruritus, photosensitization. Periarteritis nodosa & SLE. Stevens-Johnson syndrome, serum sickness syndrome, myocarditis. Neurotoxicity (psychosis, neuritis), hepatic toxicity. Blood dyscrasias, usually agranulocytosis. Crystalluria. Nausea & vomiting, headache, dizziness, lassitude, mental depression, acidosis, sulfhemoglobin. Hemolytic anemia in G6PD deficient & unstable hemoglobins (Hb Zurich). Do not use in newborn infants or in women near term, ↑ frequency of kernicterus (binds to albumin, blocking binding of bilirubin to albumin).
Tinidazole (Tindamax)	Tabs 250, 500 mg. **Dose for giardiasis: 2 gm po times 1 with food. Cost: 500 mg $18.24**	**Adverse reactions:** metallic taste 3.7%, nausea 3.2%, anorexia/vomiting 1.5%. All higher with multi-day dosing.
Trimethoprim (Trimpex, Proloprim, and others)	**100 mg po q12h or 200 mg po q24h.** Cost: 100 mg NB $0.90, G $0.15	Frequent side-effects are rash and pruritus. Rash in 3% pts at 100 mg bid; 6.7% at 200 mg q24h. Rare reports of photosensitivity, exfoliative dermatitis, Stevens-Johnson syndrome, toxic epidermal necrosis, and aseptic meningitis (CID 19:431, 1994). Check drug interaction with phenytoin. Increases serum K+ (see TMP-SMX Comments). TMP can ↑ homocysteine blood levels (Ln 352:1827, 1998).
Trimethoprim (TMP)-Sulfamethoxazole (SMX) (Bactrim, Septra, Sulfatrim, Cotrimoxazole) Single-strength (SS) is 80 TMP/400 SMX, double-strength (DS) 160 TMP/800 SMX. Ref.: AnM 163:402, 2003	**Standard po rx (UTI, otitis media): 1 DS tab bid. P. carinii: see Table 13, page 125. IV rx (base on TMP component): standard 8-10 mg per kg per day divided q6h, q8h, or q12h. For shigellosis: 2.5 mg per kg IV q6h.** Cost: 160/800 po G $1.15, NB $2; 160/800 IV $11.21 Peds susp. 200/800 mg: 100 ml $12.63	Adverse reactions in 10%: GI: nausea, vomiting, anorexia. Skin: Rash, urticaria, photosensitivity. More serious (1–10%): Stevens-Johnson syndrome & toxic epidermal necrolysis. Skin reactions may represent toxic metabolites of SMX rather than allergy (AnPharmacotherapy 32:381, 1998). Daily ascorbic acid 0.5–1.0 gm may promote detoxification (AIDS 36:1041, 2004). Rare hypoglycemia, esp AIDS pts. (LnID 6:178, 2006) TMP competes with creatinine for tubular secretion, serum creatinine can ↑; TMP also blocks distal renal tubule secretion of K+: ↑ serum K+ in 21% of pts (AnIM 124:316, 1996). TMP one etiology of aseptic meningitis (CID 19:431, 1994). TMP-SMX contains sulfites and may trigger asthma in sulfite-sensitive pts. Frequent drug cause of thrombocytopenia (AnIM 129:886, 1998). No cross allergenicity with other sulfonamide non-antibiotic drugs (NEJM 349:1628, 2003).

Rapid Oral TMP-SMX Desensitization:

Hour	Dose TMP/SMX (mg)	Hour	Dose TMP/SMX (mg)
0	0.004/0.02	3	4/20
1	0.04/0.2	4	40/200
2	0.4/2	5	160/180

Comment: Perform in hospital or clinic. Use oral suspension [40 mg TMP/ 200 mg SMX per 5 mL (tsp)]. Take 6 oz water after each dose. Corticosteroids, antihistamines NOT used. Refs.: CID 20:849, 1995; AIDS 5:311, 1991

---

* NOTE: all dosage recommendations are for adults (unless otherwise indicated) & assume normal renal function.
† Cost = average wholesale price from 2006 Drug Topics Red Book, Medical Economics
(See page 2 for abbreviations)

TABLE 10D – AMINOGLYCOSIDE ONCE-DAILY AND MULTIPLE DAILY DOSING REGIMENS
(See Table 17, page 169, if estimated creatinine clearance <90 mL per min.)

General: Dosage given as both once-daily (OD) and multiple daily dose (MDD) regimens.

Pertinent formulae: (1) Estimated creatinine clearance (CrCl): [140−age]/(ideal body weight in kg) = CrCl for men in ml per min; multiply answer times 0.85 for CrCl of women
(72)(serum creatinine) Alternative method to calculate CrCl; see NEJM 354:2473, 2006

(2) Ideal body weight (IBW)— Females: 45.5 kg + 2.3 kg per inch over 5 = weight in kg
Males: 50 kg + 2.3 kg per inch over 5 = weight in kg

(3) Obesity adjustment: use if actual body weight (ABW) is ≥30% above IBW. To calculate adj dosing weight in kg: IBW + 0.4(ABW−IBW) = adjusted weight

DRUG	MDD AND OD IV REGIMENS/ TARGETED PEAK (P) AND TROUGH (T) SERUM LEVELS	COST[1] Name Brand (NB), Generic (G)	COMMENTS For more data on once-daily dosing, see AJM 105:182, 1998, and Table 17, page 169
Gentamicin (Garamycin), **Tobramycin** (Nebcin)	MDD: 2 mg per kg load, then 1.7 mg per kg q8h - - - P: 4–10 mcg/ml, T: 1–2 mcg per ml - - - OD: 5.1 (if critically ill) mg per kg q24h - - - P: 16–24 mcg per ml, T: <1 mcg per ml - - -	Gentamicin: 80 mg $5.30 Tobramycin: 80 mg NB $7.28, G $4.20	**All aminoglycosides have potential to cause tubular necrosis and renal failure, deafness due to cochlear toxicity, vertigo due to damage to vestibular organs, and rarely neuromuscular blockade.** Risk minimal with oral (or topical) application due to small % absorption unless tissues altered by disease. Risk of nephrotoxicity ↑ with concomitant administration of cyclosporine, vancomycin, ampho B, radiocontrast Risk of nephrotoxicity ↓ by concomitant AP Pen and perhaps by once-daily dosing method (especially if baseline renal function normal).
Kanamycin (Kantrex), **Amikacin** (Amikin), Streptomycin	MDD: 7.5 mg per kg q12h - - - P: 15–30 mcg per ml, T: 5–10 mcg per ml - - - OD: 15 mg per kg q24h - - - P: 56–64 mcg per ml, T: <1 mcg per ml - - -	Kanamycin: 1 gm $13.12 Amikacin: 500 mg NB $34.26, G $7.80 Streptomycin: 1 gm $9.10	In general, same factors influence risk of ototoxicity. **NOTE: There is no known method to eliminate risk of aminoglycoside nephro/ototoxicity. Proper rx attempts to ↓ the % risk.**
Netilmicin[NUS]	MDD: 2 mg per kg q8h - - - P: 4–10 mcg per ml, T: 1–2 mcg per ml - - - OD: 6.5 mg per kg q24h - - - P: 22–30 mcg per ml, T: <1 mcg per ml - - -		The clinical trial data of OD aminoglycosides have been re- viewed extensively by meta-analysis (CID 24:816, 1997). **Serum levels:** Collect serum for a peak serum level (PSL) exactly 1 hr after the start of the infusion of the 3rd dose. In critically ill pts, it is reasonable to measure the PSL after the 1st dose as well as later doses as volume of distribution and renal function may change rapidly.
Isepamicin[NUS]	Only OD: Severe infections 15 mg per kg q24h, less severe 8 mg per kg q24h	2 gm NB $34.06	Other dosing methods and references: For once-daily 7 mg per kg per day of gentamicin—Hartford Hospital method, see AAC 39:650, 1995.
Spectinomycin (Trobicin)[NUS]	2 gm IM times 1 gonococcal infections	500 mg $1.24	
Neomycin—oral	Prophylaxis GI surgery[1]: 1 gm po times 3 with erythro, see Table 15B, page 160 For hepatic coma: 4–12 gm per day po		
Tobramycin—inhaled (Tobi). See Cystic fibrosis, Table 1, page 39. Adverse effects few: transient voice alteration (13%) and transient tinnitus (3%). Cost: 300 mg $72.00			
Paromomycin—oral. See Entamoeba and Cryptosporidia, Table 13, page 122. Cost: 250 mg $2.72			

---

[1] Estimated CrCl invalid if serum creatinine <0.6 mg per dL. Consultation suggested.
§ Cost = average wholesale price from 2006 DRUG TOPICS RED BOOK, Medical Economics.

TABLE 11A– TREATMENT OF FUNGAL, ACTINOMYCOTIC, AND NOCARDIAL INFECTIONS—ANTIMICROBIAL AGENTS OF CHOICE*
(See Table 11B for Amphotericin B Preparations and Adverse Effects)

TYPE OF INFECTION/ORGANISM/ SITE OF INFECTION	ANTIMICROBIAL AGENTS OF CHOICE		COMMENTS
	PRIMARY	ALTERNATIVE	
Actinomycosis (A. israelii most common, also A. naeslundii, A. viscosus, A. odontolyticus, A. meyeri, A. gerencseriae) Cervicofacial, pulmonary, abdominal, cerebral, & rarely pericarditis (IDCP 12:233, 2004) Classically abdominal actino presents as intraabdominal or pelvic mass with surgical draining tract (Dis Colon Rectum 48:575, 2005) yrs after surgery, may mimic cancer (World J Gastro 11:1722, 2005). Fine needle aspirate of cervicofacial actino estab dx in 15 pts in Spain (Med Oral Patol Oral Cir Bucal 9:467, 2004).	**Ampicillin** 50 mg/kg per day IV times 4-6wks, then 0.5gm **amoxicillin** po tid **OR Penicillin G** 10–20 mill units/day IV x 4-6 wks, then **penicillin V** 2-4gm/day po. Duration individualized, esp. with surgical debulking, but duration 3-6mo usually adequate for thoracic & abdominal & 3-6wks for cervicofacial (CID 38:444, 2004).	**Doxycycline** or **ceftriaxone** or **clindamycin** or **erythromycin**. **Chloramphenicol** 12.5–15mg/kg IV/po q6h has been recommended for CNS infection in pen-allergic pts.	Tuboovarian abscesses may complicate IUDs. Removal of IUD is primary rx. With abscesses, inflammatory mass or fistulae, surgery often required. While penicillin G and ampicillin IV have been effective, with home IV therapy, agents given q24h, e.g., ceftriaxone, are more practical (An Thor Surg 74:185, 2002).
Aspergillosis (A. fumigatus most common, also A. flavus and others)			
Allergic bronchopulmonary aspergillosis (ABPA) Semin Respir Crit Care Med 27:185, 2006 ABPA found in 1–2% of pts with asthma & 1–15% with cystic fibrosis (Chest 130:222,2006). (CID 37 (Suppl 3):37, 2003). Clinical manifestations: wheezing, pulmonary infiltrates, bronchiectasis & fibrosis. Airway colonization assoc. with ↑ blood eosinophils, ↑ serum IgE, and positive skin test.	Acute asthma attacks associated with ABPA. **Corticosteroids**	Rx of ABPA. **Itraconazole¹** 200mg po q24h times 16wks or longer (Allergy 60:1004, 2005)	In 2 PRCTs², itra ↓ number of exacerbations requiring corticosteroids (p <0.03). Improved immunological markers (eosinophilia in sputum & ↓ serum IgE levels), & in 1 study improved lung function & exercise tolerance (NEJM 342:756, 2000; Cochrane Database Syst Rev 3:CD001108, 2004).
Allergic fungal sinusitis: relapsing chronic sinusitis; nasal polyps without bony invasion, allergic rhinitis, eczema or allergic rhinitis; ↑ IgE levels and isolation of Aspergillus sp. or other dematiaceous sp. (Alternaria, Cladosporium, etc.)	Rx controversial: systemic cor- ticosteroids + surgical debride- ment (80% respond but 2/3 relapse) (Otolaryn Head Neck Surg 131:704, 2004)	For failures try **itra¹** 200 mg po bid times12 mos. (CID 31: 203, 2000). Flucon nasal spray benefited 12/6 pts (LInD 4:349, 2004).	In 1 report, fungal elements identified by histopathology in up to 93% of cases of "chronic sinusitis" & in a DBPCT in 24 pts, intranasal ampho was assoc. with a ↑ in mucosal thickening of 8.8% by CT scan vs ↑ of 2.5% in placebo (LInD 4:257, 2004). Controversial area.
Aspergilloma (fungus ball) (J Resp Dis 23:360, 2002)	Efficacy of antimicrobial agents not proven. **Itraconazole** (po) benefit reported sporadically (J Am Acad Derm 45:607, 1990).		Aspergillus may complicate pulmonary sequestration (Eur J Cardio Thor Surg 27:28, 2005). Parasinusal fungus balls respond to surgery;172 of 175 cases (Med Mycol 44:61, 2006)
Invasive, pulmonary (IPA) or extrapulmonary. (See COID 18:314, 2005, Am J Respir Crit Care Med 173:707, 2006). Good website doctorfungus.org Post-transplantation and post-chemotherapy in neutropenic pts (PMN <500 per mm³) but may also present in immunocompetent recovery (Mycopathologia 150:181, 2005). Most common pneumonia in (continued on next page)	**Voriconazole** 6mg/kg IV q12h on day 1; then either (4mg/kg IV q12h) or (200mg po) q12h for body weight 240kg; but 100mg po q12h for body weight <40kg **OR** Lipid-based ampho B (ABLC) may be as effective and less nephrotoxic than standard ampho B but much more expensive (see Dosage footnote below). Some authorities favor voriconazole over standard ampho B as initial rx (CID 32: 415, 2003).	For ABPA, **Itraconazole** B **but much more expensive** (see Dosage footnote below). Low doses of itraconazole itself may survive treatment and may progress to invasive infect (Eur J Haemato 73:50, 2004). 40% of salvage therapy for refractory infect survived with vori alone (Eur J Haematol 73:50, 2004). Uni survived with vori alone results in 11/20 pts with bone involvement (18 for salvage), follow-up avg of 3mo (CID) (continued on next page)	

¹ Oral solution preferred to tablets because of ↑ absorption (see Table 11B, page 96).

² **PRCTs** = Prospective randomized controlled trials

³ **Dosages: ABLC** 5mg/kg per day IV over 2 hrs, **ABCC** 3–4mg/kg per day IV given over 1hrs, **liposomal Ampho B** 3-5mg/kg per day (AWP).

* From 2006 Drug Topics Red Book, Medical Economics Data and Hospital Formulary Pricing Guide. **Price** is average wholesale price (AWP).
See page 2 for abbreviations. All dosage recommendations are for adults (unless otherwise indicated) and assume normal renal function

TABLE 11A (2)

TYPE OF INFECTION/ORGANISM/ SITE OF INFECTION	ANTIMICROBIAL AGENTS OF CHOICE		COMMENTS
	PRIMARY	ALTERNATIVE	
Aspergillosis (continued)			
(continued from previous page) transplant recipients. Usually a late (≥100 days) complication in allogeneic bone marrow & liver transplantation: median survival 36 days, but **overall mortality rates vary from 78–94%** *(CID 36:46, 2003)*. May complicate COPD when corticosteroids used *(Clin Micro Inf 12:e1)* *(CID 37:S265, 2003)*. **Typical x-ray/CT lung lesions** (halo sign, cavitation, or mycotic lung sequestration) have 90% positive predictive value for invasive pulmonary aspergillosis in pts with hematologic malignancies *(CID 31:859, 2000)*. An immunologic test that detects circulating galact-omannan is available for dx of invasive aspergillosis. A recent article reviews the strengths & weaknesses of the test *(CID 42:1417, 2006)*. **False-pos. tests consistently found in serum from pts receiving PIP-TZ & AM-CL** *(J Clin Micro 43:2548, 2005)*. Concomitant antifungal rx may also ↓ sensitivity *(CID 40:1762, 2005)*. (MiraVista: 1-866-647-2847). Graft vs host disease of GI tract also associated with positives without evidence of infection (personal experience)	*(continued from previous page)* **OR** **Some clinicians start with Voriconazole. If it fails to respond clinically in 7–10 days then switch to Lipid-based Ampho B** **Ampho B** (see footnote¹). Rapid increase to 1 mg/kg (1–1.25 mg/kg at near-max dose per day). Total dose of 2–2.5 gm inc by some but data to support this lacking. **OR** **Combination rx: Vori** *(in above dosages)* **+ caspo** *(dosage below)* are currently used as initial treatment in many bone marrow transplant units, esp. in pts receiving high doses of corticosteroids *(Abstracts in Heme & Onc 8:11, 2006)*. **Alternative: Caspofungin** 70 mg IV on day 1, then 50 mg IV q24h (reduce to 35 mg with moderate hepatic insufficiency). (Approved for salvage therapy of Aspergillosis) For all regimens: If response good may switch to oral Vori after 2–3 wks. (See on page 94) **(Micafungin, anidulafungin,** and **posaconazole** all have activity against Aspergillosis but have not yet been approved for that indication.)	*(continued from previous page)* *40:1141, 2005* & with subclude IPA &, chronic pulmonary Aspergillosis: 43 & *10% success. (Am J Med 119:527, 2006)*. **44% of 398 pts receiving ABLC cured/improved, 21% stabilized; most failed to respond to prior antifungal rx** *(CID 40:S392, 2005)*. **Ampho B overall success rate 34–42%** *(CID 32:358, 2001)* in pulmonary aspergillosis in pts >14 days. Success dependent on bone marrow engraftment. In early trans, 54% neutropenic leukemia, 33% bone marrow trans, 20% liver trans. *(CID 23:608, 1996)*. **A. terreus infec esp resist to ampho B: 83 cases, 73.4% mortality ampho B rx vs 55.8% vori rx (p<0.01) (CID 39:192, 2004). Use vori!** **Caspo:** Among 83 pts with IPA incl in primary (MITT) analysis, 37 (45%) had favorable response following salvage rx with caspo monotherapy. In pts receiving >7 days of caspo, response rate to monotherapy, 50% *(37/66)* responded favorably *(CID 39:1563, 2004)*. Response in compassionate use program 44% *(J Int 50:196, 2005)*. Minimal toxicity reported *(Transpl Int Dis 1:25, 2002)*. **Micafungin:** 57% clinical response in an open-label study of "deep-seated" infections *(ICAAC Abstract #669, 2004)*. **Posaconazole** showed 42% success in 107 pts with IPA vs 26% in 86 historical controls in "refractory IA" *(ICAAC abstract #669, 2004)* **Combo therapy:** To date no controlled trials, they are needed *(CID 39:803, 2004)*. No acting between triazoles *(vori & itra, posa)*, echinocandins (caspo, mica), & ampho B. Synergy demonstrated vs echinocandins in vitro, & animal models between triazoles & caspo. In retrospective eval of bone marrow trans pts with IPA who failed ampho B, vori + caspo superior to vori alone *(CID 39:797, 2004)*. Another study of 40 solid organ trans rx with vori & caspo compared with historical controls receiving Lipid-based Ampho B no overall survival benefit found but a subset analysis showed no. sig. benefit in combo in A fumigatus infections and in those with renal insufficiency *(Transplantation 81:320, 2006)*. **Is combo rx better that Vori alone? Don't know yet!**
Blastomycosis (Blastomyces dermatitidis) Cutaneous, pulmonary or extrapulmonary. Outbreaks with humans & dogs reported *(Emerg Inf Dis 12:1242, 2006)*. For blood/urine antigen, call 1-866-647-2847.	**Itraconazole**¹ oral solution 200–400 mg/day po for 6mo **OR** **Ampho B**¹ (0.7–1 mg/kg/day to total dose of ≥1.5gm for very sick) pts	**Fluconazole** 400–800 mg per day for at least 6 mos. 85%+ effective for non-life-threatening disease *(CID 25:200, 1997)*	Itra in patients treated for ≥2mo, 95% cure *(AJM 93: 489, 1992)*. Ampho B successful in >90% *(CID 22:S102, 1996)*. Vori successful in rx of 1 pt with cerebral blastomycosis *(CID 40:e69, 2005)*. Another rx with Lipid-Amphotericin B followed by vori *(Pediatr Infect. Dis J 25:377,2006)*

¹ Hydration before and after infusion with 500 cc saline has been shown to reduce renal toxicity.

² **Oral solution preferred to tablets because of ↑ absorption** *(see Table 11B, page 96)*.

TABLE 11A (3)

TYPE OF INFECTION/ORGANISM/ SITE OF INFECTION	ANTIMICROBIAL AGENTS OF CHOICE		COMMENTS
	PRIMARY	ALTERNATIVE	

Candidiasis: Candidemia in US is 3rd most common nosocomial blood stream infection with 10-15% mortality, 10-21 day inc length of stay and $40K-$92K inc charges (CID 41:1232, 2005) A decrease in C. albicans and increase in non-albicans species continues. The latter show ↓ susceptibility to antifungal agents (esp. fluconazole). These changes predominantly in immunocompromised pts wherein antifungal prophylaxis (esp. fluconazole) is widely used (JCM 43:2729, 2005, COID 18:490, 2005). For example patients known to be colonized with C. glabrata or C. krusei, fluconazole should be avoided for therapy. (CID 42:244, 2006). While in vitro susceptibility testing for disseminated candidiasis while receiving flu are likely to be infected with an azole-resistant strain. Fluconazole susceptibility profiles help select empiric antifungal rx.
- Fluconazole still preferred here because of impressive efficacy in randomized studies, favorable safety profile and very low cost (CID 42:249, 2006; JAC 57:384,2006)

Blood cultures clinically stable with or without venous catheter: & C. glabrata or C. krusei unlikely (no flu in 30 days) (*IDSA Guidelines: CID 42:249,2006*).	Fluconazole 26 mg/kg per day or Echinocandin (see caspo, anidula, mica below)	400mg q24h IV or po times 7 days + blood culture	
All positive blood cultures require therapy!			
• Fail to respond to flu or deteriorating (Critical to respond to flu over a wk!*) (*CID 36:1221, 2003; Scand J Inf Dis 37:111, 2005; J Clin Micro 43:1829, 2005*), esp. in non-neutropenic: mortality 21% vs 4% if catheter not removed.			
• Remove & replace venous catheter* (*not over a wire*)			
• Treat for 2wk after last pos. blood culture & resolution of signs & symptoms of infection			The echinocandins appear to have similar efficacy, vs candida including candidemia and safety profiles and decisions on use made on the basis of cost. A randomized study (277 pts, 16% were neutropenic) found caspofungin equivalent to ampho B (0.6-1 mg per day) for invasive candidiasis. For candidemia 71.7% with caspo vs 62.8% with ampho B had successful outcomes but caspo had significantly less toxicity (NEJM 347:2020, 2002). Caspo had 70% favorable response vs 55% for ampho B in 58 cancer pts with candidemia (J Int 50:443, 2005). In 119 pts with candidemia, micafungin effective in 88% with new infection, 76% with reinfection (Eur J Clin Inf Dis 24:654, 2005; CID 42:1171, 2006). Preliminary data from a randomized double-blind study (n=245) suggests anidulafungin was superior to flu for invasive candidiasis/candidemia. Data in FDA-approved label but not yet published in peer review journal. Global response (clinical + micro) at end of IV rx, 75.6% with anidula vs 60.2% with flu had successful outcomes. Tolerability was comparable (ICAAC 2005; IDSA 2005, #259). Voriconazole was found non-inferior to ampho B followed by flu in a non-neutropenic candidemia (Lancet 366:1435, 2005). However cross resistance between vori and flu reported in 9 of 28 candida isolates (J Clin Micro 44:529,2006) especially with C. glabrata. (J Clin Micro 44:1740, 2006). Would not recommend as initial rx in those with extensive azole exposure.
Bloodstream: unstable • Fail to respond to flu or deteriorating (Critical to remove intravenous catheter) • Hemodynamic instability (sepsis) • C. glabrata or C. krusei likely • Neutropenia (continuous) Observational studies (continuous) use of ampho B are still effective in neutropenic pts (*IDSA Guidelines, 2003*). **Mortality rates inc with delay in initiation of therapy:** 15% day 1, 24% day 1, 37% day 2 & 41% >day 4-p<.0009 (CID 43:25, 2006)	**Caspofungin** 70 mg IV on day 1, followed by 50mg IV q24h (reduce to 35mg IV q24h with moderate hepatic insufficiency) **OR** **Micafungin** 100 mg IV q24h **OR** **Anidulafungin** 200 mg IV times 1, then 100 mg q24h (no dosage adjustments for renal or hepatic insufficiency)	**Ampho B** 0.7 mg/kg IV q24h; (>7mg/kg/d IV for C. glabrata, krusei) **Lipid-based Amphotericin 3-5 mg/kd** **OR** **Voriconazole** 6 mg per kg IV q12h times 2 doses, then maintenance doses of 3 mg per kg IV q12h; after at least 3 days of IV therapy **OR** **Combination of fluconazole** 800 mg per day + ampho B 0.7 mg per kg per day for first 5-6 days, then switch to flu 400 mg per day po	

(continued on next page)

---

* From 2006 Drug Topics Red Book, Medical Economics Data and Hospital Formulary Pricing Guide. **Price** is **a**verage **w**holesale **p**rice (AWP). See page 2 for abbreviations. All dosage recommendations are for adults (unless otherwise indicated) and assume normal renal/hepatic function

TABLE 11A (4)

TYPE OF INFECTION/ORGANISM/ SITE OF INFECTION	ANTIMICROBIAL AGENTS OF CHOICE		COMMENTS
	PRIMARY	ALTERNATIVE	
Candidiasis/Bloodstream: clinically stable with or without venous catheter (continued)			
			(continued from previous page) In a randomized trial of 219 pts with non-neutropenic candidemia, fluconazole (800 mg per day) + ampho B (0.7 mg per kg per day for the 1st 5 days) was slightly better than flu alone: Primary analysis, success rate on day 30 was 69% vs 57% (p = .08) respectively, overall success rate 69% vs 56% (p = .045), clearance of fungemia 94% vs 83% (p = .02), & renal toxicity in combination greater (23% vs 3%, p < .001) (CID 36:1221, 2003). Given difficulty with interpretation of this study, the editors reserve combination of flu + ampho B for only the sickest candidemic patient.
Cutaneous (including paronychia, Table 1, page 24)	Apply topical **ampho B, clotrimazole, econazole, miconazole,** or **nystatin** 3-4 x daily for 7-14 days or **ketoconazole** 400 mg po once daily x 14 days.		Cost (30 gm tube cream): Clo $13, Eco $28, Mic $50, Nys $4
Endocarditis Causes: C. albicans 24%, non-albicans Candida sp. 24%, Aspergillus sp. 24%, others 27% (CID 32:50, 2001). Surgery may not always be required (Scand J Inf Dis 32:66, 2000 & 37:320, 2005).	**Ciclopirox olamine** 1% cream/lotion, 5&8% topically bid x 7-14 days. **(Ampho B** 0.6mg/kg per day IV for 7 days, then 0.8mg/kg IV every other day or **lipid-based ampho B** 3-5mg/kg per day. Continue 6-8 wks after surgery. **+ flucytosine** 25-37.5mg/kg po q6h) + surgical resection	**Fluconazole** 200-400 mg per day for chronic suppression may be of value when valve cannot be replaced (Chest 122:302, 2002) + Surgical resection	Clo $19 **Adjust flucy dose and interval to produce serum levels; peak 70-80 mg per L, trough 30-40 mg per L. Caspofungin** cidal vs candida; several reports of cure (CID 39:1044-470-3, 2004; CID 40:e-72, 2005). Cure of refractory candidal meningitis with caspo (J Clin Micro 42:5950, 2004).
Endophthalmitis (IDSA Guidelines: CID 38:161,2004) • Occurs in 10% of candidemia (PIDJ 23:635, 2004), thus ophthalmological consult for all pts • Diagnosis: typical white exudates on retinal exam and/or isolation by vitrectomy	**Ampho B** or **lipid-based ampho B** (ABLC 4.5mg/kg per day)] **OR fluconazole** 400mg/day IV or po either as initial rx or follow-up after ampho B. Role of intravitreal ampho B not well defined but commonly used in pts with substantial vision loss (CID 27:1130, 1998). Treat 6-12 wk		Treatment results mixed in small series. Fluconazole (CID 20:657, 1995), ABLC (J Inf 40:92, 2000), and vitrectomy (CID 27:1130, 1998). Von successful alone or with caspo (Korean J Ophthal 19:73, 2005; Am J Ophthal 139:135, 2005). No clinical trials available.
Oral (thrush)—not AIDS patient (See below for vaginitis)	**Fluconazole** 200mg single dose or 100mg/day po x 14 days **OR Itraconazole** oral solution 200mg (20 mL) po q24h without food x 7 days.	**Nystatin pastilles** (200,000 units) or lozenge qid, 500,000 units (swish & swallow) qid or 2 (500,000 units) tabs tid for 14 days **OR Clotrimazole** 1 troche (10 mg) 5x/day x 14 days.	Maintenance not required in non-AIDS pts. Usually improves in 3-4 days, longer & ↓ relapse. Fluconazole-resistant C. krusei fungemia reported in flucon-rx pts (NEJM 325:1315, 1991).

---

* From 2006 Drug Topics Red Book, Medical Economics Data and Hospital Formulary Pricing Guide. **Price is average wholesale price (AWP).** See page 2 for abbreviations. All dosage recommendations are for adults (unless otherwise indicated) and assume normal renal/hepatic function.

TABLE 11A (5)

TYPE OF INFECTION/ORGANISM/ SITE OF INFECTION	ANTIMICROBIAL AGENTS OF CHOICE		COMMENTS
	PRIMARY	ALTERNATIVE	
Candidiasis (continued)			
AIDS patient Stomatitis, esophagitis Oral colonization with candida correlates with HIV & with CD4 counts ↓ (JID 180:534, 1999). HAART has resulted in dramatic ↓ in prevalence of oropharyngeal & esophageal candidiasis & ↓ in refractory disease. See MMWR 53(RR-15):97, 2004	**Oropharyngeal**, initial episodes (7–14d rx): • **Fluconazole** 100mg po q24h; OR • **Itraconazole** oral solution 200mg po q24h; OR • **clotrimazole** troches 10mg po 5x/day; OR • **nystatin** suspension 100,000u/ml, 1ml po q6h; or 1–2 flavored pastilles 4–5x/day. **Esophageal** (14–21d): • **Flucon** 100mg (up to 400mg) po or IV q24h; OR • **Itra** oral solution 200mg po q24h; OR • **caspofungin** 50mg IV q24h; OR • **micafungin** 150 mg IV q24h or **anidulafungin** 100 mg IV day 1 followed by 50 mg per day	**Fluconazole-refractory oropharyngeal:** • **Itra** oral solution ≥200mg po q24h; OR • **ampho B** suspension (100mg/ml) 1 ml po q6h; or • **ampho B** 0.3mg/kg IV q24h **Fluconazole-refractory esophageal:** • **Caspofungin** 50mg IV q24h; or • **vori** 200mg IV q12h; or • **ampho B** 0.3–0.7mg/kg IV q24h; or • **ampho B lipid complex** 3–5mg/kg IV q24h	**Fluconazole-refractory disease remains uncommon** (4% in ACTG 816) & is seen in pts with low CD4 counts (<50/mm³). **Flu** superior to oral suspension of **nystatin** in 41/74 (55%) pts unresponsive to flu (AIDS Res Hum Retrovir 15:1413, 1999). **Itra** 100mg po q12h x14d achieved clinical response in 41/74 (55%) pts unresponsive to flu (AIDS Res Hum Retrovir 15:1413, 1999). **Ampho B oral suspension** gave 42.6% response rate in 54 pts refractory to flu, but 76% of those relapsed (AIDS 14:845, 2000). For esophagitis, **caspofungin** as effective as ampho B IV but less toxic (CID 33:1529, 2001; AAC 46:451, 2002; J AIDS 31:183, 2002). **Voriconazole** as effective as **fluconazole** for esophagitis (CID 33:1447, 2007). **Micafungin** 100 mg IV or 150 mg IV per day equal to flu 200 mg per day; relapse rates similar 15 vs 11% (CID 39:842, 2004; Aliment Pharmacol 21:899, 2005). **Anidulafungin** 100 mg IV day 1 followed by 50 mg per day vs flu 200 mg on day 1 followed by 100 mg per day in 494 pts: cure rate 97% vs 98.8% (CID 39:770, 2004) but relapse rate higher (53% vs 19%).
Vulvovaginitis Common among healthy young females & unrelated to HIV status.	• **Topical azoles** (clotrimazole, buto, mico, tico, or tercon) x3–7d; or • topical **nystatin** 100,000units/day as vaginal tablet x14d; or • oral **flucon** 150 mg x1 dose.	• **Itra** oral solution 200mg po q24h x3d; or • oral **fluon** 150 mg x1 dose	
Peritonitis (Chronic Ambulatory Peritoneal Dialysis) See Table 19, page 176	**Fluconazole** 400mg po q24h x 2–3wks or **caspofungin** 70mg IV on day 1 followed by 50mg IV q24h for 14 days	**Ampho B**, continuous IP dosing at 1.5mg/L of dialysis fluid times 4–6wk	Remove cath immediately or if no clinical improvement in 4–7 days. In 1 study, all 8 pts with candida peritonitis who received caspo responded favorably (as compared to 7/8 pts on ampho B) (NEJM 347:2020, 2002).
Urinary: Candiduria • Usually colonization of urinary catheter, a benign event • Rarely may be source of dissemination if pt has obstructive uropathy or marker of acute hematogenous dissemination • Persistent candiduria in immunocompromised pt warrants ultrasound or CT of kidneys	**Remove urinary catheter or stent** if has symptoms of UTI, neutropenic, low birth-weight infant, or is undergoing urologic manipulation. Then: **fluconazole** 200 mg per day po or IV times 7–14 days OR **ampho B** 0.5 mg per kg per day IV times 7–14 days.	Antifungal rx not indicated unless pt has symptoms of UTI, neutropenic, low birth-weight infant, has renal allograft or is undergoing urologic manipulation. (CID 30:14, 2000)	**Fluconazole:** In placebo-controlled trial, candiduria cleared more rapidly with flu but, at 2 weeks, clearance rates not different than placebo group (CID 30:15, 2000). **Bladder washout** with ampho B not recommended; will not treat upper tract infection. 5FC may be of value in non-albicans UTI but resistance develops rapidly. **Caspofungin** effective in clearing candiduria in 12 pts (most with candidemia) but urine levels low (IDSA 2003, Abst. 135). **NOTE:** Vori not in urine in any form.

* From 2006 Drug Topics Red Book, Medical Economics Data and Hospital Formulary Pricing Guide. Price is average wholesale price (AWP). See page 2 for abbreviations. All dosage recommendations are for adults (unless otherwise indicated) and assume normal renal function.

TABLE 11A (6)

TYPE OF INFECTION/ORGANISM/ SITE OF INFECTION	ANTIMICROBIAL AGENTS OF CHOICE		COMMENTS
	PRIMARY	ALTERNATIVE	
Candidiasis *(continued)*			
Vaginitis—Non-AIDS patients. *Review article: MMWR 51 (RR-6), 2002. (Candida vaginitis in AIDS patients; see Stomatitis, vaginitis above). (See Table 1, page 23)*			**In general, oral & vaginal rx are similarly effective.** Rx aided by avoiding tight clothing, e.g., pantyhose. Oral drugs ↓ rectal candida & may ↓ relapses.
Sporadic/infrequent	**Oral: Fluconazole** 150mg po x 1 OR **Itraconazole** 200mg po bid x 1 day.** ** For over-the-counter preparations, see below in footnote[1]	**Intravaginally:** Multiple **imidazoles** with 85-90% cure rates. See footnote[1]	**Ampho B** vaginal 50mg suppository effective in non-albicans candida infec. when other rx failed *(Am J Ob Gyn 192:2069 & 2012, 2005).*
Chronic recurrent (5–8%) >4 episodes/yr	**Fluconazole** 150 mg q72h x 3 times, then 150 mg po q wk	**Itraconazole** 100 mg po q24h x18 months (oral until response)[HDAF] Fluconazole experience disappointing.	After 6 mos. >90% of 170 women free of disease vs 21.9% who received placebo. By 6 mos. of rx, 42.9% free of disease vs 21.9% w/ rx with itra *(Mycosis 48:165, 2005)*. Significance: *NEJM 351:2554, 2004.* Only 76.9% cured 1 mo. following 3-day rx with itra *(Mycosis 48:165, 2005)*
Ref: *NEJM 351:876, 2004*			
Chromoblastomycosis *(J Am Acad Derm 44:585, 2001)* (Cladosporium or Fonsecaea). Cutaneous (usually feet, legs): raised scaly lesions, most common in tropical areas	If lesions small & few: **surgical excision or cryosurgery with liquid nitrogen** *(Int J Dermatol 42:408, 2003).* If lesions extensive, burrowing: **Itraconazole**	**Itraconazole** 100 mg po q24h times 13/13 patients rx itra responded *(CID 15:553, 1992)*. **Terbinafine**[HDAF] impressive in 35 pts rx 12 mos. (800 mg per day)—86% mycologic cures *(J Derm Treat 9:529, 1998)*. In 4 pts resistance to itra developed on rx with 2 clinical failures *(Mycosis 47:216, 2004)*. 5/6 responded to **posaconazole** *(Drugs 65:1560, 2005; RevInsMed TropSaoPaulo 47:339, 2005)*.
Coccidioidomycosis *(Coccidioides immitis) (ID Clin No.Amer 17:41, 2003; Medicine 83: 149, 2004) (IDSA Guidelines 2005: CID 41:1217, 2005)*			**Ampho B cure rate 50–70%. Responses to azoles are similar.** Itra may have slight advantage esp. in bone/soft tissue infection. Relapse rates after rx 40%. *Relapse rate ↑ if ↑ CF titer ≥1:256 (RR=4.7) (CID 25:1205, 1997)*. Following CF titers after completion of rx important: rising titers warrant readministration of rx *(CID 25: 1211, 1997)*. In an RDBS[3] of 198 pts with progressive non-meningeal cocci, 57% responded to fluo to itra (p=0.05). *(AWM 133:676, 2000)*. **Vori** effective in 1 case of widely disseminated cocci *(CID 36:1619, 2003)*. **Caspofungin** successful in a renal transplant pt *(CID 39:879, 2004)*. **Posaconazole** successful in 5/6 pts with refractory non-meningeal cocci *(CID 40:1770, 2005)* & 11/16 cases successful reported overall *(Drugs 65:1559, 2005)*.
Primary pulmonary (San Joaquin or Valley Fever): Pts low risk persistence/complication	**Antifungal rx not generally recommended.** Treat if fever, wt loss and/or infiltrate do not clear within several wks to 2mo (see below)		
Primary pulmonary in pts with ↑ risk for complications or dissemination. Rx indicated:	**Mild to moderate severity:** **Itraconazole** solution 200mg po or IV bid OR **Fluconazole** 400mg po q24h for 3–12mo		Uncomplicated pulmonary in normal host recovers spontaneously. Influenza-like illness of 1–2wk duration. *(Emerg Infect Dis 12:958, 2006)*
• Immunosuppressive disease, AIDS *(CID 41:1174, 2005)*, post-transplantation *(Am J Transp 6:340, 2006)*, hematological malignancies *(AJM 165:113, 2004)* or therapies (steroids, TNF-α antagonists) *(Arth Rheum 50:1959, 2004)*	**Locally severe or disseminated disease** **Ampho B** 0.6–1mg/kg per day x 7 days then 0.8mg/kg every other day OR **Lipid-based Ampho** *(CID 33:876, 2000)*. Switch to **itra** or **flu** for at least 1 year.		
• Pregnancy in 3rd trimester • Diabetes • CF antibody >1:16 • Pulmonary infiltrates • Dissemination (identification of spherules or culture of organism from ulcer, joint effusion, pus from abscess or bone Rx, etc.)	**Some use combination of Ampho B & Flu for progressive severe disease,** controlled series lacking *(CID 41:1177, 2005)*. **Consultation with specialist recommended:** surgery may be required. **Lifetime suppression in HIV+ patients or until CD4 >250 & infection controlled:** flu 200 mg po bid or itra 200mg po bid *(Mycosis 46:42, 2003)*		

---

[1] From 2006 Drug Topics Red Book, Medical Economics Data and Hospital Formulary Pricing Guide. *Price is average wholesale price (AWP).* See page 2 for abbreviations. All dosage recommendations are for adults (unless otherwise indicated) and assume normal renal/renal function

Butoconazole 2% cream (5gm) q24h x 3 days** or 2% cream SR 5gm x 1; or **clotrimazole** 100mg vaginal tabs (2 at bedtime times 7 days (14 days may) ↑ cure rate) or 100mg vaginal tab x 7 days or 500mg vaginal tab x1; or **miconazole** 200mg vaginal suppos (1 at bedtime x 3 days** or 100mg vaginal suppos. q24h x 7 days or 2% cream (5gm) at bedtime x 7 days** or **terconazole** 80mg vaginal supp (1 at bedtime x 3 days) or 0.4% cream (5gm) at bedtime x 3 days; or **tioconazole** q24h x 3 days; or **tioconazole** 6.5% vag. ointment x 1 dose**. ** = over-the-counter product.

TABLE 11A (7)

TYPE OF INFECTION/ORGANISM/ SITE OF INFECTION	ANTIMICROBIAL AGENTS OF CHOICE		COMMENTS
	PRIMARY	ALTERNATIVE	
Coccidioidomycosis (continued)			
Meningitis: occurs in 1/3 to 1/2 of pts with disseminated coccidioidomycosis			
Adult (see CID 42:103, 2006)	Fluconazole 400–1,000mg po q24h indefinitely	Ampho B IV as for pulmonary (above) + 0.1–0.3mg daily intrathecal (intraventricular) via reservoir device. OR Itra 400–800mg q24h OR voriconazole (see Comment)	80% relapse rate, **continue flucon indefinitely.** Voriconazole successful in high doses (6mg/kg IV q12h) followed by oral suppression (400mg po q12h) (CID 36:1619, 2003; AAC 48: 2341, 2004). **Caspofungin** also used (AAC 54: 292, 2004) & failed in another case (CID 39:879, 2004).
Child	Fluconazole (po) (Pediatric dose not established, 6mg per kg q24h used)		
Cryptococcosis (CID 30:710, 2000). Excellent review: Brit Med Bull 72:99, 2005			
Non-meningeal (non-AIDS) Risk: 57% in organ transplant (Transpl Inf Dis 4:183, 2002 & 7:26, 2005) & those receiving other forms of immunosuppressive agents (alemtuzumab—Transplant Proc 37:934, 2005).	Fluconazole 400mg/day IV or po OR **For more severe disease:** Ampho B 0.5–0.8mg/kg per day (will response then change to **fluconazole** 400mg po q24h for 8–10wk course	Itraconazole 200–400mg solution q24h for 6–12wk OR Ampho B (3mg/kg per day IV + flucytosine 37.5mg/kg po qid times 6wk	**Flucon alone 90% effective for meningeal and non-meningeal forms.** Fluconazole as effective as ampho B (CID 32:E145, 2001). Addition of interferon-γ (IFN-γ-1b 50 mcg per wk x 9wk) to liposomal ampho B assoc. with response in pt failing antifungal rx (CID 38: 910, 2004).
Meningitis (non-AIDS)	Ampho B 0.5–0.8mg/kg per day IV + flucytosine 37.5mg/kg po q6h until pt afebrile & cultures neg (~6wk) (NEJM 301:126, 1979), then stop ampho B/flucyt, start **fluconazole** 200mg po q24h (AnIM 113:183, 1990) OR Fluconazole 400mg po q24h x 8–10wk: Some recommend flu for 1yr to reduce relapse rate (CID 28:297, 1999).	[Fluconazole 400–800mg/day po or IV for less severe disease OR Fluconazole 400–800mg/day po or IV + flucytosine 25mg/kg po q6h x4–6wks **Then Consolidation therapy:** Fluconazole 400mg po q24h to complete a 10-wk course or until CSF culture sterile, then suppression (see below).]	**Fluconazole alone used successfully,** comparative clinical trials lacking (NEJM 330:263, 1994). Hydrocephalus may be successfully rx with VP or VA shunting (CID 28:629, 1999); poor response of pts in coma (CID 37:673, 2003).
HIV+/AIDS: Cryptococcaemia and/or Meningitis Treatment (see CID 30:710, 2000 & Table 11) ↓ in res of HAART (Neurol 56:257, 2001; CID 36:789, 2003) but still common when pt presents with AIDS & HIV status unknown (AIDS 18:555, 2004). Cryptococcus in blood may manifest by positive blood culture or positive test of serum for cryptococcal antigen (CRAG: >95% sens.), no help in monitoring therapy. With HAART, symptoms of acute meningitis may return: Immune reconstitution Syndrome (see Table 14D). ↑ CSF pressure associated with high mortality, lower with CSF removal (CID 38:134, 2004). If frequent LPs not possible, ventriculoperitoneal shunts an option (Surg Neurol 63:529 & 531, 2005).	[Ampho B 0.7mg/kg IV q24h + flucytosine[1] 25mg/kg po q6h x2wks **or** Liposomal amphotericin B 4mg/kg IV q24h + flucytosine 25mg/kg po q6h x2wks] **Then Consolidation therapy:** Fluconazole 400mg po q24h (see below). Start Highly Active Antiretroviral Therapy (HAART) if possible.		**Ampho B + 5FC treatment:** 29/235 pts died within 1st 2 wks & 62 (28%) by 10wks; only 129 (55%) were alive & culture-neg at 10wks (CID 28:82, 1999). In 64 pts, ampho + 5FC + crypto CFUs more rapidly than ampho + flu or combination of all 3 drugs (p <0.001) (Ln 363:1764, 2004). Monitor 5-FC levels: peak 70–80 mg/L, trough 30–40 mg/L. Higher levels assoc. with bone marrow toxicity. If normal mental status, >20 cells/mm³, CSF, & CSF crypto antigen < 1:1024, flucon alone is reasonable (CID 22:322, 1996). ...survival was 85%, 6 months after discharge from hospital & receiving flucon suppression in Uganda (IDSA 2003, Abst 630). Failure of flu may rarely be due to resistant organism (Clin Micro 9:441, 2003; JAC 54:563, 2004). Successful outcomes were observed in 14/29 (48%) subjects with cryptococcal meningitis treated with posaconazole in Uganda. Voriconazole effective in 7 of 18 but statused disease in 10 more (CID 36:1122, 2003).

---

[1] Some experts would reduce to 25 mg per kg q6h

² **VP** = ventriculoperitoneal; **VA** = ventriculoatrial

³ **Flucytosine** = 5-FC

TABLE 11A (B)

TYPE OF INFECTION/ORGANISM/ SITE OF INFECTION	ANTIMICROBIAL AGENTS OF CHOICE		COMMENTS
	PRIMARY	ALTERNATIVE	
Cryptococcosis: HIV-/AIDS: Cryptococcemia and/or Meningitis (continued)			
Suppression (chronic maintenance therapy) Discontinuation of antifungal rx can be considered among pts who remain asymptomatic with CD4 >100-200/mm³ on effective antiretroviral rx, some authorities now say for >6 months. Some might consider suppressive rx. See www.hivatis.org. Authors would only dc if CSF culture negative.	**Fluconazole** 200mg/day po [if CD4 count rises to >100/mm³ with effective antiretroviral rx, consider discontinuation of maintenance rx. Reappearance of pos. serum CRAG may predict relapse	**Itraconazole** 200mg po q12h rx. Intolerant or failure	Itraconazole not as effective as fluconazole. 13/57 (23%) pts relapsed vs 2/51 (4%) receiving fluconazole (p = 0.006) (CID 28:291, 1999) altho at doses of 600mg/day rx to flu as consol-dation rx in 35 pts in Thai (J Med Assoc Thai 86:293, 2003). No recurrences of crypto meningitis in 22 pts who dc flu suppression with >100 CD4 & undetectable VL x3mos. in Thailand (CID 36:1329, 2003) & 1 SS relapses/100 person-yrs in 100 pts in a European study (CID 38:565, 2004).
Dermatophytosis (See Superficial fungal infections, Ln 364:1173, 2004) **Onychomycosis** (Tinea unguium) (Derm Ther 17:517, 2004; Brit J Derm 149:402, 2003; Am J Clin Derm 5:225, 2004; Cutis 74:516, 2004) Topical nail lacquer (ciclopirox) approved bu cure in only 5-9% (Med Lett 42:51, 2000) but¹ to 50% cure in another study (Cutis 73:81, 2004). Maw venereal oral rx (Cutis 74:55, 2004; J Eur Acad Dermat's Venereal 19:21, 2005). Terbinafine appears to be the most cost-effective (Manag Care 12:47, 2003; Manag Care Interface 18:5E, 2005). Overall cure rate from 18 randomized controlled trials, 76% (J Drugs Derm 4:302, 2005).	**Fingernail Rx Options: Terbinafine**[1] 250mg po q24h [children <20kg: 67.5mg/day; 20-40kg: 125mg/day; >40kg: 250mg/day] x 6wk (79% effective) OR **Itraconazole**[1] 200mg po q24h x 3mo;[NFDA] or **Itraconazole**[1] 200mg po bid x 1wk/mo x 2mo; or **Fluconazole**[1] 150-300mg po q wk x 3-6mo.[NFDA] **NOTE:** For side-effects, see footnotes 1 & 2		**Toenail Rx Options: Terbinafine**[1] 250mg po q24h [children <20kg: 67.5mg/day; 20-40kg 125mg/day; >40kg 250mg/day] x 12wks (76% effective) OR **Itraconazole**[1] 200mg po q24h x 3mo (59% effective) OR **Itraconazole**[1] 200mg po q24h x 3mo OR **Fluconazole** 150-300mg po q wk x 6-12mo (48% effective)[NFDA] [Data reflect cure rate from meta-analysis of all randomized controlled trials (Brit J Derm 150:537, 2004).]
Tinea capitis (Tinea tonsurans) Trichophyton tonsurans; Microsporum canis. N. America, other sp. elsewhere (PIDJ 18:191, 1999)	**Terbinafine**[1] 250mg po q24h x 4wk for T. tonsurans; 4-8 wk for Micro-sporum canis[NFDA] Children 125mg (or 6-12mg/kg per day) po q24h. (COID 17:97, 2004; Exp Opin Pharm Ther 5:219, 2004; J Eur Acad Dermatol Venereol 18:155, 2004).	**Itraconazole**[2] 3-5mg/kg per day for 30 days[NFDA] OR **Fluconazole** 8mg/kg q wk x 8-12wk.[NFDA] Cap at 150mg/kg per q24h adults **Griseofulvin** adults 500mg po q24h x 4-6wks, children 10-20mg/kg per day until hair regrows, 6-8wk.	All agents with similar cure rates (66-100%) in clinical studies (Ped Derm 17:304, 2000). Griseofulvin considered drug of choice by some although concerns for resistance and toxicity. Addition of topical ketoconazole or selenium sulfate shampoo reduces transmissibility (Int J Dermatol 39:261, 2000).

---

[1] **Serious but rare cases of hepatic failure** have been reported in pts receiving terbinafine & should not be used in those with chronic or active liver disease ALT & AST before prescribing (Am J Health Sys Pharm 58:1076, 2001). Suggest checking

[2] Use of itraconazole has been associated with myocardial dysfunction and with onset of congestive heart failure (see Table 11B, page 96).

* From 2006 Drug Topics Red Book, Medical Economics Data and Hospital Formulary Pricing Guide. **Price is average wholesale price (AWP).** See page 2 for abbreviations. All dosage recommendations are for adults (unless otherwise indicated) and assume normal renal function

TABLE 11A (9)

TYPE OF INFECTION/ORGANISM/ SITE OF INFECTION	ANTIMICROBIAL AGENTS OF CHOICE		COMMENTS
	PRIMARY	ALTERNATIVE	
Dermatophytosis (continued) **Tinea corporis, cruris, or pedis** (Trichophyton rubrum, T. mentagrophytes, Epidermophyton floccosum) *Athlete's foot, jock itch,* and *ringworm*	**Topical rx:** Generally applied 2x/day. Available as creams, ointments, sprays, by prescription & "over the counter." Apply 2x/day for 2–3wks. See Comments & prices. Recommend: *Lotrimin Ultra* or *Lamisil AT*: contain butenafine & terbinafine—both are fungicidal	**Terbinafine** 250 mg po q24h x 2 wks[NFRA] **OR ketoconazole** 200 mg po q24h x 4 wks **OR fluconazole** 150 mg po 1x/wk for 2–4 wks[NFRA] **Griseofulvin:** adults 500 mg po q24h times 4–6 wks, children 10–20 mg/kg per day. Duration: 2–4 wks for corporis, 4–8 wks for pedis.	Keto po often effective in severe recalcitrant infection. Follow for hepatotoxicity. Terbinafine: 87% achieved mycological cure in double-blind study (32 pts) (J Med Assoc Thai 76:388, 1993; Brit J Derm 130(S43):22, 1994) and fluconazole 78% (J Am Acad Derm 40:S31, 1999).
Tinea versicolor (Malassezia furfur or Pityrosporum orbiculare) Rule out erythrasma—see Table 1, page 49	**Ketoconazole** (400mg po single dose)[NFRA] or (200mg po q24h x 7 days) or (2% cream 1x q24h x 2wks)	**Fluconazole** 400mg po single dose or **itraconazole** 400mg po q24h x 3–7 days	Keto (po) times 1 97% effective in 1 study. Another alternative: Selenium sulfide (Selsun). 2.5% lotion, apply as lather, leave on 10min then wash off. 1/day x 7 day or 3–5/wk times 2–4wks
Fusariosis Infections in eye, skin, sinus & disseminated diseases—↑ in HSCT/BM transplant & cancer pts (COID 17:527, 2004)	**Voriconazole** 6mg/kg IV q12h on day 1, then either (4mg/kg q12h) or (200mg po q12h for body weight ≥40kg, but 100mg po q12h for body weight <40kg)	**Ampho B** 1–1.2mg/kg IV q24h or **lipid-associated ampho B** or **Posa** 400 mg po bid with meals (if not taking meals, 200 mg po qid).	Voriconazole successful in 50% (CID 36:1122, 2003) Posaconazole 800 mg/d in divided doses was effective in 50% in 20 pts who failed Ampho B and 67% that recovered from myelosuppression (CID 42:1398, 2006)
Histoplasmosis (Histoplasma capsulatum): See CID 30:688, 2000; ID Clin No. Amer 17:1, 2003. Best diagnostic test 2nd generation is urinary, serum, or CSF histoplasma antigen. MiraVista Diagnostics (1-866-647-2847)			
Immunocompetent patient: Pulmonary, localized, disseminated Definition of severe—Temp >39.5°C, Karnofsky <60, albumin <3 gm per dL, hepatic enzymes >5 times normal, WBC <500, platelets <50,000, creatinine >6 mg per dL	**Minimal disease: No rx** **Moderate: Itraconazole** 200mg/day solution po for 9mo. If life-threatening initially for 3 days, then 200mg po bid until response.[SFRA] If IV rx necessary: Dose 200mg IV bid x 4 doses followed by 200mg IV q24h (see Table 11B). **Severe, inc. meningitis: Liposomal ampho B** 4 mg/kg per day IV x 7 days, then switch to **itra** 200mg/day for 9mo. **Itra not recommended for meningitis** (See CID 38:463, 2004)		**With >2 months itra, 86% success in chronic pulmonary & extrapulmonary** (AJM 93:489, 1992). Meningitis is difficult to rx & no prospective studies. **Liposomal ampho B** recommended because of ↑ CSF levels vs ampho B. Histo antigen in CSF should fall to undetectable levels before in rx (See CID 40:844, 2005). **Flu less effective than itra.**

[1] Drug name (trade name) & wholesale price for 15 gm; All are applied to affected area bid. **Prescription drugs:** butenafine (Mentax) $40, ciclopirox (Loprox) $23, clotrimazole (Lotrimin) $19, Mycelex $11), econazole (Spectazole) $22, ketoconazole (Nizoral) $25, miconazole (Monistat) $21, naftifine (Naftin) $27, oxiconazole (Oxistat) $13, terconazole (Terazol) $26, sulconazole (Exelderm) $13, terbinafine (Lamisil) $31, Mycelex $11), sertaconazole (Ertaczo) $47. **Non-prescription (over-the-counter):** Tolnaftate (Tinactin $5, Ting or Tolnate $2), undecylenic acid (Cruex $5, Desenex $5), Lotrimin 1% 12 gm $6.17, Lamisil AT 1%, 12 gm $6.79.

[2] **Oral solution preferred to tablets because of ↑ absorption** (see Table 11B, page 96).

* From 2006 Drug Topics Red Book, Medical Economics Data and Hospital Formulary Pricing Guide. Price is **average wholesale price (AWP).**
See page 2 for abbreviations. All dosage recommendations are for adults (unless otherwise indicated) and assume normal renal function

TABLE 11A (10)

TYPE OF INFECTION/ORGANISM/ SITE OF INFECTION	ANTIMICROBIAL AGENTS OF CHOICE		COMMENTS
	PRIMARY	ALTERNATIVE	

Histoplasmosis (Histoplasma capsulatum) *(continued)*

Immunocompromised patient (AIDS) (CID 30:688, 2000; & 32:1215, 2001) Risk factors for death: dyspnea, platelet count <100,000 per mm³ & LDH >2 times upper limit normal (CID 38:134, 2004). In 1 study suppression was safely dc after 12 mos. of antifungal rx & 6 mos. of HAART with CD4 >150, 0 relapses after 2 yrs follow-up in 32 pts (CID 38:1485, 2004).	**Primary prophylaxis:** Consider for pts from endemic area with CD4 <150/mcL. If used, **itraconazole 200mg po q24h.** **Severe disseminated:** **Acute phase** (3–10 days or until clinically improved): • **Ampho B** 0.7mg/kg IV q24h; or • **liposomal ampho B** 4mg/kg IV q24h **Continuation phase** (1/2 wks): **Itra** 200mg po q12h **Less severe disseminated:** **Itra** 200mg po q8h x 3 days, then 200mg po q12h x 12wks. **Meningitis:** **Suppression:** Insufficient data to rec. dc with ↑ CD4 from HAART but consider indef. **Itra** 200mg po q24h indef	**Severe disseminated:** **Acute phase:** • **Itra** 400mg IV q24h **Continuation phase:** • **Itra** oral solution 200mg po q12h; or • **flucon** 800 mg po q24h **Mild disseminated:** **Fluconazole** 800mg po q24h **Ampho B or liposomal ampho B** x 12–16wks. **Amphotericin B** 1mg/kg IV weekly or biweekly indefinitely	CD4 <500/mm³ might require no rx. Acute pulmonary histoplasmosis among HIV-1 infected pts with CD4 counts <500/mm³ might require no rx. **Liposomal ampho B** superior to ampho B (88% vs ampho B (88% vs 64% clinical success) in 81 pts with ↓ nephrotoxicity (97% vs 37%) (AnIM 137:105, 2002). **Itra** (ACTG 120) 50/59 (85%) pts responded, cleared fungemia with only 5% toxicity. Avoid rifampin, reduces itra serum concentration (AJM 98:336, 1995). Mortality 12.5% in 110 cases of disseminated histo + AIDS receiving ampho B up to 1gm followed by itra in Panama (CID 40:1199, 2005). **Itra best drug for suppression at 200 mg q24h** but 3/46 had probable hepatic toxicity (J AIDS & HR 16:100, 1997). Flu less effective than itra & induces flu & vori resistance (CID 33:1910, 2001; AAC57:1235, 2006). Posaconazole effective in 6/6 hts who failed ampho, flu, itra & vori (J. Infect July 4, 2006) There are no prospective studies addressing the management of CNS histoplasmosis (CID 40:844, 2005).

Madura foot (See Nocardia & Scedosporium, below)

Mucormycosis & other **Zygomycosis**—Rhizopus, Rhizomucor, Absidia. **Invasive:** Eur J Clin Microbiol Infect Dis 25:215, 2006 Key to successful rx: early dx with symptoms suggestive of sinusitis (or lateral facial pain or numbness): think mucor with palatal ulcers, &/or black eschars, onset unilateral blindness in immunocompromised or diabetic pt (J Otolaryn 34:166, 2005). Rapidly fatal without rx. Dx by culture of tissue or stain: wide ribbon-like, non-septate(ish) with variation in diameter & right angle branching (ClinMicro&Infect 12:7, 2006)	**Ampho B** Increase rapidly to 0.8–1.5mg/kg per day IV, when improving, then every other day. Total dose usually 2.5–3gm. **OR** **Lipid-based Ampho B** **OR** **Posaconazole** 400 mg po bid with meals (if not taking meals, 200 mg po qid).	Cure dependent on: (1) surgical debridement, (2) rx of hyperglycemia, correction of neutropenia, or reduction in immunosuppression; (3) antifungal rx: liposomal amphotericin (J Clin Micro 43:2012, 2005)—striking improvement reported, 54–70% overall success in refractory zygomycosis vs 25% or less with amphotericin or lipid ampho B (Drugs 65:1553, 2005) and 19 of 24 successful; 11 with microbiological rx successful (AAC 50:126, 2006). Prolonged use of Voriconazole prophylaxis predisposes to zygomycetes infections all resistant to vori. (Lancet ID 5:594, 2006).

---

* From 2006 Drug Topics Red Book, Medical Economics Data and Hospital Formulary Pricing Guide. **Price is average wholesale price (AWP).** See page 2 for abbreviations. All dosage recommendations are for adults (unless otherwise indicated) and assume normal renal function

TABLE 11A (11)

TYPE OF INFECTION/ORGANISM/ SITE OF INFECTION	ANTIMICROBIAL AGENTS OF CHOICE		COMMENTS
	PRIMARY	ALTERNATIVE	
Nocardiosis (N. asteroides & N. brasiliensis): Culture & sensitivies may be valuable in refractory cases; Reference Labs, R.J. Wallace (903) 877-7680 or CDC (404) 639-3158. **Cutaneous and lymphocutaneous** (sporotrichoid)	**TMP-SMX** 5–10mg/kg per day of TMP & 25–50mg/kg per day of SMX in 2–4 div. doses/day, po or IV	**Sulfisoxazole** 2gm po qid or **minocycline** 100–200mg po bid	**Linezolid** 300–600mg po/IV bid x 3-24mos. successful in 6/6 pts, 4 with disseminated disease of whom 2 had brain abscesses cured (CID 36: 313, 2003; Eur J Neurol 12:536, 2005).
Pulmonary, disseminated, brain abscess Duration of rx generally 3mo for immunocompetent host (88%) & 6mos for immunocompromised host (61%), even longer if CNS involvement. High incidence of relapse if organ transplant, malignancy, chronic lung disease, diabetes, ETOH use, steroid rx, AIDS, & infliximab rx (Canad Med J 171:1063, 2004).	**TMP-SMX** Initially 15mg/kg per day of TMP & 75mg/kg per day of SMX IV or po, div. in 2–4 doses. After 3–4wk, ↓ dose to 10mg/kg per day TMP in 2–4 doses po. Do serum level (see Comment)	**IMP** 500mg IV q6h) + (**amikacin** 7.5mg/kg IV q12h) times 3–4wk & then po regimen	Survival improved when sulfa-containing regimen used (Medicine 68:38, 1989). **Prosthetic valve endocarditis** with N. asteroides cured with IMP + amikacin times 2mo followed by TMP-SMX times 4 mos. (AJM 115:330, 2003). Measure sulfonamide blood levels: Peak of 100–150mcg/mL 2hrs post-po dose. Increasing sulfa resistance—recommend sensitivity testing (Eur J Clin Micro Inf Dis 24:142, 2005; AAC 48:832, 2004).
Paracoccidioidomycosis (South American blastomycosis)/ P. brasiliensis	**Itraconazole** 200mg/day x 6mo or **Ketoconazole** 400mg/day po for 6–18mo	**Ampho B** 0.4–0.5mg/kg per day IV to total dose of 1.5–2.5gm or **sulfonamides** (dose: see Comment) or **ampho B**	Improvement in >90% pts on itra or keto. HIV+ **Sulfa** 4–6gm/day for 3 weeks, then 500mg/day for 3–5yr also used (CID 14 (Suppl.):S-68, 1992). Low-dose itra (50–100mg/day), keto (200–400mg/day) & sulfadiazine (up to 6mg/day) showed similar clinical responses in 4-mno in a randomized study (Med Mycol 40: 411, 2002). HIV+ TMP-SMX suppressive rx indefinitely (CID 21:1275, 1995).
Lobomycosis (keloidal blastomycosis)/P. loboi	Surgical excision, clofazimine		
Penicilliosis (Penicillium marneffei): Common disseminated fungal infection in AIDS pts in SE Asia (esp. Thailand & Vietnam) (CID 24:1080, 1997; Intl J Inf Dis 3:48, 1998)	**Ampho B** 0.5–1mg/kg per day times 2wks followed by **itraconazole** 400mg/day po then **itraconazole** 200mg/day po **indefinitely for HIV+ infected pts** (CID 26:1107, 1998). See Comment	For less sick patients **itra** 200mg po tid x 3 days, then 200mg po bid x 12wks. (if able to take 200mg po q24h? (IV if unable to take po)	3° most common OI in AIDS following TB- and cryptococcal meningitis. Prolonged fever, wt loss, hepatomegaly. Skin nodules umbilicated (mimic cryptococcal infection or molluscum contagiosum). In AIDS pts, suppression with itra is effective in **preventing relapses** (NEJM 339:1739, 1998).
Phaeohyphomycosis, Black molds, Dematiaceous fungi (See CID 41:521, 2005; CID 43:53, 2006) Sinuses, skin. bone & joint, brain abscess, endocarditis, emerging especially in h-HSCT pts with disseminated disease **Species: Scedosporium prolificans** – Bipolaris, Wangiella, Curvularia, Exophiala, Phialemonium, Scytalidium, Alternaria	**Surgery + Itraconazole** 400mg/day po, duration not defined, probably 6mo [AWP]	**Voriconazole** has in vitro activity, but clinical experience limited vs S. prolificans (CID 17:527, 2004). OR **Itraconazole + terbinafine** synergistic against S. prolificans (AAC 44:470, 2000. No clinical data & combination could show ↑ toxicity (see Table 11B, page 96)	**Notoriously resistant to antifungal rx including amphotericin & azoles** (CID 34:899, 2002). **Mortality >80%. Posaconazole** successful in case of brain abscess (CID 34:1648, 2002). Posaconazole accounted for 10% of mycelial infections post-transplant (CID 37:221, 2003).
Scedosporium apiospermum (Pseudallescheria boydii) (not considered a true dematiaceous mold) (Medicine 81:333, 2002). Skin, subcut (Madura foot), brain abscess, recurrent meningitis. May appear after near-drowning incidents. Also emerging especially in h-HSCT pts with disseminated disease	**Voriconazole** 6mg/kg IV q12h on day 1, then either (4mg/kg IV q12h) or (200mg po q12h for body weight ≥40 g, but 100mg po q12h for body weight <40g) (PIDJ 21:240, 2002)	**Surgery + itraconazole** 200mg po bid. (Many species now resistant or refractory to Itra) OR **Posa** 400 mg po bid with meals (if not taking meals, 200 mg po qid)	**Notoriously resistant to antifungal drugs including amphotericin.** In vitro voriconazole more active than itra (J Clin Micro 39: 954, 2001). Case reports of successful rx in disseminated S. boydii disease with voriconazole (Clin Micro Inf Dis 9:750, 2003; EJCMID 22:408, 2003) but only 10 to 18 successful in one study (CID 36:1122, 2003). Posaconazole active in vitro and successful in several case reports.

---

¹ **Oral solution preferred to tablets because of ↑ absorption** (see Table 11B, page 96).

* From 2006 Drug Topics Red Book, Medical Economics Data and Hospital Formulary Pricing Guide. **Price is average wholesale price (AWP).** See page 2 for abbreviations. *All dosage recommendations are for adults (unless otherwise indicated) and assume normal renal function.*

TABLE 11A (12)

TYPE OF INFECTION/ORGANISM/ SITE OF INFECTION	ANTIMICROBIAL AGENTS OF CHOICE		COMMENTS
	PRIMARY	ALTERNATIVE	
Sporotrichosis (CID 36:34, 2003; ID Clin No. Amer 17:59, 2003; Derm Ther 17:59, 2004)			
Cutaneous/Lymphonodular	Itraconazole 100–200mg/day solution tps times 3-6mo (then 100mg po bid long-term for HIV-infected pts)[NFGH]	Fluconazole 400mg po q24h x 6mo OR Sat. soln. potassium iodide (SSKI) (1gm of KI in 1mL of H₂O). Start with 5-10 drops tid or 1⁰ to 40–50 drops tid for 3-6mo. Take after meals.	Itra rx: CID 17:210, 1993. Some authorities use ampho B as primary therapy. Ampho B resistant strains reported (AJM 95: 279, 1993). Itra rx for up to 24 months effective in multifocal osteoarticular infection (CID 36:1403, 1996). SSKI with 5-10 drops tid, 1⁰ 1st dose is fast). Infusion duration gradually, 1⁰ to 40-50 drops tid x 3-6mo. SSKI side-effects: nausea, rash, fever, metallic taste, salivary gland swelling.
Osteoarticular, pulmonary	Itraconazole 300mg po bid x 6-12mo, then 200mg po bid (long-term for HIV+ pts) (IV if unable to take po)	**Disseminated, meningeal:** Ampho B 0.5mg/kg per day to total 1-2gm, followed by itra 200mg po q24h	
Extracutaneous: Osteoarticular, disseminated, meningeal			

TABLE 11B – ANTIFUNGAL DRUGS: ADVERSE EFFECTS, COMMENTS, COST

DRUG NAME, GENERIC (TRADE)/USUAL DOSAGE/COST*	ADVERSE EFFECTS/COMMENTS
Non-lipid amphotericin B **Amphotericin B deoxycholate** (Fungizone) 0.3–1mg/kg per day as single infusion 50mg $11.64 Mixing ampho B with lipid emulsion results in precipitation and is discouraged (Am J Hlth Pharm 52:1463, 1995)	**Admin:** Ampho B is a colloidal suspension that must be prepared in electrolyte-free D5W at 0.1mg/mL to avoid precipitation. No need to protect suspensions from light. Infusions cause chills/fever, myalgia, anorexia, nausea, rarely hemodynamic collapse/hypotension. Postulated that histamine is the mediator of these reactions (severe dyspnea & hypotension). Postulated to be histamine release (Pharmaco 23:966, 2003). Manufacturer recommends test dose of 1mg, but often not done (1st few mL of 1st dose is test). Infusion duration usu. 4 + hrs. No difference found in 1 vs 4hr infus. (AAC 34:1402, 1992) except chills/fever occurred sooner with 1hr infus. Febrile reactions ↓ with repeat doses. Rare pulmonary reactions (severe dyspnea & local infiltrates) suggest ampho-related edema) assoc. with rapid infus (CID 33:75, 2001). Severe rigors respond to morphine (25–50mg) or meperidine (25-50mg). Premedication with acetaminophen, diphenhydramine, hydrocortisone (25–50mg) and heparin (1000 units/mg) had no influence on rigors/fever (CID 707:55, 1995). If cytokine (postulate correct), NSAIDs or high-dose steroids may prove efficacious but their use may risk worsening infection under rx or increased risk of nephrotoxicity (CID 26:334, 1998). **Toxicity:** Major concern is nephrotoxicity (15% of 7/8 pts surveyed). Manifest initially by kaliuresis and hypokalemia, then fall in serum bicarbonate (may accompany distal renal tubular acidosis), ↓ in renal erythropoietin and anemia, and rising BUN/serum creatinine. Hypomagnesemia may occur. Can reduce risk of renal injury by (a) **pre- & post-infusion hydration with 500mL saline (if clinical status allows salt load)**, (b) avoidance of other nephrotoxins, eg, radiocontrast, aminoglycosides, cis-platinum, (c) use of lipid prep of ampho B (see below). Low-dose dopamine did not significantly ↓ renal toxicity (AAC 42:3103, 1996). In single randomized controlled trial of 80 neutropenic pts with refractory severe & suspected CID proven invasive fungal infection. 0.6mg/kg/day ampho **continuously infused over 4hr** compared to classic **rapid infusion over 24hr period** compared to classic rapid infusion produced less nephrotoxicity [26% ↓ in max. serum Cr (p=0.005)] ↓ in fever, chills & vomiting (p < 0.0003) & appeared as effective as rapid infusion but in very few proven fungal infections (7 & 3, respectively) (BMJ 3221:1, 2001). Continuous infusion allows a dramatic ↑ in administered dosage without sig. toxicity (CID 36:943, 2003). It is disturbing that these & other controlled continuous infusion observations have not led to controlled trials examining efficacy in rx of life-threatening fungal infections (CID 36:952, 2003). Await trials of efficacy in rx of proven or higher number of proven fungal infection!
Lipid-based ampho B products: **Amphotericin B lipid complex (ABLC) (Abelcet):** 5mg/kg per day 100mg $190.28 [Published Cost § cost ratios] **(except liposomal ampho B was more expensive)**[1] Relationship between Abelcet & AmBisome in serum creatinine were observed in 1/3 of both (BU Hemat 103:198, 1998; Focus on Fungal Tx 20:39, 1997, CID 26:1383, 1998).	**Admin:** Consists of ampho B complexed with 2 lipid bilayer ribbons. Compared to standard ampho B: larger volume of distribution, rapid blood clearance and high tissue concentrations (liver, spleen, lung). Dosage: **5mg/kg per day.** Infuse at 2.5mg/kg per hr; adult and ped. dose the same. Do NOT use an in-line filter. Do not dilute with saline or mix with other drugs or electrolytes[2]. **Toxicity:** Fever and chills in 14–18%; nausea 9%, vomiting 8%; serum creatinine ↑ in 11%, renal failure 5%, anemia 4%. A fatal case of fat embolism reported following ABLC infusion (Exp Mol Path 177:246, 2004). Relationship of ABLC to conventional ampho B deoxycholate (Fungizone). **None of the lipid ampho B preps have shown superior efficacy compared to ampho B in prospective trials** (AJM 137:105, 2002; DJ 37:415, 2003). **Dosage equivalency has not been established** (CID 36:1500, 2003). Compared with all lipid ampho B preps: ABLC has higher frequency of mild hepatic toxicity with AmBisome (59% vs 38%, p=0.05). In disseminated histoplasmosis at 2 wks (NEJM 340:764, 1999).

From 2006 Drug Topics Red Book, Medical Economics Data and Hospital Formulary Pricing Guide. Price is average wholesale price (AWP).
§ Dosage recommendations are for adults (unless otherwise indicated) and assume normal renal function.
See page 2 for abbreviations.

TABLE 11B (2)

DRUG NAME, GENERIC (TRADE) NAME/ USUAL DOSAGE/COST*	ADVERSE EFFECTS/COMMENTS
Liposomal amphotericin B (L-AmB, AmBisome): 1-5mg/kg per day as single infusion. 50mg $157	**Admin:** Consists of vesicular bilayer liposome with ampho intercalated within the membrane. Dosage: **3-5mg/kg per day** (IV as single dose infused over a period of approx. 120min. If well tolerated, infusion time can be reduced to 60min. (see footnote 2, page 96) 1mg/kg per day was as effective as 4mg/kg per day (6mo survival rates 43% vs 37%, respectively) in pts with invasive aspergillosis complicating bone marrow transplant &/or neutropenia from malignancy (CID 27:1406, 1998). Tolerated well in elderly pts (J Inf 50:277, 2005). **Major tox:** less than other ampho B. Nephrotox 18.7% vs 33.7% for ampho B, chills 47% vs 75%, nausea 39.7% vs 38.7%, vomiting 31.8% vs 43.9%, rash 24% for both. Ca 18.4% vs 20.9%, ↓ K 20.4% vs 25.6%. Acute infusion-related reactions common with liposomal ampho B. 20–40%. 86% occur within 5min of infusion, incl chest pain, dyspnea, hypoxia or severe abdom, flank or leg pain; 14% dev flushing & urticaria near end of 4hr infusion. All responded to diphenhydramine (1mg/kg) & interruption of infusion. Reactions may be due to complement activation by liposome (CID 36:1213, 2003).
Amphotericin B cholesteryl complex (amphotericin B colloidal dispersion, ABCD, Amphotec): 3-4mg/kg per day as single infusion. 100mg $160	**Admin:** Consists of ampho B deoxycholate stabilized with cholesteryl sulfate resulting in a disc-shaped colloidal complex. Compared to standard ampho B, larger volume of distribution, rapid blood clearance, high tissue concentrations. Dosage: Initial dose for adults & children: **3–4mg/kg per day.** If necessary, can ↑ to 6mg/kg per day. Dilute in D5W & infuse at 1mg/kg per hr. Do NOT use in-line filter. **Toxicity:** Chills 50%, fever 33%, ↑ serum creatinine 12–20%, ↓ Ca 8%, ↓ K 17%. Hepatotoxicity more common (incidence 1.5) in bone marrow transplant pts than ampho B (inc. 0.78/100 pt days) (CID 41:1384-1387, 2005).
Caspofungin (Cancidas) 70mg IV on day 1 followed by 50mg IV q24h (reduce to 35mg IV q24h with moderate hepatic insufficiency) 70mg $509. 50mg $395	An echinocandin which inhibits synthesis of β-(1,3)-D-glucan. Fungicidal against candida (MIC <2mcg/mL) & active against aspergillus (MIC 0.4–2.7mcg/mL). In some preclinical studies very high drug concentrations found less effective clinically. Approved indications for caspo incl: empirical rx for febrile, neutropenic pts; rx of candidemia, candida intraabdominal abscesses, peritonitis, & pleural space infections, esophageal candidiasis; & invasive aspergillosis in pts refractory to or intolerant of other therapies. Serum levels on rec: dosages = peak 12, trough 1.3 (24hrs) mcg/mL. **Toxicity** (similar to fluconazole): rare (Mycosis 48:227, 2005). Only 2% of 263 pts in double-blind trial dc drug due to drug-related adverse event (transpl Inf Dis 7:55, 2002). 14% had ↓ transaminases (similar to triazoles). Most common adverse effect: pruritus at infusion site & headache, & rash. Drug interacts: ↑ level on cyclosporine in 8% on caspo vs 3%, short-course ampho B in 422 pts with candidemia (Ln, Oct 12, 2005, online). Drug metab ↓ in liver & dosage ↑ to 35mg in moderate to severe hepatic failure. Class C for preg (embryotoxic in rats & rabbits). See Table 22, page 184 for drug-drug interactions, esp. cyclosporine (hepatic toxicity) & tacrolimus (drug level monitoring recommended). Reversible thrombocytopenia reported (Pharmacotherap 24:1408, 2004).
Micafungin (Mycamine) 50mg/day for prophylaxis post-bone marrow stem cell trans: $157/day.	The 2nd echinocandin approved by FDA (Mar 2005) for rx of esophageal candidiasis & prophylaxis against candida infections in HSCT recipients (CID 39:1407, 2004). Active against most strains of candida sp. & aspergillus sp., incl those resist to fluconazole such as C. glabrata & C. krusei. No antagonism seen when combo with other antifungal drugs & co-synergism with ampho B & voriconazole (AAC 49:2994, 2005). No dosage adjust for severe renal impairment. Watch for ↑ LFTs during rx in pts with mild to moderate hepatic impairment. Monitor for ↓ hepatic or renal function. Few drug-drug interactions; can ↑ sirolimus 21% & nifedipine blood level 18%. Common adverse events incl nausea 7.8%, vomiting 2.4%, & headache 2.4%. Transient ↑ LFTs, BUN, creatinine reported; rare cases of significant hepatitis & renal insufficiency (pkg insert for micafungin). See CID 42:1171, 2006
Anidulafungin (Eraxis) For Candidemia: 200mg IV on day 1 followed by 100mg/day IV). Rx forEC: 100 mg IV x 1, then 50mg IV onceID: $90.00/d	An echinocandin with antifungal activity (cidal) against candida sp. & aspergillus sp. including ampho B- & triazole-resistant strains. FDA approved for treatment of esophageal candidiasis (EC), candidemia, and other invasive Candida infections. Effective in clinical trials of esophageal candidiasis & in 1 trial was superior to fluconazole in rx of invasive candidiasis/candidemia in 245 pts (75.6% vs 60.2%) (ICAAC 2005). Like other echinocandins, remarkably non-toxic; most common side-effects: nausea, vomiting, ↓ Mg, ↓ K, & diarrhea assoc with infusion. Few drug-drug interactions (see Table 22). Pregnancy Cat C. See CID 43:215, 2006
Fluconazole (Diflucan) 100mg tabs NB $16, G $0.90. 150mg tabs NB $16, G $2.80. 200mg tabs NB $16, G $2.00. 400mg IV NB $170, G $84. Oral suspension: 50mg per 5mL, $40/35mL bottle--NB	IV-oral dose because of excellent bioavailability. **Pharmacology:** absorbed po, water solubility enables IV. Peak serum levels (see Table 9, page 77), 1/2 30hr (range 20–50hr), protein bound <12%. CSF levels 50-90% of serum in normals in meningitis. No effect on mammalian steroid metabolism. **Drug-drug interactions common, see Table 22.** CSF levels 50–90% of serum. AEs: Nausea 3.7%, headache 1.9%, skin rash 1.8%, abdominal pain 1.7%, vomiting 1.7%, diarrhea 1.5%. ↑ SGOT 5% [more common in HIV+ pts (21%)]. Nausea 3.7%. headache 1.9%, skin rash 1.9%, alopecia (scalp, pubic crest) in 12–20% pts on ≥400mg po q24h after median of 3mo (reversible in approx. 6mo) (AnIM 123:354, 1995). Rare: severe hepatotoxicity (CID 41:301, 2005), exfoliative dermatitis. Anaphylaxis (BMJ 302:1341, 1991). Ref: AJM 330:263, 1994
Flucytosine (Ancobon) 500 mg/day $0.50	AEs: Overall 30%. GI 6% (diarrhea, anorexia, nausea, vomiting); hematologic 22% [leukopenia, thrombocytopenia, when serum level >100mcg/mL, esp. in azotemic pts]; hepatotoxicity (asymptomatic) ↑ SGOT (reversible); skin rash 7%, aplastic anemia (rare—2 or 3 cases). False ↑ in serum creatinine on EKTACHEM analyzer. (JAC 26:171, 2000)

TABLE 11B (3)

DRUG NAME, GENERIC (TRADE)/USUAL DOSAGE/COST*	ADVERSE EFFECTS/COMMENTS
Griseofulvin (Fulvicin, Grifulvin, Grisactin) 500mg G $2.70, susp 125mg/mL: 120mL $42	Photosensitivity, urticaria, GI upset, fatigue, leukopenia (rare). Interferes with warfarin drugs. Increases blood and urine porphyrins, should not be used in patients with porphyria. Minor disulfiram-like reactions. Exacerbation of systemic lupus erythematosus.
Imidazoles, topical For vaginal and/or skin use	Not recommended in 1st trimester of pregnancy. Local reactions: 0.5-1.5%: dyspareunia, mild vaginal or vulvar erythema, burning, pruritus, urticaria, rash. Rarely similar symptoms in sexual partner.
Itraconazole (Sporanox) 100 mg cap $10 10mg/mL oral solution (fasting state) (150 mL: $141) *(AAC 42:1862, 1998)* IV usual dose 200mg bid x 4 doses followed by 200mg q24h for a max of 14 days ($213/250 mg)	**Itraconazole tablet & solution forms not interchangeable, solution preferred.** Many authorities recommend measuring drug serum concentration after 2wk to ensure satisfactory absorption. To obtain highest plasma concentration, tablet is given with food & acidic drinks (e.g., cola) while solution is taken in fasted state; under these conditions, the peak conc. of capsule is approx. 3mcg/mL & of solution 5.4mcg/mL. Peak levels reached faster (2.2 vs 5hrs) with solution. **Peak plasma concentrations after IV injection (200mg) compared to oral capsule (200mg): 2.8mcg/mL (on day 7 of rx) vs 2mcg/mL (on day 36 of rx).** Protein-binding for both preparations is over 99%, which explains virtual absence of penetration into CSF **(do not use to treat meningitis)**. Most common adverse effects are dose-related nausea 10%, diarrhea 8%, vomiting 6%, & abdominal discomfort 5.7%. Allergic rash 8.6%, ↑ bilirubin 6%, edema 3.5%, & hepatitis 2.7% reported. ↑ doses may produce hypokalemia 8% & ↑ blood pressure 3.2%. Delirium & peripheral neuropathy reported *(Psychosomatics 44:260, 2003; Diabetes Care 28:225, 2005)*. **Reported to produce impairment in cardiac function** *(see footnote 2 page 80)*. Severe liver failure req transplant in pts receiving pulse rx for onychomycosis: FDA reports 24 cases with 11 deaths out of 50mill people who received the drug prior to 2001 *(Eur Acad Derm & Venereol 19:205, 2005)*. Other concern, as with fluconazole and ketoconazole, is **drug-drug interactions; see *Table 22***. Some can be life-threatening.
Ketoconazole (Nizoral) 200mg tab $2.25	Gastric acid required for absorption—cimetidine, omeprazole, antacids block absorption. In achlorhydria, dissolve tablet in 4 mL 0.2N HCl, drink with a straw. Coca-Cola ↑ absorption by 65% *(AAC 39:1671, 1995)*. CSF levels "none". **Drug-drug interactions important, see *Table 22*. Some interactions can be life-threatening. Dose- dependent nausea and vomiting.** Liver toxicity of hepatocellular type reported in about 1:10,000 exposed pts—usually after several days to weeks of exposure. At doses of ≥800 mg per day serum testosterone and plasma cortisol levels fall. With high doses, adrenal (Addisonian) crisis reported.
Miconazole (Monistat IV) 200mg—*not available in U.S.*	IV miconazole indicated in patient critically ill with Scedosporium (Pseudallescheria boydii) infection. Very toxic due to vehicle needed to get drug into solution.
Nystatin (Mycostatin) 30gm cream NB $30, G $4 500,000 units oral tab $0.70	Topical: virtually no adverse effects. Less effective than imidazoles and triazoles. PO: large doses give occasional GI distress and diarrhea.
Posaconazole *(Noxafil)* 400mg po bid with meals (if not taking meals, 200mg qid). No cost data available. *(See Drugs 65:1552, 2005)* 200mg po TID (with food) for prophylaxis	An oral triazole with activity against a wide range of fungi refractory to other antifungal rx including: aspergillosis, zygomycosis, fusariosis, Scedosporium (Pseudallescheria), phaeohyphomycosis, histoplasmosis, refractory candidiasis, refractory coccidioidomycosis, refractory cryptococcosis, & refractory chromoblastomycosis. Approved for prophylaxis. Clinical response in 75% of 176 AIDS pts with azole-refractory oral/esophageal candidiasis. Posaconazole has similar toxicities as other triazoles: nausea 9%, vomiting 6%, abd. pain 5%, headache 5%, diarrhea, ↑ ALT, AST, & rash (3% each). In pts rx for >6 mos., serious side-effects have included adrenal insufficiency, nephrotoxicity, & QTc interval prolongation. Significant drug-drug interactions; inhibits CYP3A4 *(see Table 22)*.
Terbinafine (Lamisil) 250mg tab $12	In pts rec terbinafine for onychomycosis, rare cases (8) of idiosyncratic & symptomatic hepatic injury & more rarely liver failure leading to death or liver transplant. The drug is **not recommended** for pts with **chronic or active liver disease;** hepatotoxicity may occur in pts with or without pre-existing disease. Pretreatment serum transaminases (ALT & AST) advised & alternate rx used for those with abnormal levels. Pts started on terbinafine should be warned about symptoms suggesting liver dysfunction (persistent nausea, anorexia, fatigue, vomiting, RUQ pain, jaundice, dark urine or pale stools). If symptoms develop, drug should be discontinued & liver function immediately evaluated. In controlled trials, changes in ocular lens and retina reported—clinical significance unknown. Major drug-drug interaction is 100% ↑ in rate of clearance by rifampin. AEs: usually mild, transient and rarely caused discontinuation of rx. % with AE, terbinafine vs placebo: nausea/diarrhea 2.6–5.6 vs 2.9; rash 5.6 vs 2.2; taste abnormality 2.8 vs 0.7. Inhibits CYP2D6 enzymes *(see Table 22)*. An acute generalized exanthematous pustulosis has been reported in 13 cases *(Brit J Derm 152:780, 2005)* & 5 cases of subacute cutaneous lupus erythematosus *(Acta Derm Venerol 84:472, 2004)*.

* *From 2006 Drug Topics Red Book, Medical Economics Data and Hospital Formulary Pricing Guide.* **Price is average wholesale price (AWP).**
See page 2 for abbreviations. All dosage recommendations are for adults (unless otherwise indicated) and assume normal renal function

TABLE 11B (4)

DRUG NAME, GENERIC (TRADE/USUAL DOSAGE/COST*	ADVERSE EFFECTS/COMMENTS
Voriconazole (Vfend) IV: Loading dose 6 mg per kg q12h times 1 day, then 4 mg per kg q12h iv for invasive aspergillosis & serious mold infections; **3 mg per kg IV q12h** for serious candida infections. 200mg IV = $116 **Oral: >40 kg body weight: 400** mg po q12h times 1 day, then 200 mg po q12h. 200mg po q. = $37 **<40 kg body weight: 200** mg po q12h times 1 day, then 100 mg po q12h **Take oral dose 1 hour before or 1 hour after eating.** Oral suspension (40 mg per mL) $45/200 mg dose. Oral suspension dosing: Same as for oral tabs. Reduce to ½ maintenance dose for moderate hepatic insufficiency	A triazole with activity against Aspergillus sp., **including Ampho resistant strains of A. terreus** (*J Clin Micro* 37:2343, 1999). Active vs Candida sp. (including krusei), Fusarium sp., & various molds. Steady state serum levels reach 2.5–4 mcg per mL. Toxicity similar to other azoles/triazoles including uncommon serious hepatic toxicity (hepatitis, cholestasis & fulminant hepatic failure. Liver function tests should be monitored during rx & drug dc'd if abnormalities develop. Rash reported in up to 20%, occ. photosensitivity & rare Stevens-Johnson. **Approx. 21% experience a transient visual disturbance** following IV or po ("altered/enhanced visual perception", blurred or colored visual change or photophobia) within 30–60 minutes. Visual changes resolve within 30–60 min. after administration & are attenuated with repeated doses (**do not drive at night for outpatient rx**). No persistence of effect reported. Cause unknown. In patients with ClCr <50 mL per min., the drug should be given orally, not IV, since the intravenous vehicle (SBECD-sulfobutyl/ether-B cyclodextrin) may accumulate. Hallucinations, hypoglycemia, electrolyte disturbance & pneumonitis attributed to ↑ drug concentrations (*CID* 39:1241, 2004). Potential for drug-drug interactions high—see *Table 22* (*CID* 36:630, 1087, 1122, 2003). **NOTE:** Not in urine in active form. **Cost:** 50 mg tab $9; 200 mg tab $35; 200 mg IV $109

Continued from top right of table: infusion reactions with fever and hypertension (*Clin Exp Dermatol* 26:648, 2001). 1 case of QT prolongation with ventricular tachycardia in a 15 y/o pt with ALL reported (*CID* 39:3864, 2004)

Table 11C – IN VITRO ACTIVITY OF SELECTED ANTIFUNGAL DRUGS AGAINST PATHOGENIC FUNGI

Microorganism	Antifungal[1-4]				
	Fluconazole[5]	Voriconazole	Posaconazole	Echinocandin	Polyenes
Candida albicans	+++	+++	+++	+++	+++
Candida glabrata	±	+	+	+++	++
Candida tropicalis	+++	+++	+++	+++	+++
Candida parapsilosis[6]	+++	+++	+++	++ (higher MIC)	+++
Candida krusei	-	++	++	+++	++
Candida guilliermondii	+++	+++	+++	++ (higher MIC)	++
Cryptococcus neoformans	+++	+++	+++	-	+++
Aspergillus fumigatus[7]	-	+++	+++	++	++
Aspergillus flavus[7]	-	+++	+++	++	++ (higher MIC)
Aspergillus terreus	-	++	++	++	-
Fusarium sp.	-	++	++	-	++ (lipid formulations)
Scedosporium apiospermum (Pseudoallescheria boydii)	-	+++	+++	±	±
Scedosporium prolificans[8]	-	±	±	-	-
Zygomycetes (e.g., Absidia, Mucor, Rhizopus)	-	-	+++	-	+++ (lipid formulations)
Dematiaceous molds[9] (e.g., Alternaria, Bipolaris, Curvularia, Exophiala)	±	+++	+++	-	+
Dimorphic Fungi[10]					
Blastomyces dermatitidis	+	++	++	-	+++
Coccidioides immitis/posadasii	+++	+++	+++	-	+++
Histoplasma capsulatum	+	++	++	-	+++
Sporothrix schenckii	+	++	++	-	+++

- = no activity; ± = possibly activity; + = active, 3rd line therapy (least active clinically)
++ = Active, 2nd line therapy (less active clinically); +++ = Active, 1st line therapy (usually active clinically)

1. Minimum inhibitory concentration values do not always predict clinical outcome.
2. Echinocandins, voriconazole, posaconazole and polyenes have poor urine penetration.
3. During severe immune suppression, success requires immune reconstitution.
4. Flucytosine has activity against Candida sp., Cryptococcus sp., and demaltiaceous molds, but is primarily used in combination therapy.
5. For infections secondary to Candida sp., patients with prior triazole therapy have higher likelihood of triazole resistance.
6. Successful treatment of infections from Candida parapsilosis requires removal of foreign body or intravascular device.
7. Lipid formulations of amphotericin may have greater activity against A. fumigatus and A. flavus (+++).
8. Scedosporium prolificans is poorly susceptible to single agents and may require combination therapy (e.g., addition of terbinafine).
9. Infections from zygomycetes, some Aspergillus spp. and dematiaceous molds often require surgical debridement.
10. For dimorphic fungi, itraconazole is first-line therapy and active clinically (+++).

TABLE 12A – TREATMENT OF MYCOBACTERIAL INFECTIONS*

Tuberculin skin test (TST). Same as PPD [MMWR 52(RR-2):15, 2003]
Criteria for positive TST after 5 tuberculin units (intermediate PPD) read at 48-72 hours:
≥5 mm induration: + HIV, immunosuppressed, recent close contact
≥10 mm induration: foreign-born, countries with high prevalence; IVDusers; low income; NH residents; chronic illness; silicosis
≥15 mm induration: otherwise healthy

Two-stage to detect sluggish positivity: If 1st PPD + but <10 mm, repeat intermediate PPD in 1wk. Response to 2nd PPD can also happen if pt received BCG in childhood.
BCG vaccine as child: If ≥10 mm induration, & from country with TBc, should be attributed to M. tuberculosis. In areas of low TB prevalence, TST reactions of ≤18mm more likely from BCG than TB [CID 40:1457, 2005]. Prior BCG may result in booster effect in 2-stage TST [AMJ 161:1760, 2001; Clin Micro Inf 10:980, 2005].
Routine anergy testing no longer recommended in HIV+ or HIV-negative patients [JAMA 283:2003, 2000].

Whole blood interferon-gamma release assay (QuantiFERON-TB [QFT]) approved by U.S. FDA as diagnostic test for TB [JAMA 286:1740, 2001; CID 34:1449 & 1457, 2002]. CDC recommends TST for TB suspects & pts at ↑ risk for progression to active TB & suggests either TST or QFT for individuals at ↑ risk for latent TB (LTBI) & for persons who warrant testing but are deemed at low risk for LTBI [MMWR 52(RR-2):15, 2003]. IFN-γ assay is better indicator of TBc risk than TST in BCG-vaccinated population [JAMA 293:2756, 2005]. A more sensitive assay based on M. tbc-specific antigens (QuantiFERON-TB GOLD) was approved by the USFDA 5/2/05 and an enzyme-linked immunospot method (ELISpot) using antigens specific for MTB (do not cross-react with BCG) is under evaluation & looks promising [Thorax 58:916, 2003; Ln 361:1168, 2003; AnlM 140:709, 2004; LnID 4:761, 2005; CID 4:761, 2005; JAMA 293:2756, 2005; MMWR 54:49, 2005].

CAUSATIVE AGENT/DISEASE	MODIFYING CIRCUMSTANCES	INITIAL THERAPY	SUGGESTED REGIMENS CONTINUATION PHASE OF THERAPY
I. Mycobacterium tuberculosis exposure but TST negative (household members & other close contacts of potentially infectious cases)	Neonate—Rx essential	INH (10mg/kg/ day for 3mo)	Repeat tuberculin skin test (TST) in 3mo. If mother's smear neg & infant's TST neg & chest x-ray (CXR) normal, stop INH. In UK, BCG is then given [Ln 2:1479, 1990], unless mother HIV+. If infant's repeat TST +&/or CXR abnormal (hilar adenopathy &/or infiltrate), INH + RIF (10-20 mg/kg/day) (or SM). Total (x 6mo. If mother is being rx, separation of infant from mother not indicated.
	Children <5 years of age— Rx indicated	As for neonate for 1-3 mos.	If repeat TST at 3mo is neg, stop. If repeat TST +, continue INH for total of 9mo. If INH not given initially, repeat TST at 3mo, if
	Older children & adults— risk 2-4% 1st yr	No rx	No rx

(Continued on next page)

* Dosages are for adults (unless otherwise indicated) and assume normal renal function   † DOT = directly observed therapy

TABLE 12A (2)

CAUSATIVE AGENT/DISEASE	MODIFYING CIRCUMSTANCES	SUGGESTED REGIMENS	
		INITIAL THERAPY	ALTERNATIVE
II. Treatment of latent infection with M. tuberculosis (formerly known as "prophylaxis) *NEJM 347:1860, 2002; NEJM 350:2060, 2004; JAMA 293:2776, 2005)* **A. INH indicated due to high-risk.** Assumes that pts susceptibly infected. INH 54–88% effective in preventing active TB for ≥2yr.	(1) + tuberculin reactor & HIV+ (risk of active TBc in HIV+ pts after INH usually due to reinfection, not INH failure (*CID 34:386, 2002*). (2) Newly infected persons (TST conversion in past 2 yrs—risk 3.3% 1st yr) (3) Past tuberculosis, not rx with adequate chemotherapy (INH, RIF or alternatives) (risk 0.5–5.0% per yr) (4) + tuberculin reactors with CXR consistent with non-progressive tuberculous disease (risk 0.5–5.0% per yr) (5) + tuberculin reactors with specific predisposing conditions: illicit IV drug use (*MMWR 38:236, 1989*), silicosis, diabetes mellitus, prolonged adrenocortical rx (>15mg/day prednisone/day), immunosuppressive rx, hematologic diseases (Hodgkin's, leukemia), or dialysis renal disease, clinical condition with rapid substantial weight loss or chronic under-nutrition, previous gastrectomy (*ARRD 134: 355, 1986*) (6) + tuberculin reactors due to start anti-TNF-(alpha) therapy. For management algorithm see *Thorax 60:800, 2005.* **NOTE: For HIV, see Sanford Guide to HIV/AIDS Therapy &/or MMWR 48:RR-10, 1999**	**INH** (5mg/kg/day, max 300mg/ day for adults; 10mg/kg/day for children). May use 2x/wk INH with DOT (*MMWR 52:735, 2003*). Optimal duration 9 mos. (includes children, HIV-, HIV+, old fibrotic lesions on chest x-ray). In some cases, 6 mos. may be given for cost-effectiveness (*AJRCCM 161:S221, 2000*. Do not use 6 mo. regimen in HIV+ persons <18yr, or those with fibrotic lesions on chest film (*NEJM 345:189, 2001*).	If compliance problem: **INH** by DOT 15mg/kg 2x/wk times 9mo. 2mo. **RIF + PZA** regimen effective in HIV- and HIV+ pts (*AJRCCM 161:S221, 2000; JAMA 281:1445, 2000*). **However, there are recent descriptions of severe & fatal hepatitis in immunocompetent pts on RIF + PZA** (*MMWR 50:289, 2001*). Monitoring for cofactors doesn't allow prediction of fatalities. (*CID 42:346, 2006*). Therefore, regimen is no longer rec for LTBI (*MMWR 52:735, 2003; CID 39:488, 2004*). Risk appears lower in HIV+ pts (*CID 39:561, 2004*). **RIF** 600mg/day po for 4mo. (HIV- and HIV+). Meta-analysis suggests 3mo of INH + RIF may be equiv to 'standard' (6-12mo) INH therapy (*CID 40:670, 2005*).
B. TST positive (organisms likely to be INH-susceptible)	Age no longer considered modifying factor (see Comments)	**INH** (5 mg per kg per day, max. 300 mg per day for adults; 10 mg per kg per day for children); 9 mos. rx of as effective as 12 mos. (65% vs 75% reduction in disease). 9 mos. is current recommendation. See I/A above for details and alternate rx.	Reanalysis of earlier studies favors **INH** prophylaxis (if INH related, hepatitis case fatality rate <1% and TB case fatality 6.7%, which appears to be the case) (*AIM 150:2517, 1990*). Recent data suggest INH positive risk-benefit ratio in pts ≥35 if monitored for hepatotoxicity (*AnIM 127:1051, 1997*). Overall risk of hepatotoxicity 0.1–0.15% (*JAMA 281:1014, 1999*).
	Pregnancy—Any risk factors (II.A above)	Treat with **INH** as above. For women at risk for progression of latent to active disease, esp. those with HIV+ or who have been recently infected, rx should not be delayed even during the first trimester.	Risk of INH hepatitis may be ↑ (*JID 346:199, 1995*)
	Pregnancy—No risk factors	No initial rx. (see Comment)	Delay rx until after delivery (*AJRCCM 149:1359, 1994*)
C. TST positive & drug resistance likely (For data on worldwide prevalence of drug resistance, see *NEJM 344:1294, 2001; JID 185:1197, 2002*)	INH-resistant (or adverse reaction to INH), RIF-sensitive organisms likely	**RIF** 600 mg per day po for 4 mos. (HIV+ or HIV-)	IDSA guideline lists rifabutin in 600 mg per day dose as another alternative; however, current recommended dose of rifabutin is 300 mg per day.
	INH- and RIF-resistant organisms likely	Efficacy of all regimens uncertain. RIF-resistant: [**PZA** 25–30 mg per kg per day + **ETB** 15–25 mg per kg per day po] times 6–12 mos.	Estimate RIF alone has protective effect of 56%, 26% of pts reported adverse effects (only 2/157 did not complete rx) (*AJRCCM 155:1735, 1997*). [**PZA** 25 mg per kg per day to max. of 2 gm + **oflox** 400 mg per kg bid] all po; times 6–12 mos. PZA + oflox associated with asymptomatic hepatitis (*CID 24:1264, 1997*).

See page 2 for abbreviations, page 1/5 for footnotes

Dosages are for adults (unless otherwise indicated) and assume normal renal function   *Indicates first choice*   † **DOT** = directly observed therapy

TABLE 12A (3)

CAUSATIVE AGENT/DISEASE	MODIFYING CIRCUMSTANCES	SUGGESTED REGIMENS					COMMENTS
		INITIAL PHASE[a]			CONTINUATION PHASE OF THERAPY[f] (in vitro susceptibility known)		
		Regimen in order of preference	Drugs	Interval/Doses[1] (min. duration)	Regimen	Drugs	Interval/Doses[1,2] (min. duration)	Range of Total Doses (min. duration)	
III. Mycobacterium tuberculosis A. Pulmonary TB [General reference on rx in adults & children: Ln 362; 887; 2003; MMWR 52(RR-11):1, 2003; CID 40(Supp1): S1, 2005] Isolation essential Pts with active TB should be isolated in single rooms, not cohorted (MMWR 54(RR-17), 2005). Older observations on infectivity of susceptible & resistant M. tbc before and after rx (ARRD 85:5111, 1962) may not be applicable to MDR M. tbc or to the HIV+ individual. Extended isolation may be appropriate. See footnotes, page 115 USE DOT REGIMENS IF POSSIBLE (continued on next page)	Rate of INH resistance known to be <4% (drug-susceptible organisms) [Modified from MMWR 52 (RR-11):1, 2003]	1 (See Figure 1, page 114)	INH RIF PZA ETB	7 days per wk times 56 doses (8 wk) or 5 days per wk times 40 doses (8 wk)[b]	1a	INH/RIF[4]	7 days per wk times 126 doses (18 wk) or 5 days per wk times 90 doses [18 wk][b]	182-130 (26 wk)	See COMMENTS FOR DOSAGE AND DIRECTLY OBSERVED THERAPY (DOT) REGIMENS
					1b	INH/RIF	2 times per wk times 36 doses (18 wk)	92-76 [26 wk][4]	
					1c[3]	INH/RFP	1 time per wk times 18 doses (18 wk)	74-58 [26 wk]	
		2 (See Figure 1, page 114)	INH RIF PZA ETB	7 days per wk times 14 doses (2 wk), then 2 times per wk times 12 doses (6 wk) or 5 days per wk times 10 doses (2 wk) then 2 times per wk times 12 doses (6 wk)[b]	2a	INH/RIF	2 times per wk times 36 doses (18 wk)	62-58 (26 wk)[4]	
					2b[3]	INH/RFP	1 time per wk times 18 doses (18 wk)	44-40 (26 wk)	
		3 (See Figure 1, page 114)	INH RIF PZA ETB	3 times per wk times 24 doses (8 wk)	3a	INH/RIF	3 times per wk times 54 doses (18 wk)	78 (26 wk)	
		4 (See Figure 1, page 114)	INH RIF PZA ETB	7 days per wk times 56 doses (8 wk) or 5 days per wk times 40 doses (8 wk)[b]	4a	INH/RIF[4]	7 days per wk times 217 doses (31 wk) or 5 days per wk times 155 doses [31 wk][b]	273-195 (39 wk)	
					4b	INH/RIF[4]	2 times per wk times 62 doses (31 wk)	118-102 (39 wk)	

COMMENTS — Doses in mg per kg (max. q24h dose):

Regimen[*]	INH	RIF	PZA	ETB	SM	RFB
Q24h:						
Child	10-20 (300)	10-20 (600)	15-30 (2000)	15-30 (1000)	20-40 (1000)	10-20 (300)
Adult	5 (300)	10 (600)	15-30 (2000)	15-25 (1000)	15 (1000)	5 (300)
2 times per wk (DOT):						
Child	20-40 (900)	10-20 (600)	50-70 (4000)	50	25-30 (1500)	10-20 (300)
Adult	15 (900)	10 (600)	50-70 (4000)	50	25-30	5 (300)
3 times per wk (DOT):						
Child	20-40 (900)	10-20 (600)	50-70 (3000)	25-30	25-30 (1500)	NA
Adult	15 (900)	10 (600)	50-70 (3000)	25-30	25-30	NA

Second-line anti-TB agents can be dosed as follows to facilitate DOT: Cycloserine 500-750 mg po q24h (5 times per wk) Ethionamide 500-750 mg po q24h (5 times per wk) Kanamycin or capreomycin 15 mg per kg IM/IV q24h (3-5 times per wk) Ciprofloxacin 750 mg po q24h (5 times per wk) Ofloxacin 600-800 mg po q24h (5 times per wk) Levofloxacin 750 mg po q24h (5 times per wk) (CID 21:1245, 1995)

Risk factors for drug-resistant TB: Recent immigration from Latin America or Asia or living in area of TB resistance (≥4%) or previous rx without RIF; exposure to known MDR TB. Incidence of MDR TB in U.S. appears to have stabilized and may be slightly decreasing in early 1990s (JAMA 278:833, 1997). Incidence of primary drug resistance is particularly high (>25%) in parts of China, Thailand, Russia, Estonia & Latvia (NEJM 344:1294, 2001; NEJM 347:1850, 2002). (continued on next page)

TABLE 12A (4)

CAUSATIVE AGENT/DISEASE	MODIFYING CIRCUMSTANCES	SUGGESTED REGIMEN[a]	DURATION OF TREATMENT (mo)	SPECIFIC COMMENTS[1]	COMMENTS
III. Mycobacterium tuberculosis A. Pulmonary TB (continued from previous page) **REFERENCE:** CID 22:683, 1996	INH (± SM) resistance	RIF, PZA, ETB (an FQ may strengthen the regimen for pts with extensive disease). Emergence of FQ resistance is a concern (LnID 3:432, 2005).	6	(continued from previous page) In British Medical Research Council trials, 6-mo. regimens have yielded >95% success rates despite resistance to INH if 4 drugs were used in the initial phase & RIF + ETB or SM was used throughout (ARRD 133: 423, 1986). Additional studies suggested that results were best if PZA was also used throughout the 6 mos (ARRD 136:1339, 1997). PZA was used & employed in 5MRC studies, it may strengthen the regimen for pts with more extensive disease. INH should be stopped in cases of INH resistance [see MMWR 52/RR-11):1, 2003 for additional discussion].	(continued from previous page) For MDR TB, consider rifabutin; ~30% RIF-resistant strains are rifabutin-susceptible). Note that CIP not as effective as PZA + ETB in multidrug regimen for susceptible TB (CID 22:287, 1996). Moxifloxacin, gatifloxacin and levofloxacin have enhanced activity compared with CIP against M. tuberculosis (AAC 46: 1022, 2002; AAC 47:2442, 2003; AAC 47:3117, 2003; JAC 53:441, 2004; JAC 48:780, 2004). FQ resistance may be seen in pts previously treated with FQ (CID 37:1448, 2003). Linezolid has excellent in vitro activity, including MDR strains (AAC 47: 416, 2003). Mortality reviewed: Ln 349:71, 1997
Multidrug-Resistant Tuberculosis (MDR TB): Defined as resistant to at least 2 drugs. Pt clusters with high mortality (AnIM 117:177, 1992; EJCMID 23: 174, 2004; MMWR 55:305, 2006). Reviews of therapy for MDR TB: JAC 54:593, 2004; Med Lett 2:83, 2004 **See footnotes, page 115**	Resistance to INH & RIF (± SM)	FQ, PZA, ETB, IA & alternative agent[7]	18-24	In such cases, extended rx is needed to ↓ the risk of relapse: in cases with extensive disease, the use of an additional agent (alternative agents) may be prudent to ↓ the risk of failure & additional acquired drug resistance. Preactional surgery may be appropriate.	Rapid (24-hr) diagnostic tests for M. tuberculosis: (1) The Amplified Mycobacterium tuberculosis Direct Test amplifies and detects M. tuberculosis ribosomal RNA. (2) The AMPLICOR Mycobacterium tuberculosis Test amplifies and detects M. tuberculosis DNA. Both tests have sensitivities & specificities >95% in sputum samples that are AFB-positive. In negative smears, specificity remains >95% while sensitivity is 40–77% (AJRCCM 155:1497, 1997). Note that MTB may grow out on standard blood agar plates in 1–2 wks (J Clin Micro 47:1710,2003).
	Resistance to INH, RIF (± INH), & ETB or PZA	FQ (ETB or PZA if active), IA, & 2 alternative agents[7]	24	Use the first-line agents to which there is susceptibility. Add 2 or more alternative agents in case of extensive disease. Surgery should be considered. Survival ↑ in pts receiving active FQ & surgical intervention (AJRCCM 169:1103, 2004).	
	Resistance to RIF	INH, ETB, FQ, supplemented with PZA for the first 2 mos. An IA may be included for the first 2-3 mos for pts with extensive disease)	12-18	Q24h & 3 times per wk regimens of INH, PZA, & SM given for 9 mos. were effective in a BMRC trial (ARRD 115:727, 1977). However, extended use of an IA may be prudent. ETB would be an effective as SM in these regimens. An all-oral regimen times 12-18 mos should be effective. But for more extensive disease &/or to shorten duration (e.g., to 12 mos.), an IA may be added in the initial 2 mos. of rx.	

CAUSATIVE AGENT/DISEASE; MODIFYING CIRCUMSTANCES	SUGGESTED REGIMENS (in vitro susceptibility known)		COMMENTS
	INITIAL THERAPY	**CONTINUATION PHASE OF THERAPY**	
B. Extrapulmonary TB	INH + RIF (or RFB) + PZA (q24h times 2 months) Authors add pyridoxine 25–50 mg po q24h to regimens that include INH.	INH + RIF (or RFB)	6mo regimens probably effective. Most experience with 9–12mo regimens. Am Acad Ped (1994) recommends 6mo rx for isolated cervical adenitis, renal and 12mo for meningitis, miliary, bone/joint. DOT useful here as well as for pulmonary tuberculosis. IDSA recommends 6mo for pulmonary TB, pleural, pericardial, disseminated disease, genitourinary & peritoneal TBc; 6–9mo for bone & joint; 9–12mo for CNS (including meningitis) TB. Corticosteroids 'strongly rec' only for pericarditis & meningeal TBc (MMWR 52/RR-11):1, 2003).
C. Tuberculous meningitis For critical appraisal of adjunctive steroids: CID 25:872, 1997	INH + RIF + ETB + PZA	May omit ETB when susceptibility to INH and RIF established. See Table 9, page 78, for CSF drug penetration. Initial reg of INH + RIF + SM + PZA also effective, even in pt with INH resistant organisms (JID 192:79, 2005).	3 drugs often rec for initial rx; we prefer 4. May sub ethionamide for ETB. Infection with MDR TB ↑ mortality & morbidity (CID 38:851, 2004; JID 192:79, 2005). Dexamethasone (for 1st mo) has been shown to ↓ complications (Pediatrics 99:226, 1997) & ↑ survival in pts >1yr old (NEJM 351:1741, 2004). PCR of CSF markedly ↑ diagnostic sensitivity and provides rapid dx (J Inf 36:597, 1998) but overall sensitivity dependent on method used (LnID 3:633, 2003). ↓survival in HIV pts (JID 192:2134, 2005)

See page 2 for abbreviations, page 115 for footnotes • Dosages are for adults (unless otherwise indicated) and assume normal renal function [1] DOT = directly observed therapy

114

TABLE 12A (5)

FIGURE 1: TREATMENT ALGORITHM FOR TUBERCULOSIS *(Modified from MMWR 52(RR-11):1, 2003)*

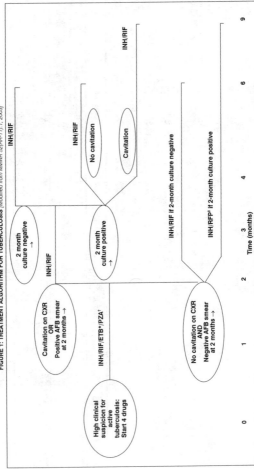

If the pt has HIV infection & the CD4 cell count is <100 per mcL, the continuation phase should consist of q24h or 3 times per wk INH & RIF for 4–7 months.
* ETB may be discontinued in <2 months if drug susceptibility testing indicate no drug resistance. † PZA may be discontinued after 2 months (56 doses). ‡ RFP should not be used in HIV patients with tuberculosis or in patients with extrapulmonary tuberculosis.

See page 2 for abbreviations

TABLE 12A (6)

CAUSATIVE AGENT/DISEASE; MODIFYING CIRCUMSTANCES	SUGGESTED REGIMENS		COMMENTS
	INITIAL THERAPY	CONTINUATION PHASE OF THERAPY (in vitro susceptibility known)	
III. Mycobacterium tuberculosis *(continued)*			
D. Tuberculosis during pregnancy	**INH + RIF + ETB** for 9mo		PZA not recommended: teratogenicity data inadequate. Because of potential ototoxicity to fetus throughout gestation (16%), SM should not be used unless other drugs contraindicated. Add pyridoxine 25 mg per day for pregnant women on INH. Breast-feeding should not be discouraged in pts on first-line drugs *(MMWR 52:RR-11):1, 2003)*
E. Treatment failure or relapse: Usually due to poor compliance or resistant organisms *(AJM 102:164, 1997)*	Directly observed therapy *(DOT)*. Check susceptibilities. *(See Section III.A, page 112 & above)*		Pts whose sputum has not converted after 5–6 mos. = treatment failures. Failures may be due to non-compliance or resistant organisms. Check susceptibilities of original isolates and obtain susceptibility on current isolates. Non-compliance common, therefore institute DOT. If isolates show resistance, use at least 2 effective agents, preferably ones which pt has not received. Surgery may be necessary in pts with TB but extra-pulmonary disease. In HIV+ patients, reinfection is a possible explanation for "failure"
	MODIFYING CIRCUMSTANCES	**SUGGESTED REGIMENS**	**COMMENTS**
		PRIMARY/ALTERNATIVE	
CAUSATIVE AGENT/DISEASE			
F. HIV Infection and AIDS—pulmonary or extrapulmonary (NOTE: 60–70% of HIV+ pts with TB have extrapulmonary disease)	**INH + RIF (or RFB) + PZA** q24h times 2 months.	**INH + RIF** (or RFB) + **PZA** q24h times 4 months (total 6 mos.). May treat up to 9 mos. in pts with delayed response.	1. Because of possibility of developing resistance to RIF in pts with low CD4 cell counts who receive wkly or biwkly (2x/wk) doses of RFB, it is recom. that such pts receive q24h (or min 3x/wk) doses of RFB for initiation & continuation phase of rx.
	(Authors add **pyridoxine** 25–50 mg per day on q24h to regimens that include INH)		2. Clinical & microbiologic response same as in HIV-neg patient although there is considerable variability in outcomes among currently available studies *(CID 32:623, 2001).*
			3. Post-treatment suppression not necessary for drug-susceptible strains.
			4. Rate of INH resistance known to <4% for ↑ rates of resistance, see Section III.A
			5. More info: see *MMWR 47(RR-20):1, 1998; CID 28:139, 1999; MMWR 52(RR-11):1, 2003*
			6. May use partially intermittent therapy: 1 dose per day for 2 weeks followed by 2–3 doses per wk for 2–6wk *(MMWR 47(RR-20), 1998)*
			7. Adjunctive prednisolone of NO benefit in HIV+ patients with TBc pleurisy *(JID 190:869, 2004).* *JID 191:856, 2005)* or in patients with TBc meningitis *(JID 190:869, 2004).*
—Concomitant protease inhibitor (PI) therapy *(Modified from MMWR 49:185, 2000, AJRCCM 152:7, 2001)*	**Initial & cont. therapy:** **INH** 300 mg + **RFB** (see below for dose) + **PZA** 25 mg per kg + **ETB** 15 mg per kg q24h times 2 mos., then **INH** + **RFB** times 4 mos. (up to 7 mos.)	**Alternative regimen:** **INH** + **SM** + **PZA** + **ETB** times 2 mo, then **INH** + **SM** + **PZA** 2–3 x per wk for 7 mo. May be prolonged up to 12 mo in pts with delayed response.	**Comments:** Rifamycins induce cytochrome CYP450 enzymes (RIF > RFB) & reduce serum levels of concomitantly administered PIs. Conversely, PIs (ritonavir > RFB) indinavir = nelfinavir > saquinavir) inhibit CYP450 & cause ↑ serum levels of RIF, RFP & RFB. If dose of RFB is not reduced, toxicity.[1] RFB/PI combinations are therapeutically effective *(CID 30:779, 2000).* RFB has no effect on nelfinavir levels at dose of 1250 mg *(Can JID 10:21B, 1999).* Although RFB is preferred, RIF can be used for rx of active TB in pts receiving PIs or ritonavir + saquinavir because drug-induced hepatitis with marked transaminase elevations has been seen in healthy volunteers receiving this regimen (Roche; www.fda.gov). **RIF should not be administered to pts who are on regimens containing efavirenz or ritonavir.**
	PI Regimen	**RFB Dose**	
	Nelfinavir 1200mg q12h or indinavir 1000mg q8h or amprenavir 1200mg q12h	150 mg q24h or 300 mg intermittently	
	Lopinavir/ritonavir‑Lopinavir/ritonavir standard dose	150 mg 2x per wk	

FOOTNOTES: [1] When DOT is used, drugs may be given 5 days/wk & necessary number of doses adjusted accordingly. Although no studies compare 5 with 7 q24h doses, extensive experience indicates that this would be an effective practice. [2] Patients with cavitation on initial chest x-ray & positive cultures at completion of 2mo of rx should receive 7mo (31 wk, either 217 doses [q24h] or 62 doses [2x/wk] continuation phase. 5 day/wk admin is always given by DOT. [3] Not recommended for HIV-infected pts with CD4 cell counts <100 cells/mcL. [4] Options 1c & 2b should be used only in HIV-neg. pts who have neg. sputum smears at the time of completion of 2mo rx & do not have cavitation on initial chest x-ray. For pts started on this regimen & found to have a positive culture from 2mo specimen, rx should be extended extra 3mo. [5] Options 4a & 4b should be considered only when options 1–3 cannot be given. Alternative agents = ethionamide, cycloserine, p-aminosalicylic acid, clarithromycin, AM-CL, linezolid. [6] Modified from *MMWR 52(RR-11):1, 2003.* See also *IDCP 11:329, 2002.* [7] Continuation regimen with INH+ETB less effective than INH/RIF *(Lancet 364:1244, 2004).*

See page 2 for abbreviations, page 115 for footnotes

Dosages are for adults (unless otherwise indicated) and assume normal renal function   † **DOT** = directly observed therapy

TABLE 12A (7)

CAUSATIVE AGENT/DISEASE	MODIFYING CIRCUMSTANCES	SUGGESTED REGIMENS		COMMENTS
		PRIMARY	ALTERNATIVE	
IV. Other Mycobacterial Disease ("Atypical") (See ATS Consensus: AJRCCM 152:51, 1997; IDC: No. Amer. March 2002; CMR 15:716, 2002; CID 42:1756, 2006)				
A. M. bovis				The M. tuberculosis complex includes M. bovis. All isolates resistant to PZA. 9–12 months of rx used by some authorities. Isolation not required.
B. Bacillus Calmette-Guerin (BCG) (derived from M. bovis)	Only fever (>38.5°C) for 12–24 hrs	**INH** 300 mg q24h times 3 months		Intravesical BCG effective in superficial bladder tumors and carcinoma in situ. Adverse effects: fever 2.9%, granulomatosis, pneumonitis, hepatitis 0.7%, sepsis 0.4% (J Urol 147:596, 1992). With sepsis, consider initial adjunctive prednisolone. Resistant to PZA. BCG may cause regional adenitis or pulmonary disease in HIV-infected children (CID 31:1226, 2000).
	Systemic illness or sepsis	**INH** 300 mg + **RIF** 600 mg + **ETB**	**INH** 300 mg + RIF 600 mg + **ETB** 1200 mg po q24h times 6 mos.	
C. M. avium-intracellulare complex (MAC, MAI, or Battey bacillus) ATS Consensus Statement: AJRCCM 156:51, 1997. Clin Chest Med 23:633, 2002	**Immunocompetent patients** with infection, usually disseminated or localized disease (subcutaneous, bone)	**Clarithro** 500 mg po bid (or **azithro** 600 mg po q24h) + **ETB** 25 mg per kg q24h times 2 mos., then 15 mg per kg po q24h + **RIF** 600 mg po q24h (or **RFB** 300 mg po q24h). May add **SM** or **AMK** 15 mg per kg 3 times per week for 2–6 mos. for severe disease. May also add **CLO** 100–200 mg po q24h (until "tan"; then 50 mg po q24h or 100 mg 3 times per week). Rx until culture neg. times 1 yr.	**Clarithro** 500 mg po bid + **ETB** 15–25 mg per kg po q24h + **RFB** 300 mg po q24h for up to 24 mos. (Curr Inf Dis Repts 2:193, 2000; CID 32:1547, 2001). Regimens dosing azithro 600 mg 3 times per week also effective (CID 32:1547, 2001)	**"Classic" pulmonary MAC:** Men 50–75, smokers, COPD. May be associated with hot tub (Am J Clin Chest Med 23:675, 2002). **"Nodular pulmonary MAC:** Women 30–70, scoliosis, mitral valve prolapse, (bronchiectasis), pectus excavatum ("Lady Windemere syndrome"). May also be associated with interferon gamma deficiency (AJM 113:756, 2002). Susceptibility testing of MAC not recommended except clarithro for isolates from pts who have failed prior clarithro rx. Alternative: **Clarithro** 500 mg po bid + **RFB** (25 mg per kg po), RFB 600 mg & initial 2 times per wk azithro (600 mg po q24h). SM may be effective in immunocompetent patients (JID 178:121, 1998; CID 30:288, 2000). Late "relapses" (following completion of therapy) after treatment with clarithro or azithro in pts with nodular bronchiectasis usually represent reinfection, not failure of rx (JID 186:266, 2002).
	Immunocompromised pts: Primary prophylaxis—Pt's CD4 count <50–100 per mm³. Discontinue when CD4 count >100 per mm³ in response to HAART (NEJM 342:1085, 2000; CID 34: 662, 2002). Guideline. AnIM 137:435, 2002	**Azithro** 1200 mg po weekly OR **Clarithro** 500 mg po bid (continued on next page)	**RFB** 300 mg po q24h OR **Azithro** 1200 mg po weekly + RIF 300 mg po q24h (continued on next page)	RFB reduces MAC infection rate by 55% (no survival benefit); clarithro by 68% (30% survival benefit); azithro by 59% (68% survival benefit) (CID 26:611, 1996). Azithro + RFB more effective than either alone but not as well tolerated (NEJM 335:392, 1996). **Many drug-drug interactions**, see Table 22, pages 186, 188. Drug-resistant MAI disease seen in 29–58% of pts in whom disease develops while taking clarithro prophylaxis & in 11% of those on azithro but has not been observed with RFB prophylaxis (J Inf 38:51, 1999). Clarithro resistance more likely in pts with extremely low CD4 counts at initiation (CID 27:807, 1998). Need to be sure no active M. tbc (NEJM 335:384 & 428, 1996).
	Either presumptive dx or after r culture of blood, bone marrow, or usually, sterile body fluids, eg liver	**Clarithro** 500 mg* po q24h or **Cla**rithro + **azithro** bid or azithro (600 mg po q24h) + (continued on next page)	**Cla**rithro or **azithro** + **ETB** + **RFB** one or more of: (continued on next page)	Median time to neg. blood culture clarithro + ETB 4.4 wks vs azithro + ETB >16 wks. At 16 wks, clearance of bacteremia seen in 37.5% of clarithro-treated pts (CID 27:1278, 1998). More recent study suggests similar clearance rates for azithro (46%) vs clarithro (56%) but wks when combined with ETB (CID 31:1245, 2000). Azithro 250 mg po q24h not effective, but azithro 600 mg po q24h as effective as 1200 mg q24h & yields fewer adverse effects (AAC 43: 2869, 1999) **† DOT** = directly observed therapy (continued on next page)

See page 2 for abbreviations.   * Dosages are for adults (unless otherwise indicated) and assume normal renal function   **†** DOT = directly observed therapy

TABLE 12A (8)

CAUSATIVE AGENT/DISEASE	MODIFYING CIRCUMSTANCES	SUGGESTED REGIMENS		COMMENTS
		PRIMARY	**ALTERNATIVE**	
IV. Other Mycobacterial Disease ("Atypical") *(Continued)* **C. M. avium-intracellulare complex** *(continued)*		*(continued from previous page)* **ETB** 15–25mg/kg/day + **RFB** 300mg/day * **Higher doses of clari (1000 mg bid) may be associated**	*(continued from previous page)* **CIP** 750 mg po bid or **Oflox** 400 mg po bid + **Amikacin** 7.5–15 mg/kg IV q24h Pts resc to protease inhibitors can use **clarithro** 500 mg bid (or + **azithro** 600 mg q24h) + **ETB** 15–25 mg/kg/day) if the pt has not had previous prophylaxis with a neomacrolide (*Johns Hopkins AIDS Report 9:2, 1997)*	*(continued from previous page)* Addition of RFB to clarithro + ETB ↓ emergence of resistance to clari, ↓ relapse rate & improves survival *(CID 37:1234, 2003).* Data on clofazimine difficult to assess. Earlier study suggested adding CLO of no value *(CID 25:621, 1997).* More recent study suggests it may be as effective as RFB in 3 drug regimens containing clari & ETB *(CID 29:125, 1999)* although it may not be as effective as RFB at preventing clari resistance *(CID 28:136, 1999).* Thus, pending more data, we still do not recommend CLO for MAI in HIV+ pts. Drug toxicity: With clarithro, 23% pts had to stop drug 2° to dose-limiting adverse reaction *(AnIM 121: 905, 1994).* Combination of clarithro, ETB and RFB led to uveitis and pseudojaundice *(NEJM 330:438, 1994);* result is reduction in max. dose of RFB to 300 mg. Treatment failure rate is high. Reasons: drug toxicity, development of drug resistance, & inadequate serum levels. Serum levels of clarithro ↓ in pts also given RIF or RFB *(JID 171:747, 1995).* If pt not responding to initial regimen after 2–4 weeks, add one or more drugs. Several anecdotal reports of pts not responding to usual primary regimen who gained weight and became afebrile with dexamethasone 2–4 mg per day po *(AAC 38:2215, 1994; CID 26:682, 1998).*
	Chronic post-treatment suppression—secondary prophylaxis	Always necessary **(Clarithro** or azithro) + **ETB** (↓ dose to 15mg/kg/day (dosage above)	**Clarithro** or **azithro** or **RFB** (dosage above)	Recurrences almost universal without chronic suppression. However, in patients on HAART with robust CD4 cell response, it is possible to discontinue chronic suppression *(JID 178:1446, 1998; NEJM 340:1301, 1999).*
D. Mycobacterium celatum	Treatment; optimal regimen not defined		May be susceptible to **clarithro**, **FQ** *(Clin Micro 37:3050, 1997).* Suggest rx "like MAI" but often resistant to RIF *(J Inf 38:157, 1999).* Most reported cases received 3 or 4 drugs, usually clarithro + ETB + CIP ± RFB *(EID 9:399, 2003)*	Isolated from pulmonary lesions and blood in AIDS patients *(CID 24:144, 1997).* Easily confused with M. xenopi (and MAC). Susceptibilities similar to MAC, but highly resistant to RIF *(CID 24:140, 1997).*
E. Mycobacterium chelonae ssp. abscessus— Mycobacterium chelonae ssp. chelonae	Treatment; Surgical excision may facilitate clarithro rx in subcutaneous abscess and is important adjunct to rx *(CID 24:1147, 1997)*		**Clarithro** 500 mg po bid times 6 mos. *(AnIM 119:482, 1993; CID 24:1147, 1997; EJCMID 19:43, 2000).* Azithro may also be effective. For serious disease add **IMP** + tobramycin + IMP for 1° 2–6 wks *(Clin Micro Rev 15:716, 2002)*	M. abscessus susceptible to AMK (70%), clarithro (95%), cefoxitin (70%), CLO, cefmetazole, IMP, azithro, cipro, doxy, mino, tigecycline *(CID 42:1756, 2006).* Single isolates of M. abscessus often resistant with disease. Clarithro-resistant strains now described *(J Clin Micro 38:2745, 2001).* M. chelonae susceptible to AMK (80%), clarithro, tobramycin (100%), IMP (60%), gatifloxacin (90%), moxifloxacin *(AAC 46:3283, 2002);* cipro, mino, doxy, linezolid (94%) *(CID 42:1756, 2006).* Resistant to cefoxitin, FQ *(CID 24:1147, 1997; AJRCCM 156:S1, 1997).*
F. Mycobacterium fortuitum	Treatment; optimal regimen not defined. Surgical excision of infected areas.		**AMK** + **cefoxitin** + **probenecid** 2–6wk, then po **TMP-SMX**, or **doxy** 2–6 mo. Usually responds to 6–12mo of oral rx with 2 drugs to which it is susceptible *(AAC 46:3283, 2002; Clin Micro Rev 15:716, 2002).* Nail salon-acquired infections respond to 4–6 mo of minocycline, doxy, or CIP *(CID 38:38, 2004).*	Resistant **to all standard anti-TBc drugs.** Sensitive to doxycycline, minocycline, cefoxitin, IMP, AMK, TMP-SMX, CIP, oflox, azithro, clarithro, gatifloxacin (80%) *(AAC 46:3283, 2002),* linezolid *(Clin Micro Rev 15:716, 2002).* May be resistant to azithromycin, rifabutin *(IJAC 39:567, 1997).*

See page 2 for abbreviations.

* Dosages are for adults (unless otherwise indicated) and assume normal renal function   † **DOT** = directly observed therapy

TABLE 12A (9)

CAUSATIVE AGENT/DISEASE; MODIFYING CIRCUMSTANCES	SUGGESTED REGIMENS		COMMENTS
	PRIMARY	ALTERNATIVE	
IV. Other Mycobacterial Disease ("Atypical") *(continued)*			
F. Mycobacterium haemophilum	Regimen(s) not defined. **clarithro + rifabutin** effective (AAC 39:2316, 1995). Combination of **CIP + RFB + clarithro** reported effective but clinical experience limited (Clin Micro Rev 9:435, 1996). Surgical debridement may be necessary (CID 26:505, 1998).		Clinical: Ulcerating skin lesions, synovitis, osteomyelitis, cervicofacial lymphadenitis in children (CID 41:1569, 2005). Lab: Requires supplemented media to isolate. Sensitive in vitro to: CIP, cycloserine, rifabutin. Over ½ resistant to: INH, RIF, ETB, PZA (AnIM 120:118, 1994).
H. Mycobacterium genavense	Regimens used include ≥2 drugs: **ETB, RIF, RFB, CLO, clarithro**. In animal model, **clarithro & RFB** (& to lesser extent amikacin & ETB) shown effective in reducing bacterial counts; CIP not effective (AAC 42:483, 1998).		Clinical: CD4 <50. Symptoms of fever, weight loss, diarrhea. Lab: Growth in BACTEC vials slow (mean 42 days). Subcultures grow only on Middlebrook 7H11 agar containing 2 mcg per ml mycobactin J—growth still insufficient for in vitro sensitivity testing (Ln 340:76, 1992; AnIM 117:586, 1992). Survival ↑ from 81 to 263 days in pts rx for at least 1 month with ≥2 drugs (AIM 155:400, 1995).
I. Mycobacterium gordonae	Regimen(s) not defined, but consider **RIF + ETB + KM** or **CIP** (J Inf 38:157, 1999)		In vitro: sensitive to ETB, RIF, AMK, CIP, clarithro, linezolid (AAC 47:1736, 2003). Resistant to INH (AAC 14:1229, 1992). Surgical excision.
J. Mycobacterium kansasii	(Q24h po. **INH** (300 mg) + **RIF** (600 mg) + **ETB** (25 mg per kg times 2 mos., then 15 mg per kg) x 18 mos. (until culture-neg sputum times 12 mos.; 15 mos. if neg times 12–15 mos. if HIV+ pt.) (See Comment)	If RIF-resistant, po q24h: **INH** (900 mg) + **pyridoxine** (50 mg) + **sulfamethox-azole** (1.0 gm tid). Rx until culture-neg. (See Comment) **ClarI + ETB = RIF** also effective in small study (CID 37:1178, 2003)	All isolates are **resistant to PZA**. Rifampentine, azithro. ETB effective alone or in combination in ethymic mice (AAC 42:417, 2001). Highly susceptible to linezolid in vitro (AAC 47:1736, 2003) and to clarithro and moxifloxacin (JAC 55:950, 2005). If HIV+ and taking protease inhibitor, substitute either clarithro (500 mg bid) or RFB (150 mg per day) for RIF (AJRCCM 156:S1, 1997). Because of variable susceptibility to INH, some substitute clarithro 500–750 mg q24h for INH. Resistance to clarithro reported (DMID 31:369, 1998), but most strains susceptible to clarithro as well as moxifloxacin (JAC 55:950, 2005) & levofloxacin (AAC 48:4562, 2004). Prognosis related to level of immunosuppression (CID 37:584, 2003).
K. Mycobacterium marinum	(**clarithro** 500 mg bid) or **minocycline** 100–200 mg q24h) or **doxycycline** 100–200 mg q24h), or **TMP-SMX** 160/800 mg po bid), or **RIF + ETB** for 3 mos. (AJRCCM 156:S1, 1997). Surgical excision.		Resistant to INH & PZA (AJRCCM 156:S1, 1997). Also susceptible to clarithro in vitro & linezolid (AAC 47:1736, 2003). CIP, gatifloxacin, moxifloxacin also show moderate in vitro activity (AAC 46:1114, 2002). Susceptible to clarithro, strep, erythromycin.
L. Mycobacterium scrofulaceum	Surgical excision. Chemotherapy seldom indicated. Although regimens not defined, **clarithro + CLO** with or **without ETB INH RIF strep + cycloserine** have also been used.		Most isolates resistant to all 1st-line anti-tbc drugs. Isolates often not clinically significant (CID 26:625, 1998).
M. Mycobacterium simiae	Regimen(s) not defined. Start 4 drugs as for disseminated MAI.		Susceptible in vitro to RIF, strep, CLO, clarithro, CIP, ofloxacin, AMK, linezolid (AAC 42:2070, 1998; JAC 45: 231, 2000; AAC 46:3193, 2002; AAC 50:192, 2006). Monotherapy with RIF selects resistant mutants in mice (AAC 47:1228, 2003). RIF + strep effective in small study (AAC 49:3182, 2005).
N. Mycobacterium ulcerans (Buruli ulcer)	**RIF + AMK** (7.5 mg per kg IM bid), or **ETB + TMP-SMX** (160/800 mg po tid) for 4–6 weeks. Surgical excision most important. WHO recommends RIF + SM for 8 weeks but overall value of drug therapy not clear (Lancet Infection 6:288, 2006; Lancet 367:1849, 2006).		Treatment generally disappointing—see review, Ln 354:1013, 1999. RIF + dapsone only slightly better (82% improved) than placebo (75%) in small study (Int J Inf Dis 5:60, 2002).
O. Mycobacterium xenopi	Regimen(s) not defined (CID 24:226 & 233, 1997). Some recommend a macrolide + RIF (or RFB) + ETB ± INH (AJRCCM 156:S1, 1997) or **RIF + INH + ETB** (Resp Med 97:439, 2003) but recent study suggests no need to treat in most pts with HIV (CID 37:1250, 2003).		In vitro: sensitive to clarithro (AAC 36:2841, 1992) and rifabutin (JAC 39:567, 1997) and many standard antimycobacterial drugs. Small studies suggest more effective than RIF/INH/ETB regimens in mice (AAC 45:3229, 2001). FQs, linezolid also active in vitro.

See page 2 for abbreviations.   * Dosages are for adults (unless otherwise indicated) and assume normal renal function   † **DOT** = directly observed therapy

TABLE 12A (10)

CAUSATIVE AGENT/DISEASE	MODIFYING CIRCUMSTANCES	SUGGESTED REGIMENS		COMMENTS
		PRIMARY	ALTERNATIVE	
Mycobacterium leprae (leprosy)	There are 2 sets of therapeutic recommendations here: one from USA (National Hansen's Disease Programs [NHDP], Baton Rouge, LA) and one from WHO. Both are based on expert recommendations and neither has been subjected to controlled clinical trial (P. Joyce & D. Scollard, Conns Current Therapy 2004; MP. Joyce, Immigration Medicine, in press 2006; J Am Acad Dermatol 51:417, 2004).			
Type of Disease	NHDP Regimen	WHO Regimen		COMMENTS
Paucibacillary Forms: (Intermediate, tuberculoid, Borderline tuberculoid)	(Dapsone 100 mg/day + RIF 600 mg/day) for 12 months	(Dapsone 100 mg/day (unsupervised) + RIF 600 mg 1x/mo (supervised)) for 6 mo		Side effects overall 0.4%
Single lesion paucibacillary	Treat as paucibacillary leprosy for 12 months.	Single dose ROM therapy: (RIF 600 mg + Oflox 400 mg + Mino 100 mg) (Ln 353:655, 1999)		
Multibacillary forms: Borderline Borderline-lepromatous Lepromatous See Comment for erythema nodosum leprosum Rev.: Lancet 363:1209, 2004	(Dapsone 100mg/day + CLO 50mg/day + RIF 600mg/day) for 24mo Alternative regimen: (Dapsone 100mg/day + RIF 600mg/day + Minocycline 100mg/day) for 24mo if CLO is refused or unavailable.	(Dapsone 100mg/day + CLO 50 mg/day (both unsupervised) + (RIF 600 mg + CLO 300 mg once monthly (supervised))). Continue regimen for 12 months.		Side-effects overall 5.1%. For erythema nodosum leprosum, prednisone 60-80mg/day or thalidomide 100-400mg/day (BMJ 44: 775, 1988; AJM 108:487, 2000). Thalidomide available in US at 1-800-4-CELGENE. Altho thalidomide effective, WHO no longer rec because of potential toxicity (JID 192:1743, 2006) however the majority of leprosy experts feel thalidomide remains drug of choice for ENL under strict supervision. CLO (Clofazimine) available from NHDP under IND protocol; contact at 1-800-642-2477. Ethionamide (250mg q24h) or prothionamide (375mg q24h) may be subbed for CLO. Oflox 400mg po q24h, bactericidal and effective clinically with 4 log ↓ in organisms in small trials (AAC 38:662, 1994; AAC 38:67, 1994). Clarithro also rapidly bactericidal (AAC 38:515, 1994; Ln 345:4, 1995). Regimens incorporating clarithro, minocycline, RIF, moxifloxacin, and/or oflox also show promise (AAC 44:2919, 2000; AAC 50:1558, 2006). High relapse rate in pts treated with (24h RIF + oflox for 4wk (AAC 41:1953, 1997). Resistance to Dapsone, RIF & oflox reported (Ln 349:103, 1997). Dapsone monotherapy has been abandoned due to emergence of resistance, but older patients previously treated with dapsone monotherapy may remain on lifelong maintenance therapy. Dapsone (or acedapsone[NA]) effective for prophylaxis in one study (J Inf 41:137, 2000).

TABLE 12B – DOSAGE, PRICE AND SELECTED ADVERSE EFFECTS OF ANTIMYCOBACTERIAL DRUGS

AGENT (TRADE NAME)[1]	USUAL DOSAGE*	ROUTE/[1] DRUG RESISTANCE (RES)[2] US$/COST**	SIDE-EFFECTS, TOXICITY AND PRECAUTIONS	SURVEILLANCE
FIRST LINE DRUGS				
Ethambutol (Myambutol)	25mg/kg/day for 2mo then 15mg/kg/day q24h as 1 dose (<10% protein binding) [Bacteriostatic to both extra-cellular & intracellular organisms]	po RES: 0.3% (0-0.7%) 400 mg tab $1.80	**Optic neuritis** with decreased visual acuity, central scotomata, and loss of green and red/green perception; peripheral neuropathy and headache (~1%), rashes (rare), arthralgia (rare), hyperuricemia (rare). Anaphylactoid reaction (rare). **Comment:** Primarily causes resistance. Disrupts outer cell membrane in M. avium with ↑ activity to other drugs.	Monthly visual acuity & red/green with dose >15mg/kg/day ≥10% loss considered significant. Usually reversible if drug discontinued.

[1] Note: Malabsorption of antimycobacterial drugs may occur in patients with AIDS enteropathy. For review of adverse effects, see AJRCCM 167:1472, 2003.

[2] **RES** = % resistance of M. tuberculosis

See page 2 for abbreviations.   * Dosages are for adults (unless otherwise indicated) and assume normal renal function.   † **DOT** = directly observed therapy

* Dosages are for adults (unless otherwise indicated) and assume normal renal function.   * See page 2 for abbreviations.

TABLE 12B (2)

AGENT (TRADE NAME) [1]	USUAL DOSAGE*	ROUTE/[1] DRUG RESISTANCE (RES) US$/COST**	SIDE-EFFECTS, TOXICITY AND PRECAUTIONS	SURVEILLANCE
FIRST LINE DRUGS				
Isoniazid (INH) (Nydrazid, Laniazid, Teebaconin)	(continued) Q24h dose: 5–10mg/kg/day up to 300mg/day as 1 dose. 2x/wk dose: 15mg/kg (900mg max dose). [Bactericidal to both extracellular and intracellular organisms] Add pyridoxine in alcoholic, pregnant, or malnourished pts.	po RES: 4.1% (2.6–8.5%) 300 mg tab (IM route not FDA-approved but has been used, see in AIDS) 100 mg in 10 ml vials. (IM) $16.64	Overall ~1%. Liver **Hep** (children 10% mild ↑ SGOT, normalizes with continued use, age <20yr rare, age 20–34yr 1.2%, age>50yr 2.3%) (less in HIV+). Severe hepatitis rare, rarely fatal, ↑ with alcohol use, other drugs (JAMA 281:1014, 2003). May be fatal. With prodromal sx, dark urine do LFTs, discontinue if SGOT >3–5x normal. **Peripheral neuropathy** (17% on 6mg/kg per day, less on 300mg, incidence ↑ in slow acetylators): **pyridoxine 10mg q24h will ↓ incidence.** other neurologic symptoms: dizziness, convulsions, optic neuritis, toxic encephalopathy, psychosis, muscle twitching, dizziness, coma (all rare); allergic skin rashes, fever, minor disulfiram-like reaction, flushing after Swiss cheese (tyramine). **Hematologic** (rare) – antinuclear (20%). **Drug-induced lupus erythematosus** (JID 349:152, 1977).	Pre-rx liver functions. Repeat if symptoms (fatigue, weakness, malaise, anorexia, nausea or vomiting) >3 days (AJRCCM 152: 1705, 1995). Some recommend SGOT at 2, 4, 6 mo esp. if age >50yr. Clinical evaluation every mo.
Pyrazinamide	25 mg per kg per day (maximum 2.5 gm per day) q24h as 1 dose [Bactericidal for intracellular organisms]	po 500 mg tab $1.09	**Arthralgia; hyperuricemia** (with or without symptoms), hepatitis (not over 2% if recommended dose not exceeded), gastric irritation; photosensitivity (rare)	Pre-rx liver functions. Monthly SGOT, uric acid. Measure serum uric acid if symptomatic gouty attack occurs.
Rifamate— combination tablet	2 tablets single dose q24h	po 1 tablet contains 150 mg INH, 300 mg RIF	As with individual drugs	As with individual drugs
Rifampin (Rifadin, Rimactane, Rifocin)	10.0 mg per kg per day up to 600 mg per day q24h as 1 dose [Bactericidal to all populations of organisms]	po (1 hr before meal) 0.1–0.3% 300 mg cap $1.90 (IV available, Merrell-Dow, Cost 600 mg $90.28)	INH+RIF dcol in ~3% for toxicity, gastrointestinal irritation, antibiotic-associated colitis, drug fever (1%) with or without skin rash (1%), anaphylactoid reactions in HIV+ pts, flu-like illness with intermittent use, hepatotoxicity (1%), hemolytic anemia, transient mental confusion, thrombocytopenia (1%), leukopenia (1%). **"Flu syndrome"** (fever, chills, headache, bone pain, shortness of breath) seen if RIF taken irregularly or if q24h dose restarted after an interval of no rx. **Discolors urine, tears, sweat, contact lens an orange-brownish color.** May cause drug-induced lupus erythematosus (JID 349:152, 1977).	As with individual drugs. PZA 25 mg per kg
Rifater[2]— combination tablet (See Side-Effects)	Wt ≤55 kg, 6 tablets single dose q24h	po 1 tab $1.96	1 tablet contains 50 mg INH, 120 mg RIF, 300 mg PZA. Used [2]. 1 ≥2 months in 4x (PZA 25 mg/kg), PZA toxicity ≈ weight lost. Rifater is convenient in dosing, compliance (AHM 122: 951, 1995) but cost 1.58 more. Side-effects = individual drugs.	
Streptomycin	15 mg per kg IM q24h, 0.75–1.0 gm per day initially for 60–90 days, then 1.0 gm 2–3 times per week (15 mg per kg per day) q24h as 1 dose	IM (or IV) RES: 3.9% (2.7–7.6%) 1.0 gm $9.10	Overall 8%. **Ototoxicity** vestibular dysfunction (vertigo), paresthesias, dizziness & nausea (all less in pts receiving 2–3 doses per week); tinnitus and high frequency loss (1%); nephrotoxicity (rare); peripheral neuropathy (rare); allergic skin rashes (4–5%); drug fever. Available from X-Gen Pharmaceuticals, 607-732-4411. Ref. re: IV—CID 19:1150, 1994. Toxicity similar with q/d vs bid dosing (CID 38:1538, 2004).	Monthly audiogram. In older pts, serum creatinine or BUN at start of rx and weekly if pt stable.
SECOND LINE DRUGS (more difficult to use and/or less effective than first line drugs)				
Amikacin (Amikin)	7.5–10.0 mg per kg q24h [Bactericidal for extracellular organisms]	IV or IM RES (test q1%) 500 mg $7.80	See Table 10, pages 80 & 83 Toxicity similar with q/d vs bid dosing (CID 38:1538, 2004).	Monthly audiogram. Serum creatinine or BUN weekly if pt stable
Capreomycin sulfate (Capastat sulfate)	15 mg per kg per day (≤1 gm per day) q24h as 1 dose	IM or IV RES: 0.1% (0–0.9%) 1 gm $25.54	Nephrotoxicity (36%), ototoxicity (auditory 11%), eosinophilia, leukopenia, skin rash, fever, hypokalemia, neuromuscular blockade.	Monthly audiogram, biweekly serum creatinine or BUN
Ciprofloxacin (Cipro)	750 mg bid	IM or IV (po) RES: 3.9% (2.7–7.6%) 750 mg (po) $5.33	TB not an FDA-approved indication for CIP. Desired CIP serum levels 4–6 mcg per mL, requires median dose 800 mg (AJRCCM 151:2006, 1995). Discontinuation rates 6–7%. CIP-resistant M. Tb identified in New York (Ln 345:1148, 1995). See Table 10, pages 83 & 84 for adverse effects.	None

*Dosages are for adults (unless otherwise indicated) and assume normal renal function.   †**DOT** = directly observed therapy

*Dosages are for abbreviations.   ** Dosages are for adults (unless otherwise indicated)

See page 2 for abbreviations.

TABLE 12B (3)

AGENT (TRADE NAME)[1]	USUAL DOSAGE*	ROUTE/[1] DRUG RESISTANCE (RES) US$/COST**	SIDE-EFFECTS, [1]%, CNS, [2]% TOXICITY AND [3]% PRECAUTIONS	SURVEILLANCE
SECOND LINE DRUGS *(continued)*				
Clofazimine (Lamprene)	50 mg per day (unsupervised) + 300 mg 1 time per month supervised or 100 mg per day	po (with meals) 50 mg $0.20	Skin: **pigmentation (pink-brownish black)** 75–100%; dryness 20%, pruritus 5% GI: abdominal pain 50% (rarely severe leading to exploratory laparoscopy), splenic infarction (VR), bowel obstruction (VR), GI bleeding (VR). Eye: conjunctival irritation, retinal crystal deposits.	None
Cycloserine (Seromycin)	750–1000 mg per day (15 mg per kg per day) 2–4 doses per day [Bacteriostatic for both extracellular & intracellular organisms]	po RES: 0.1% (0–0.3%) 250 mg cap $3.50	Convulsions, **psychoses** (5–10% of those receiving 1.0 gm per day), headache, somnolence, hyperreflexia, increased CSF protein and pressure, **peripheral neuropathy**. 100 mg pyridoxine (or more) q24h should be given concomitantly. Contraindicated in epileptics.	None
Dapsone	100 mg per day	po 100 mg $0.20	Blood: ↓ hemoglobin (1–2 gm) & [4] retics (2–12%), in most pts. Hemolysis in G6PD deficiency. **Methemoglobinemia**. CNS: peripheral neuropathy (rare). GI: nausea, vomiting. Renal: albuminuria, nephrotic syndrome. Erythema nodosum leprosum in pts rx for leprosy (½ pts 1+ year)	None
Ethionamide (Trecator-SC)	500–1000 mg per day (15–20 mg per kg per day) 1–3 doses per day [Bacteriostatic for extracellular organisms only]	po RES: 0.8% (0–1.5%) 250 mg tab $3.09	**Gastrointestinal irritation** (up to 50% on large dose); goiter; peripheral neuropathy (rare); convulsions (rare); changes in affect (rare); difficulty in diabetes control; rashes; hepatitis; purpura; stomatitis; gynecomastia; menstrual irregularity. Give drug with meals or antacids; 50–100 mg pyridoxine per day concomitantly, SGOT monthly. Possibly teratogenic.	
Ofloxacin (Floxin)	400 mg bid	po, IV 400 mg (po) $4.2	Not FDA-approved indication. Overall adverse effects 11%, 4% discontinued due to side-effects. GI: nausea 3%, diarrhea 1%. **CNS**: insomnia 3%, headache 1%, dizziness 1%	None
Para-aminosalicylic acid (PAS, Paser) (Na+ or K+ salt)	4–6 gm (200 mg per kg per day) [Bacteriostatic for extracellular organisms only]	po RES: 0.8% (0–1.5%) 450 mg tab $0.08 (see Comment)	**Gastrointestinal irritation** (10–15%); goitrogenic action (rare); depressed prothrombin activity (rare); G6PD-mediated hemolytic anemia (rare); drug fever, rashes, hepatitis, myalgia, arthralgia. Retards hepatic enzyme induction, may ↓ INH hepatotoxicity. Available from CDC. (404) 639-3670, Jacobus Pharm. Co. (609) 921-7447.	None
Rifabutin (Mycobutin)	300 mg (prophylaxis or treatment)	po 150 mg $7. 19	Polymyalgia, polyarthralgia, leukopenia, granulocytopenia. Anterior uveitis when given with concomitant clarithromycin; avoid 600 mg dose (NEJM 330:438, 1994). Uveitis reported with 450 mg per day (AIHM 12:510, 1994). Reddish urine, orange skin (pseudojaundice).	None
Rifapentine (Priftin)	600 mg twice weekly for 1st 2 mos., then 600 mg q week	po 150 mg $3.00	Similar to other rifamycins. (See RIF, RFB). Hyperuricemia seen in 21%. Causes red-orange discoloration of body fluids. Note [5] prevalence of RIF resistance in pts on weekly rx (Ln 1843:1843, 1999)	None
Thalidomide (Thalomid)	100–300 mg po q24h (may use up to 400 mg po q24h for severe erythema nodosum leprosum)	po 50 mg $42.36	**Contraindicated in pregnancy. Causes severe life-threatening birth defects. Both male and female patients must use barrier contraceptive methods (Pregnancy Category X).** Frequently causes drowsiness or somnolence. **May cause peripheral neuropathy.** (AJM 108:487, 2000) For review, see Ln 363:1803, 2004	Available only through pharmacists participating in System for Thalidomide Education and Prescribing Safety (S.T.E.P.S.)

* Adult dosage only;   [1] Mean (range) (higher in Hispanics, Asians, and patients <10 years old);   ** Average wholesale price according to 2006 DRUG TOPICS RED BOOK, Medical Economics

* Adult dosage only;   [1] Mean (range)   * Dosages are for adults (*unless otherwise indicated*) and assume normal renal function   [1] **DOT** = directly observed therapy

See page 2 for abbreviations.

TABLE 13A – TREATMENT OF PARASITIC INFECTIONS*

Many of the drugs suggested are not licensed in the US. The following are helpful resources available through the Center for Disease Control and Prevention (CDC) in Atlanta. Website is www.cdc.gov.
General advice for parasitic diseases other than malaria: (770) 488-7760 or (770) 488-7775.
For CDC Drug Service: 8:00 a.m.–4:30 p.m. EST: (404) 639-3670 (or -2888); emergency after hours: (404) 639-2888; fax: (404) 639-3717.
For malaria: Prophylaxis advice (770) 488-7788 or (877) 394-8747; treatment (770) 488-7788, or after hours (770) 488-7100; website: www.cdc.gov/travel, fax (888) 232-3299
NOTE: All dosage regimens are for adults with normal renal function unless otherwise stated.
For licensed drugs, suggest checking package inserts to verify dosage and side-effects. Occasionally, post-licensure data may alter dosage as compared to package inserts.
For abbreviations of journal titles, see page 3. **Reference with peds dosages: Med Letter on-line version: www.medletter.com (August 2004). General resource: www.gideononline.com**

INFECTING ORGANISM	SUGGESTED REGIMENS		COMMENTS
	PRIMARY	**ALTERNATIVE**	
PROTOZOA—INTESTINAL (non-pathogenic: E. hartmanni, E. dispar, E. coli, Iodamoeba butschii, Endolimax nana, Chilomastix mesnili)			
Balantidium coli	**Tetracycline** 500mg po tid times 5 days	**Metronidazole** 750mg po tid times 5 days	See Table 10C for side-effects.
Blastocystis hominis: Role as pathogen controversial	**Nitazoxanide:** Adults 500mg tabs (children 200mg oral suspension)—both po q12h x 3 days (TRSM 91:701, 1997)	**Metronidazole** 1.5gm po as single dose 1x/day x 10 d (placebo-controlled trial) Travel Med 10:128, 2003). **Alternatives: Iodoquinol** 650mg po tid x 20 days or **TMP-SMX-DS**, one bid x 7 days	**Nitazoxanide:** Approved in liquid formulation for rx of children & 500mg tabs for adults. Ref. CID 40:1173, 2005. E. hominis assoc. with 1 in post-infection dx & joint pain, recurrent headache, & dizzy spells (CID 39:504, 2004).
Cryptosporidium parvum & hominis Treatment is unsatisfactory Ref. CID 39:504, 2004	**Immunocompetent—No HIV: Nitazoxanide** 500mg po bid x3 days	**HIV with immunodeficiency:** (1) Effective anti-retroviral therapy best therapy; (2) **Nitazoxanide** 500mg po bid x 14 days in adults (60% response) Not effective in non-HIV children.	If sulfa-allergic: **CIP** 500mg po bid x7 days & then 1 tab po 3x/wk x 2wk.
Cyclospora cayetanensis	Immunocompetent pts: **TMP-SMX-DS** tab 1 po bid X 7–10 days	AIDS Pts: **TMP-SMX-DS** tab 1 po qid x 10 days; then tab 1 po 3x/wk.	Other alternatives: doxy 100mg po bid x7 days; paromomycin 500mg po tid x 7 days
Dientamoeba fragilis	**Iodoquinol** 650mg po tid x 20 days	**Tetracycline** 500 mg po qid x 10 days OR **Metronidazole** 500-750 mg po tid x 10 days	
Entamoeba histolytica; amebiasis Reviews: Lancet 361:1025, 2003; NEJM 348:1563, 2003.			
Asymptomatic cyst passer	**Paromomycin** (aminosidine A) x 500mg po tid x 7 days OR **Iodoquinol** 650mg po tid x20 days	**Diloxanide furoate**[NUS] (Furamide) 500mg po tid x 10 days (Source: Panorama Compound. Pharm., 800-247-9767).	Metronidazole not effective vs cysts.
Patient with diarrhea/dysentery; mild/moderate disease. Oral rx possible	**Metronidazole** 500–750mg po tid x 10 days or **tinidazole** 2gm 1x/day x3 days followed by	**Tinidazole** 2gm po q12h x 3 days) or **ornidazole**[NUS] 500 mg po q12h x 5 days) followed by	Drug side-effects in Table 10C. Colitis can mimic ulcerative colitis; ameboma can mimic adenocarcinoma of colon.
	Either **paromomycin** 500mg po tid x 7 days] or **iodoquinol** 650mg po tid x 20 days	**paromomycin** 500mg po tid x 7 days] or **iodoquinol** (was diiodohydroxyquin) 650mg po tid x 20 days	**Dx:** antigen detection & PCR better than O&P (Clin Micro Rev 16:713, 2003). Watch out for non-pathogenic E. dispar (J 351:1672, 1998)
Severe or extraintestinal infection, e.g., hepatic abscess	**(Metronidazole** 750mg IV or PO tid x10 days or **tinidazole** 2gm 1x/day x 5 days) followed by **paromomycin** 500mg po tid x 7 days	**Metronidazole** 500-750mg po tid x 5 days (high frequency of GI side-effects). See Comment Rx if assoc. **Paromomycin** 500mg 4x/day x7 days	**Serology positive** (antibody present) with extraintestinal disease.
Giardia lamblia; giardiasis	**(Tinidazole** 2gm po x 1) OR **(nitazoxanide** 500mg po bid x3 days)	**Pyrimethamine** 75mg/day po + **folinic acid** 10mg/day po] x 14 days OR **CIP** 500mg po bid x 7 days—87% response (AnIM 132:885, 2000)	**Paromomycin** 500 mg po x 3 days, or (**quinacrine**[1] 100mg po) both 3x/day x 5wk. Ref. CID 33:22, 2001. Nitazoxanide ref. CID 40:1173, 2005.
Isospora belli	**TMP-SMX-DS** 1 po bid x 10 days; if AIDS pt: TMP-SMX-DS x10 days & then 1 bid x 3wk.		Chronic suppression in AIDS pts: either 1 TMP-SMX-DS tab 3x/wk OR (pyrimethamine 25mg/day po + folinic acid 5mg/day po)

---

[1] **Drugs available from CDC Drug Service:** 404-639-2888 or –3670 or www.cdc.gov/ncidod/srp/drugs/formulary.html: Bithionol, dehydroemetine, diethylcarbamazine (DEC), melarsoprol, nifurtimox, stibogluconate (Pentostam), suramin.

[2] Quinacrine available from Panorama Compounding Pharmacy, (800) 247-9767, (818) 988-7979.

* See page 2 for abbreviations. All dosage recommendations are for adults (unless otherwise indicated) and assume normal renal function.

TABLE 13A (2)

INFECTING ORGANISM	SUGGESTED REGIMENS		COMMENTS
	PRIMARY	**ALTERNATIVE**	
PROTOZOA—INTESTINAL (continued)			
Microsporidiosis			
Ocular: Encephalitozoon hellum or. cuniculi, Vittaforma (Nosema) corneae, Nosema oculorum.	For HIV pts: antiretroviral therapy key. **Albendazole** 400mg po bid x 3wk	In HIV+ pts, reports of response of E. hellum to **fumagillin** eyedrops (see Comment). For V. corneae, may need keratoplasty.	To obtain fumagillin: 800-292-6773 or www.leiterrx.com. Neutropenia & thrombocytopenia serious adverse events. Dx: Most labs use modified trichrome stain. Need electron micrographs for species identification. FA and PCR methods in development.
intestinal (diarrhea): Enterocytozoon bieneusi, Encephalitozoon (Septata) intestinalis	**Albendazole** 400mg po bid x 3wk; peds dose: 15mg/kg per day div. into 2 daily doses x7 days	For V. corneae, may need keratoplasty. Oral **fumagillin 20mg po bid** reported effective for E. bieneusi (NEJM 346:1963, 2002)—see Comment	Peds dose ref. PIDJ 23:915, 2004
Disseminated: E. hellum, cuniculi or intestinalis; Pleistophora sp. otherson Comment	**Albendazole** 400mg po bid x 3wk	No established rx for Pleistophora sp.	For Trachipleistophora sp., try itraconazole + albendazole (NEJM 351:42, 2004). Other pathogens: Brachiola vesiculatum & algerae (NEJM 351:42, 2004).
PROTOZOA—EXTRAINTESTINAL			
Amebic meningoencephalitis			
Acanthamoeba sp — no proven rx Rev.: Clin Micro Rev 16:273, 2003	Success with IV **pentamidine**, topical **chlorhexidine** & 2% **ketoconazole** cream & then po rx: **TMP-SMX** + **rifampin** + **keto** (NEJM 331:85, 1994). 2 children responded to po rx: **flucon** + **itra** (CID 37:1304, 2003; Arch Path Lab Med 128:466, 2004).		For treatment of keratitis, see Table 1, page 12
Balamuthia mandrillaris	A cause of chronic granulomatous meningitis		
Naegleria fowleri, >95% mortality. Sappinia diploidea	**Pentamidine** + **clarithro** + **flucon** + **sulfadiazine** + **flucytosine** (CID 35:e131, 2002). Or **Ampho B** 1.5mg/kg per day in 2 div. doses & then 1mg/kg per day IV x 6 days **Azithro + pentamidine + itra + flucytosine** (JAMA 285:2450, 2001)		Case report: Ampho, micronazole, & RIF (NEJM 306:346, 1982).
Babesia microti; babesiosis (CID 22:1117, 2001)	**Atovaquone** 750mg bid po x 7–10 days + **azithro** 600mg po daily x 7–10 days (NEJM 343:1454, 2000)	(**Clindamycin** 600mg po tid) + (**quinine** 650mg po tid) x 7–10 days For adults, can give **clinda** IV as 1.2gm bid.	Can cause overwhelming infection in asplenic patients. Reported in Washington State (EID 10:622, 2004).
Ehrlichiosis—See Table 1, page 51			
Leishmaniasis Refs: Ln366:1561, 2005 & LnID 6:342, 2006			
Cutaneous (C), mucocutaneous (MC) **New World (Mexico/Cen./S. Amer.)** L. viana Includes braziliensi (C, MC), guyanensis (C,MC), panamensis (C,MC), peruviana (C) & L. mexicana Includes mexicana (C), amazonensis (C), venezolensis (C). NOTE: antimony resistance of L. viana reported JID 193, 1345, 2006	**Sodium stibogluconate (Pentosam)** from CDC drug service (404-639-3670) or **meglumine antimoniate (Glucantime)** in France & Latin America. Dose: 20 mg/kg/d in 2 divided doses IV/IM x 28 d. Dilute in 120ml of D5W & infuse over 2 hr. Ideally, monitor EKG. Note: only antimony drugs efficacious vs L. braziliensis	**Amphotericin B** 1mg/kg IV q.o.d. x 20 doses **or Liposomal ampho (Ambisome)** 3 mg/kg per day x 6 d for cutaneous & 3 wks for mucocutaneous. **Or miltefosine** effective vs L. panamensis, marginal vs L. mexicana, failed vs L. braziliensis. Obtain from Zentaris, Germany; Impavido @ Zentaris.de. Dose 2.5mg/kg p.o. once daily x 28 d.	Concern for species that disseminate to mucosa. Method of choice for speciation is pCR - not widely available; so empirically treat for species with potential to disseminate. Spontaneous resolution varies by species: L. mexicana: 75% in 3 mo; L. braziliensis: 10% in 3 mo; L. major 90% in 2-4 mo; L. tropica: 90% in 6-15 mo. For antimony AEs - see Table 13 B(1). Primary treatment for L. guyanensis in French Guiana is **pentamidine** 3 mg/kg IV q.o.d. x 4 for cutaneous & 15 for mucocutaneous.
Old World (Europe, Asia, Africa) L. major, L. tropica, L. aethiopica, L. infantum, L. chagas	**Stibogluconate or meglumine antimoniate** as above: 20mg/kg/d x 10 d	**Fluconazole** 200mg po once daily x 6wk effective vs L. major in Saudi Arabia (NEJM 346: 891, 2002)	

* See page 2 for abbreviations. All dosage recommendations are for adults (unless otherwise indicated) and assume normal renal function.

TABLE 13A (3)

INFECTING ORGANISM	SUGGESTED REGIMENS		COMMENTS
	PRIMARY	ALTERNATIVE	
PROTOZOA—EXTRAINTESTINAL *(continued)*			
Visceral leishmaniasis – Kala-Azar – New World & Old World *L. donovani:* India, Africa *L. infantum:* Mediterranean *L. chagasi:* New World	Everywhere except Bihar State, India & Southern Europe: **Stibogluconate or meglumine antimonite** as above. Dose: 20 mg/kg/d IV/IM in 2 divided doses 28-30 d [see Table 13 B(1)].	Bihar, India: **Ampho B** 1 mg/kg IV q.o.d. x 15 days or daily x 20 days or liposomal ampho B 1-3 mg/kg/d IV x 5 d (or 57.5 mg/kg IV x 1 dose or [paromomycin as above in comment]. Mediterranean: **liposomal ampho B** 3 mg/kg per day IV x 5 d, no drug x 5 d, then 10 mg/kg per day IV x 2 d. CID 43:917, 2006]	Other options for Bihar, India: 1) **Paromomycin** 16-20 mg/kg/d IM x 21 d, 2) **miltefosine** 2.5 mg/kg/d po x 28 d.
Malaria (Plasmodium species)—NOTE: CDC Malaria info—prophylaxis (877) 394-8747; treatment (770) 488-7788. After hours: 770-488-7100. **Websites:** www.cdc.gov/ncidod/dpd/parasites/malaria/default.htm, www.cdc.gov/malaria.			
	Prophylaxis: Chloroquine (CQ) plus personal protection measures, nets, 30-35% DEET skin repellent (avoid 95% products in children). Permethrin spray on clothing and nets **For areas free** of chloroquine (CQ)-resistant P. falciparum: Haiti, Dom. Republic, Cen. America west & north of the Panama Canal, & parts of Middle East.	**CQ** 500mg (300mg base) po per wk starting 1-2wk before travel, during travel, & 4 wks post-travel or **AP** 1 adult tab per day (1 day prior to, during, & 7 days post-travel). Note: May exacerbate psoriasis.	**CQ Peds dose:** 8.3mg/kg (5mg/kg of base) po 1x/wk up to 300mg (base) max. dose or **AP** by weight (peds tabs): 11-20kg, 1 tab; 21-30kg, 2 tabs; 31-40kg, 3 tabs; >40kg, 1 adult tab per day	CQ safe during pregnancy. **The areas free of CQ-resistant falciparum malaria continue to shrink:** Central America west of the Panama Canal, Haiti, and parts of Middle East. CQ-resistant falciparum malaria reported from Saudi Arabia, Yemen, Oman, & Iran.
	For areas with CQ-resistant P. falciparum	**Atovaquone** 250mg—**proguanil** 100mg (Malarone), 1 comb. tablet, 1 per day with food 1-2 days prior to, during, & 7 days post-travel. Peds dose in footnote.¹ Cost per 2wks: \$125.	**Doxycycline** 100mg po daily or tabs & children 2wks. Cost per 2wks: \$30. **OR** **Mefloquine (MQ)** 250mg (228mg base) po per wk, 1 wk before, during, & for 4 wks after travel. Cost per 2wks: \$80	**Pregnancy: Avoid current best option.** Insufficient data with **Malarone. Avoid doxycycline and primaquine.** Primaquine. Used only if prolonged exposure to endemic area (e.g., Peace Corps). **Can cause hemolytic anemia if G6PD deficiency present.**
	CDC info on prophylaxis: (770) 488-7788 or website: www.cdc.gov & LnID 6:139, 2006	Another option for adults: **primaquine** (PO) 30mg base po daily in non-pregnant G6PD-neg. travelers 88% protective vs P. falciparum & >92% vs P. vivax (CID 33:1990, 2001)	MQ dose in footnote.¹ Primaquine dose in footnote.¹	**MQ not recommended** if cardiac conduction abnormalities, seizures, or psychiatric disorders, e.g. depression, psychosis. MQ outside U.S.: 275mg tab, contains 250mg of base. MQ CDC Hotline: 770-488-7788.

Treatment—Based on CDC Guidelines for drugs available in US. Artesunate drugs of major import in SE Asia & Africa but presently **not available in US.**

Suggested Treatment Regimens (Drug)

Clinical Severity/ Plasmodia sp.	Region Acquired	Primary—Adults	Alternative & Peds	Comments
Uncomplicated:¹ P. falciparum (or not identified)	Cen. Amer., west of Panama Canal, Haiti, Dom. Republic, & most of Mid East—**CQ-sensitive**	**CQ** 1 gm salt (600mg base), then 0.5gm (6hrs, then) 0.5gm daily x 2 days. Total: 2500mg salt.	**Peds: CQ** 10mg/kg of base po, then 5mg/kg of base at 6, 24, & 48 hrs. Total: 25mg/kg base.	Peds dose should never exceed adult dose.
	CQ-resistant or unknown resistance	**QS** 650mg po tid x 3 days + [(**Doxy** 100mg po bid) or **tetra** 250mg po qid or **clinda** 20mg/kg/d divided t.id]) x 7 days **OR** **Atovaquone-proguanil** 1 gm—400mg (4 adult tabs) po 1x/day x 3 days w/ food or mefloquine 750mg po x 1 dose, then 500mg po x 1 dose 6-12hr later.	**Peds: QS** 650mg po, then 500mg po in 12 hrs. **Peds: QS** 10mg/kg po tid) + **clinda** 20mg/kg per day (div. t.id) — both x 7 days	Can substitute clinda for doxy/tetra: 20mg/kg per day po div. tid x 7 days. MQ alternative due to neuropsych. reactions. Avoid if malaria acquired in SE Asia due to resistance.
Uncomplicated:¹ P. malariae	All regions	**CQ** as above: adults & peds		

---

¹ **Peds prophylaxis dosages.** (Ref.: *CID* 34:493, 2002): **Mefloquine** weekly dose by **weight** in kg: <15 = 5 mg/kg; 15-19 = ¼ adult dose; 20-30 = ½ adult dose; 31-45 = ¾ adult dose; >45 = adult dose.
Atovaquone/proguanil by **weight** in kg, single daily dose using peds tab (62.5 mg atovaquone & 25 mg proguanil): <11 kg—do not use; 11-20 kg, 1 tab; 21-30 kg, 2 tabs; 31-40 kg, 3 tabs; ≥41 kg = adult dose.
one adult tab. **Doxycycline**, ages >8-12 yrs: 2 mg per kg per day up to 100 mg/day
* See page 2 for abbreviations. All dosage recommendations are for adults (unless otherwise indicated) and assume normal renal function.

TABLE 13A (4)

INFECTING ORGANISM	SUGGESTED REGIMENS		COMMENTS
	PRIMARY	ALTERNATIVE	

PROTOZOA—EXTRAINTESTINAL/Malaria/Treatment (continued)

Clinical Severity/ Plasmodium sp.	Region Acquired	Suggested Treatment Regimens (Drug)		Comments
		Primary—Adults	**Alternative—Adults**	
Uncomplicated/ P. vivax or P. ovale	All except Papua, New Guinea & Indonesia (CQ-resistant)	**CQ** as above + **PQ** base: 30mg po once daily x 14 days	**Peds: CQ** as above + **PQ** base: 0.5mg/kg base once daily x 14 days	PQ added to eradicate latent parasites in liver. Screen for G6PD def. before starting PQ, if G6PD positive, dose PQ as 45mg po once weekly x 8wk.
Uncomplicated/ P. vivax	CQ-resistant: Papua, New Guinea & Indonesia	**QS + (doxy or tetra) + PQ** as above	**MQ + PQ** as above. **Peds** <8yrs old: **QS** alone x 7 days or **MQ** alone. If latter fail, add **doxy** or **tetra**	Doxy or tetra used if benefits outweigh risks.
Uncomplicated/ Pregnancy	CQ-sensitive areas	**CQ** as above		No controlled studies of AP in pregnancy. Possible association of MQ & ↑ number of stillbirths.
	CQ-resistant P. falciparum	**QS + clinda** as above	If failing or intolerant, **QS + doxy**	If P. vivax or P. ovale, after pregnancy check for G6PD & give PQ 30mg po daily times 14 days.
	CQ-resistant P. vivax	**QS** 650mg po tid x 7 days		During quinidine IV: monitor BP, EKG (prolongation of QTc), & blood glucose (hypoglycemia).
Severe malaria, i.e., impaired consciousness, severe anemia, renal failure, pulmonary edema, ARDS, DIC, jaundice, acidosis, seizures, parasitemia >5%. One or more of latter. Almost always P. falciparum	All regions	**Quinidine gluconate** in normal saline: 10mg/kg (salt) IV over 1hr then 0.02mg/kg/min by constant infusion OR 24mg/kg IV over 4hrs & then 12mg/kg IV over 4hrs q8h x (continue until parasite density <1% & can take po) **PLUS** **Doxy** 100mg IV q12h x 7 days) OR **clinda** 10mg/kg IV load & then 5mg/kg IV q8h x 7 days)	**Peds: Quinidine gluconate** IV—same mg/kg dose as for adults **PLUS** **Doxy** (if <48kg, 4 mg per kg IV q12h; if >48kg, dose as for adults) OR **Clinda**, same mg/kg dose as for adults	Consider exchange transfusion if parasitemia > 10%. Switch to oral QS, doxy, & clinda when patient able. Steroids not recommended for cerebral malaria. **Outside US, artemisinins (artemether, artesunate) are widely used in combo because of efficacy vs resistant plasmodia, modest cost, & relative safety**, e.g. artesunate 2mg/kg iv q8h + clinda (CID 40:1777, 2005). For more info: NEJM 352:1565, 2005 & WHO article & www.rbm/WHO int. Not available to date in US
Malaria—self-initiated treatment: Only for emergency situation where medical care not available		**Atovaquone-proguanil (AP)** 4 adult tabs (1gm/400mg) po x 3 days	**Peds**: Using adult AP tabs for 3 consecutive days: 11–20kg, 1 tab; 21–30kg, 2 tabs; 31–40kg, 3 tabs; >41 kg, 4 tabs.	Do not use for renal insufficiency pts. Do not use if weight <11kg, pregnant, or breast-feeding.
Pneumocystis carinii pneumonia (PCP). New name is **Pneumocystis jiroveci** (yes—row wiki ex). Refs.: CID 40(Suppl 3):S131, 2005; 41:1752 & 1756, 2005; 42:1208, 2006				
Not acutely ill, able to take po meds. PaO₂ >70 mmHg		(**TMP-SMX-DS**, 2 tabs po q8h x 21 days) OR (**Dapsone** 100mg po q24h + **trimethoprim** 5mg/kg po tid x 21 days)	(**Clindamycin** 300-450mg po q6h + **primaquine** 15mg base po q24h) x 21 days OR **Atovaquone** suspension 750mg po bid with food x 21 days	Mutations in gene of the enzyme target (dihydropteroate synthetase) of sulfamethoxazole result in resistance. Unclear whether mutations result in resist to TMP-SMX or dapsone → TMP resist (EID 10:1721, 2004). Dapsone ref.: CID 27:191, 1998.
		NOTE: Concomitant use of corticosteroids usually reserved for sicker pts with PaO₂ <70 (see below)		After 21 days, chronic suppression in AIDS pts (see below)
Acutely ill, po rx not possible. PaO₂ <70 mmHg		**Prednisone** (15–30 min. before TMP-SMX): 40 mg po bid times 5 days, then 40 mg q24h times 5 days, then 20 mg po q24h times 11 days) + **TMP-SMX** (15 mg of TMP component per kg per day IV div q6–8h x 21 days) Can substitute IV prednisolone (reduce dose 25%) for prednisone	**Prednisone** as in primary + PLUS (**Clinda** (600 mg IV q8h) + **primaquine** 30 mg base po q24h) times 21 days OR **Pentamidine** 4 mg per kg per day IV times 21 days. Caspofungin active in animal models: CID 36:1445, 2003	After 21 days, chronic suppression of HIV infection & steroids (CID 25:215 & 219, 1997). **PCP can occur in absence of HIV infection** (CID 25:215 & 219, 1997). Wait at least 4–8 days before declaring treatment failure & switching to clinda + primaquine or pentamidine. See above regarding gene mutations.

* See page 2 for abbreviations. All dosage recommendations are for adults (unless otherwise indicated) and assume normal renal function.

TABLE 13A (5)

INFECTING ORGANISM	SUGGESTED REGIMENS		COMMENTS
	PRIMARY	ALTERNATIVE	
PROTOZOA—EXTRAINTESTINAL / Pneumocystis carinii pneumonia (PCP) (continued)			
Primary prophylaxis and post-treatment suppression	**TMP-SMX-DS or -SS.** 1 tab po q24h or 1 DS 3x/wk. **Dapsone** 100mg po q24h or DS 3x/wk then CD4 >200x/3mo (NEJM 344:159, 2001).	**Pentamidine** 300mg nebul. in 6mL sterile water by special of aero q3wk. **Dapsone** 200mg po + **pyrimethamine** 75mg po + **folinic acid** 25mg po —**all once a week**) or **atovaquone** 1500mg po q24h with food.	TMP-SMX-DS regimen provides cross-protection vs toxo and other bacterial infections. Dapsone + pyrimethamine po protects vs toxo. Atovaquone suspension 1500 mg once daily as effective as daily dapsone (NEJM 339:1889, 1998) or inhaled pentamidine (JID 180:369, 1999).
Toxoplasma gondii (Reference: Ln 363:1965, 2004)			
Immunologically normal patients (For pediatric doses, see reference)			
Acute illness w/ lymphadenopathy	No specific rx unless severe/persistent symptoms or evidence of vital organ damage		
Acq. via transfusion (lab accident)	Treat as for active chorioretinitis		
Active chorioretinitis: meningitis; lowered resistance due to steroids or cytotoxic drugs	**Pyrimethamine** (pyri) 200mg po x 1 day, then 50–75 mg po q24h + **sulfadiazine** (see footnote*) 1–1.5gm po q6h) + **leucovorin** (folinic acid) 5–20mg 3x/wk — **see Comment**. Treat 1–2wk beyond resolution of signs/symptoms; continue leucovorin 1wk after stopping pyri.		For congenital toxo, toxo meningitis in adults, & chorioretinitis, **add prednisone 1mg/kg/day in 2 div. doses** until CSF protein conc. falls or vision-threatening inflammation subsides. Adjust folinic acid dose by following CBC results. IgG avidity test of help in 1st trimester (J Clin Micro 42:941, 2004).
Acute in pregnant woman	**Spiramycin** [From FDA, (301) 827-2335] 3gm po q6h (w/o food) until term or until fetal infection. NOTE: Use caution interpreting commercial tests for toxoplasma IgM antibody; for help, FDA Advisory, (301) 594-3060, Toxoplasma Serology Lab, Palo Alto Med. Found., (650) 853-4828.		Details in Ln 363:1965, 2004. **Consultation advisable.**
Fetal/congenital	Mgmt complex. Combo rx with pyrimethamine + sulfadiazine + leucovorin—see Comment		
Acquired immunodeficiency syndrome (AIDS)			
Cerebral toxoplasmosis Ref.: Ln 363:1965, 2004; CID 40(Suppl-3):S131, 2005	**Pyrimethamine** (pyri) 200mg x 1 po, then 50–75mg/day + **sulfadiazine** 1–1.5gm po q6h + **folinic acid** 10–20mg/day po) for 4–6wks after resolution of signs/symptoms, and then suppressive rx (see below) OR **TMP-SMX** 10/50mg/kg per day po or IV div q12h x 30 days (AAC 42:1346, 1998)	**Pyri + folinic acid** (as in primary regimen) + 1 of the following: (1) **Clinda** 600mg po/IV q6h or q12 (2) **clarithro** 1gm po bid or (3) **azithro** 1.2–1.5gm po q24h or (4) **atovaquone** 750mg po q6h. Treat 4–6 wks after resolution of signs/symptoms, then suppression.	Use alternative regimen for pts with severe sulfa allergy. If multiple ring-enhancing brain lesions (CT or MRI), >85% of pts respond to 7–10 days of empiric rx; if no response, suggest brain biopsy. Pyri penetrates brain even if no inflammation; folinic acid prevents pyrimethamine hematologic toxicity.
Primary prophylaxis. AIDS pts—IgG toxo antibody + CD4 count <100 per mcL	**TMP-SMX-DS.** 1 tab po q24h) or (**TMP-SMX-SS.** 1 tab po q24h)	**(Dapsone** 50mg po q24h) + **(pyri** 50mg po q wk) + **folinic acid** 25mg po q wk). OR (**Dapsone** 200mg po q24h + pyri 75mg po q24h + folinic acid 25mg po q wk) OR **atovaquone** 750mg po q6-12h	Prophylaxis for pneumocystis also effective vs toxo. Refs: MMWR 51(RR-8), 6/14/2002; ArlM 137:435, 2002
Suppression after rx of cerebral toxo	**Sulfadiazine** 500–1000mg po 4x/day + (**pyri** 25–50mg po q24h) + (**folinic acid** 10–25mg po q24h). DC if CD4 count >200 x 3mo	**(Clinda** 300–450mg po q6-8h) + **pyri** 25–50mg po q24h) + **folinic acid** 10–25mg po q24h) OR **atovaquone** 750mg po q6-12h	(Pyri + sulfa) prevents PCP and toxo; (clinda + pyri) prevents toxo only.
Trichomonas vaginalis	See Vaginitis, Table 1, page 23		
Trypanosomiasis. Ref.: Ln 362:1469, 2003			
West African sleeping sickness (T. brucei gambiense)			
Early: Blood/lymphatic–CNS OK	**Pentamidine** 4mg/kg IM daily x 10 days	**Suramin** 100mg IV (test dose), then 1gm IV on days 1,3,7,14,21	
Late: Encephalitis	**Melarsoprol** 2.2mg/kg per day IV x 10 days	**Eflornithine** 100mg/kg q6h IV x 14 days (CID 41:748, 2005)	Melarsoprol trial data: JID 191:1793 & 1922, 2005
Prophylaxis	**Pentamidine** 3mg/kg IM q6 mos.	Not for casual visitor	

---

† Sulfonamides now commercially available. Sulfadiazine much less effective.
* See page 2 for abbreviations. All dosage recommendations are for adults (unless otherwise indicated) and assume normal renal function.

TABLE 13A (6)

INFECTING ORGANISM	SUGGESTED REGIMENS		COMMENTS
	PRIMARY	**ALTERNATIVE**	
PROTOZOA—EXTRAINTESTINAL/Trypanosomiasis (continued)			
East African sleeping sickness (T. brucei rhodesiense)			
Early: Blood/lymphatic	**Suramin** 100mg IV (test dose), then 1gm IV on days 1,3,7,14, & 21	None	
Late: Encephalitis	**Melarsoprol** [1] 2-3.6mg/kg per day IV x 3 days; repeat after 7 days & for 3rd time 7 days after 2nd course	Prednisone may prevent/attenuate encephalopathy	
T. cruzi—**Chagas disease** or acute American trypanosomiasis Ref: Ln 357:1521, 2001 For chronic disease: see Comment.	**Nifurtimox** [1] 8-10mg/kg per day po div. 4x/day after meals x 120 days Ages 11-16yrs: 12.5-15mg/kg per day div. qid x 90 days Children <11yrs: 15-20mg/kg per day div. qid x 90 days	**Benznidazole** [N1] [5] 5-7mg/kg per day po div. 2x/day (A7MH 63:11, 2000). NOTE: Avoid tetracycline and steroids.	Chronic disease: 1) Immunosuppression for heart transplant can reactivate chronic Chagas disease. 2) Reduced progression with 30 d of benznidazole 5 mg/kg per day. AnIM 144:724, 2006
NEMATODES—INTESTINAL (Roundworms) Eosinophilia? Think Strongyloides, Schistosomiasis and Filariasis: CID 34:407, 2005; 42:1781 & 1655, 2006			
Ascaris lumbricoides (**ascariasis**) Ln 367:1521, 2006	**Albendazole** 400mg po x 1 dose or **mebendazole** 100mg po bid x 3 days or 500mg po x 1 dose	**Ivermectin** 150-200mcg/kg po x 1 dose or **Nitazoxanide: Adults**—500mg po bid x 3 days; **children 4-11**—200mg oral susp. po q12h	Can present with intestinal obstruction.
Capillaria philippinensis (**capillariasis**)	**Mebendazole** 200mg po bid x 20 days	**Albendazole** 200mg po bid x 10 days	
Enterobius vermicularis (**pinworm**)	**Albendazole** 400mg po x 1, repeat in 2wks OR **mebendazole** 100mg po x 1, repeat in 2wks	**Pyrantel pamoate** 11mg/kg (to max. dose of 1gm) po x 1 dose; repeat every 2wks x 2.	Side-effects in Table 13B, pages 124, 124
Hookworm (Necator americanus and Ancylostoma duodenale)	**Albendazole** 400mg po x 1 dose or **mebendazole** 500mg po x 1 dose	**Pyrantel pamoate** 11mg/kg (to max. dose of 1gm) po daily x 3 days	NOTE: Ivermectin not effective. Eosinophilia may be absent but eggs in stool (NEJM 351:799, 2004).
Strongyloides stercoralis (**strongyloidiasis**)	**Ivermectin** 200mcg/kg per day po x 2 days	**Albendazole** 400mg po bid x 2 days (7-10 days for hyperinfection syndrome)	Case report of ivermectin failure in pt with hypogamma-globulinemia (Am J Med Sci 311:178, 1996)
Trichostrongylus orientalis	**Albendazole** 400mg po x 1 dose	**Pyrantel pamoate** 11mg/kg (max. 1gm) po x 1	**Mebendazole** 100mg po bid x 3 days
Trichuris trichiura (**whipworm**) Ln 367:1521, 2006	**Albendazole** 400mg po 1x/day x 3 days	**Mebendazole** 100mg po bid x 3 days or 500mg po once	**Ivermectin** 200mcg/kg daily po x 3 days
Angiostrongylus cantonensis—a cause of eosinophilic meningitis	Supportive care. Serial LPs to ↓ intracranial pressure	Anthelminth therapy may worsen meningitis (NEJM 346:668, 2002). Prednisone may help.	Mortality rate <1%. Ref: AJM 114:217, 2003)
Anisakis simplex (**anisakiasis**) CID 41:1297, 2005; UnD 4:294, 2004	Physical removal: endoscope or surgery IgE antibody test vs A. simplex may help diagnosis.	Anecdotal reports of possible treatment benefit from albendazole (Ln 360:54, 2002; CID 41:1825, 2005)	Anisakiasis acquired by eating raw fish: herring, salmon, mackerel, cod, squid. Similar illness due to Pseudoterranova species acquired from cod, halibut, red snapper.
Ancylostoma braziliense & caninum: causes **cutaneous larva migrans**	**Ivermectin** 200mcg/kg po x 1 dose/day x 1-2 days	**Albendazole** 200mg po bid x 3 days	Also called "creeping eruption," dog and cat hookworm. Ivermectin cure rate 77% (1 dose) to 97% (2-3 doses) CID 31:493, 2000).
Baylisascariasis (Raccoon ascaris)	No drug proven efficacious. Try po **albendazole**. Both x 10 days	**Peds**: 25-50mg/kg per day; **Adults**: 400mg po bid	Some add steroids (CID 39:1484, 2004).
Dracunculus medinensis: **Guinea worm**	Slow extraction of pre-emergent worm	**Metronidazole** 250mg po tid x 10 days used to ↓ inflammatory response and facilitate removal. Immersion in warm water promotes worm emergence. Mebendazole 400-800mg/day x 6 days may kill worm.	

[1] Available from CDC Drug Service; see footnote 1 page 122

* See page 2 for abbreviations. All dosage recommendations are for adults (unless otherwise indicated) and assume normal renal function.

TABLE 13A (7)

INFECTING ORGANISM	SUGGESTED REGIMENS		COMMENTS
	PRIMARY	ALTERNATIVE	
NEMATODES—INTESTINAL (Roundworms) *(continued)*			
Filariasis. Wolbachia bacteria needed for filarial development. Rx with doxy 100-200mg/day ×4-6wks × number of worms/ number of wolbachia & number of microfilaria (*BMJ* 326:207, 2003)			
Lymphatic (**Elephantiasis**): Wuchereria bancrofti or Brugia malayi or B. timori	**Doxycycline** 100mg po t.i.d. x 3 wks & then of: Albendazole 400mg po + ivermectin 150mg/kg po) (*CID 42:1*(081 & 1090, 2006)	**Diethylcarbamazine**[1,2] (DEC) 6mg/kg po once — similar effect as multiple doses. Induces inflammatory response due to release of microfilaria & Wolbachia.	**Diethylcarbamazine**[1,2] (DEC): po over 14 days: Day 1, 50 mg; day 2, 50mg tid; day 3, 100mg tid; days 4-14, 2mg/kg tid. NOTE: DEC & ivermectin could cause irreversible eye damage if concomitant onchocerciasis.
Cutaneous			
Loiasis: **Loa loa, eyeworm disease** (*Ln 360:203, 2002*)	**Diethylcarbamazine** (DEC)[2,4]—6mg/kg po times 1 dose	**Ivermectin** 150mcg/kg po times 1 dose; repeat q6mo to suppress dermal & ocular microfilariae.	DEC 300mg/Wk po effective prophylaxis. Ivermectin ↓ number of microfilariae in skin and impairs female worm fertility; does not kill adult worms (nothing does). Ivermectin OK in pregnancy.
Onchocerca volvulus (**onchocerciasis**)—river blindness	**Ivermectin** 150mcg/kg po times 1 dose; if eye involved, start **prednisone** 1mg/kg po several days before ivermectin. NOTE: Worm survival requires symbiotic bacteria Wolbachia (*Science 296:1365, 2002*).		
Body cavity			
Mansonella perstans (dipetalonemiasis)	**Mebendazole**[1] 100mg po bid x 30 days or **albendazole** 400mg po bid x 10 days	Usually no or vague allergic symptoms + eosinophilia. Ivermectin has no activity against this species.	
Mansonella streptocerca	**Diethylcarbamazine**[2,4] as above for Wuchereria OR **Ivermectin** 150mcg/kg x 1	Chronic pruritic hypopigmented lesions that may be confused with leprosy. Can be asymptomatic.	
Mansonella ozzardi	**Ivermectin** 200mcg/kg x 1 dose may be effective	Usually asymptomatic. Articular pain, pruritus, lymphadenopathy reported. May have allergic reaction from dying organisms.	
Dirofilariasis: **Heartworms**			
D. immitis, dog heartworm	No effective drugs; surgical removal only option		Can lodge in pulmonary artery → coin lesion. Eosinophilia rare.
D. tenuis (raccoon), D. ursi (bear), D. repens (dogs, cats)	No effective drugs	Worms migrate to conjunctivae, subcutaneous tissue, scrotum, breasts, extremities	
Gnathostoma spinigerum: eosinophilic myeloencephalitis	**Albendazole** 400 mg po q24h or bid times 21 days		**Ivermectin** 200 mcg per kg per day times 2 days
Toxocariasis: *Clin Micro Rev 16:265, 2003*	**Rx directed at relief of symptoms as infection self-limited, e.g., steroids & antihistamines; use of anthelminthics controversial.**		
Visceral larval migrans	**Albendazole** 400mg po bid x 5 days	**Mebendazole** 100-200 mg po bid times 5 days	Severe lung, heart or CNS disease may warrant steroids. Differential dx of larval migrans syndromes: Toxocara canis & cati, Ancylostoma spp., Gnathostoma spp., Strongyloides spp.
Ocular larval migrans	First 4 wks of illness: (Oral **prednisone** 30-60mg po q24h) + subtenon **triamcinolone** 40mg/Wk x 2Wk		No added benefit of anthelminthic drugs. Rx of little effect after 4Wk.
Trichinella spiralis (**trichinosis**)—muscle infection	**Albendazole** 400mg po bid x 8-14 days	**Mebendazole** 200-400mg po tid x 3 days, then 400-500mg po tid x 10 days	Use albendazole/mebendazole with caution during pregnancy
	Concomitant **prednisone** 40-60mg po q24h		

---

[1] Available from CDC Drug Service, see footnote 1 page 122

[2] May need antihistamine or corticosteroid for allergic reaction from disintegrating organisms

[3] Available from CDC Drug Service; see footnote 1 page 122

[4] May need antihistamine or corticosteroid for allergic reaction from disintegrating organisms

* See page 2 for abbreviations. *All dosage recommendations are for adults (unless otherwise indicated) and assume normal renal function.*

TABLE 13A (B)

INFECTING ORGANISM	SUGGESTED REGIMENS		COMMENTS
	PRIMARY	ALTERNATIVE	
TREMATODES (Flukes)			
Clonorchis sinensis (liver fluke)	**Praziquantel** 25mg/kg po tid x 1 day	or **albendazole** 10mg/kg per day po x 7 days	Same dose in children
Fasciola buski (intestinal fluke)	**Praziquantel** 25mg/kg po tid x 1 day		Same dose in children
Fasciola hepatica (sheep liver fluke)	**Triclabendazole**[1] (Fasinex; Novartis Agribusiness) 10mg/kg po x 1 dose. Ref. CID 32:1, 2001		**Bithionol**[1] Adults and children: 30-50mg/kg (max. dose 2gm/day) every other day times 10-15 doses
Heterophyes heterophyes (intestinal fluke); Metagonimus yokogawai (intestinal fluke); Opisthorchis viverrini (liver fluke)	**Praziquantel** 25mg/kg po tid x 1 day		Same dose in children. Same regimen for **Metorchis conjunctus (North American liver fluke)**; **Nanophyetus salmincola:** Praziquantel 20mg/kg po tid x 1 day
Paragonimus westermani (lung fluke)	**Praziquantel** 25mg/kg po tid x 2 days or **bithionol**[1] 30-50mg/kg po x 1 every other day x 10 days		Same dose in children. Alternative: mefinfonate 10mg/kg per dose po q2 wks for 3 doses.
Schistosoma haematobium: GU bilharziasis. (NEJM 346:1212, 2002)	**Praziquantel** 20mg/kg po bid x 1 day (2 doses)		Same dose in children
Schistosoma intercalatum.	**Praziquantel** 20mg/kg po bid x 1 day (2 doses)		Same dose in children
Schistosoma japonicum: Oriental schisto. NEJM 346:1212, 2002	**Praziquantel** 20mg/kg po **tid** x 1 day **(3 doses)**		Same dose in children. Cures 60-90% pts.
Schistosoma mansoni (intestinal bilharziasis)	**Praziquantel** 20mg/kg po bid x 1 day (2 doses)	**Oxamniquine** [4a] single dose of 15mg/kg po once; In North and East Africa 20mg/kg po daily x 3 days Do not use during pregnancy.	Same dose for children. Cures 60-90% pts. Report of success treating myeloradiculopathy with single po dose of praziquantel, 50mg/kg, + prednisone for 6mo (CID 39:1618, 2004).
Possible praziquantel resistance (JID 176:304, 1997) (NEJM 346:1212, 2002)			
Schistosoma mekongi	**Praziquantel** 20 mg per kg po **tid** times 1 day **(3 doses)**		Same dose for children
Toxemic schisto: Katayama fever	**Praziquantel** 25 mg per kg po q4h with food times 3 doses		Massive infection with either S. japonicum or S. mansoni
CESTODES (Tapeworms)			
Echinococcus granulosus (hydatid disease) CID 37:1073, 2003; CID 362:1295 2003)	Meta-analysis supports percutaneous aspiration-injection-reaspiration (PAIR) + albendazole. Before & after drainage: **albendazole** ≥60kg, 400mg po bid or <60kg, 15mg/kg per day div. bid, with meals. Then: Puncture (P) & needle aspirate (A) cyst content. Instill (I) hypertonic saline (15–30%) or absolute alcohol, wait 20–30min, then re-aspirate (R) with final irrigation. **Continue albendazole x 28 days** Cure in 96% as comp to 90% with surgical resection.		
Echinococcus multilocularis (alveolar cyst disease) (CID 16:437, 2003)	**Albendazole** efficacy not clearly demonstrated, can try in dosages used for hydatid disease. Wide surgical resection only reliable rx; technique evolving (Radiology 198:259, 1996).		
Intestinal tapeworms			
Diphyllobothrium latum (fish); Dipylidium caninum (dog); Taenia saginata (beef); & Taenia solium (pork)	**Praziquantel** 5-10mg/kg po x 1 dose for children and adults. **Alternative was Niclosamide** 2gm po x 1, however, drug no longer available.		
Hymenolepis diminuta (rats) and H. nana (humans)	**Praziquantel** 25 mg/kg po x 1 dose for children and adults. Alternativewas **Niclosamide** 500mg po q24h x 3 days; however, drug no longer available.		
Neurocysticercosis (NCC): Larval form of T. solium Ref.: AJTMH 72:3, 2005	**NOTE: Treat T. solium intestinal tapeworms,** if present, with **praziquantel** 5-10 mg/kg po x 1 dose for children & adults.		

[1] Available from CDC Drug Service; see footnote 1, page 122

* See page 2 for abbreviations. All dosage recommendations are for adults (unless otherwise indicated) and assume normal renal function.

TABLE 13A (9)

INFECTING ORGANISM	SUGGESTED REGIMENS		COMMENTS
	PRIMARY	**ALTERNATIVE**	

CESTODES (Tapeworms) / Neurocysticercosis (NCC) *(continued)*

INFECTING ORGANISM	PRIMARY	ALTERNATIVE	COMMENTS
Parenchymal NCC "Viable" cysts by CT/MRI Meta-analysis: Treatment assoc with cyst resolution, ↓ seizures, and ↓ seizure recurrence. *AnIM 145:43, 2006.*	**[Albendazole ≥60 kg: 400mg bid with meals or <60 kg: 15mg/kg per day in 2 div. doses (max. 800mg/day) +** Anti-seizure medication] — all x 8 days **Dexamethasone** 0.1mg/kg per day ± Anti-seizure medication] — all x 15 days.	**(Praziquantel** 50–100mg/kg per day in 3 div. doses + **Dexamethasone** 0.1mg/kg per day ±** Anti-seizure medication) See Comment	Albendazole assoc. with 46% ↓ in seizures *(NEJM 350:249, 2004).* Praziquantel less cysticidal activity. Steroids decrease serum levels of praziquantel. NIH reports success substituting methotrexate for dexamethasone.
"Degenerating" cysts	**Albendazole + dexamethasone** as above		Treatment improves prognosis of associated seizures.
Dead calcified cysts	No treatment indicated		
Subarachnoid NCC	**(Albendazole + steroids** as above) + shunting for hydrocephalus. Without shunt, 50% died within 9yrs *(J Neurosurg 66:686, 1987).*		
intraventricular NCC	**Albendazole + dexamethasone** as above		
Sparganosis (Spirometra mansonoides) Larval cysts; source—frogs/snakes	Surgical resection or ethanol injection of subcutaneous masses *(NEJM 330:1887, 1994).*		

DISEASE	INFECTING ORGANISM	SUGGESTED REGIMENS		COMMENTS
		PRIMARY	**ALTERNATIVE**	

ECTOPARASITES Ref.: *CID 36:1355, 2003; Ln 363:889, 2004.* NOTE: Due to potential neurotoxicity, lindane not recommended.

DISEASE	INFECTING ORGANISM	PRIMARY	ALTERNATIVE	COMMENTS
Head lice *Med Lett 47:68, 2005*	Pediculus humanus var. capitis	**Permethrin** 1% (generic lotion or cream rinse [Nix]): Apply to shampooed dried hair for 10min.; repeat in 1 wk. **OR Malathion** 0.5% (Ovide): Apply to dry hair for 8–14 hrs, then shampoo.	**Ivermectin** 200–400mcg/kg po once; repeat in 7–10 days	**Permethrin** success in 78%. Extra combing of no benefit. Resistance increasing. No advantage to 5% permethrin. **Malathion:** Report that 1–2 20-min. applications 98% effective *Ped Derm 21:670, 2004),* in alcohol—potentially flammable.
Pubic lice (crabs)	Phthirus pubis	**Pubic hair: Permethrin OR malathion** as for head lice	**Eyelids: Petroleum jelly** applied qid x 10 days OR **yellow oxide of mercury** 1% qid x 14 days	Costs: Permethrin 1% lotion/cream $8–9 Malathion 0.5% lotion $119 Ivermectin $20
Body lice	Pediculus humanus var. corporis	No drugs for pt; treat the clothing. Organism lives in & deposits eggs in seams of clothing. Discard clothing. If not possible, treat clothing with 1% malathion powder or 10% DDT powder. Success with ivermectin in home shelter 12mg po on days 0, 7, & 14 *(JID 193:474, 2006)*		
Scabies Immunocompetent patients *Rds: 367:1767, 2006; NEJM 354:1718, 2006.* (Norwegian scabies—see Comments)	Sarcoptes scabiei	**Primary: Permethrin** 5% cream (ELIMITE). Apply entire skin from chin to toes. Leave on 8–14hr. Repeat in 1wk. Safe for children >2mo old. **Alternative: Ivermectin** 200mcg/kg po x 1; 2nd dose 14 days later. For Norwegian scabies: **Permethrin** 5% as above on day 1, then 6% sulfur in petrolatum daily on days 2–7, then repeat times several weeks. **Ivermectin** 200mcg/kg po x 1 reported effective.		Trim fingernails. Reapply to hands after handwashing. Pruritus may persist times 2wk after mites gone. Less effective: Crotamiton 10% cream, apply x 24 hr, rinse off, then reapply x 24 hr. Norwegian scabies in AIDS pts: Extensive, crusted. Can mimic psoriasis. Not pruritic. ELIMITE: 60 gm $18.60; Ivermectin $19.62 Highly contagious—isolate!
AIDS patients, CD4 <150 per mm³ (Norwegian scabies—see Comments)				
Myiasis Due to larvae of flies		Usually cutaneous/subcutaneous nodule with central punctum. Treatment: Occlude punctum to prevent gas exchange with petrolatum, fingernail polish, makeup, cream or bacon. When larva migrates, loosely remove.		

* See page 2 for abbreviations. All dosage recommendations are for adults (unless otherwise indicated) and assume normal renal function.

TABLE 13B – DOSAGE, PRICE, AND SELECTED ADVERSE EFFECTS OF ANTIPARASITIC DRUGS

NOTE: Drugs available from CDC Drug Service indicated by "CDC". Call (404) 639-3670 (or -2888).
Doses vary with indication. For convenience, drugs divided by type of parasite; some drugs used for multiple types of parasites, e.g. albendazole.
COMMENT: Cost data represent average wholesale prices as listed in 2006 Drug Topics Red Book, Medical Economics.

CLASS, AGENT, GENERIC NAME (TRADE NAME)	USUAL ADULT DOSAGE (Cost)	ADVERSE REACTIONS/COMMENTS
Antiprotozoan Drugs		
Intestinal Parasites		
Albendazole (Albenza)	Doses vary with indication. 200-400mg bid po 200mg tab $1.58	Teratogenic. Pregnancy Cat. C; give after negative pregnancy test. Abdominal pain, nausea/vomiting, alopecia, ↑ serum transaminase. Rare leukopenia.
Dehydroemetine (CDC)*	1.5mg/kg per day to max. of 90mg IM	Local pain, ECG changes, cardiac arrhythmias, precordial pain, paresthesias, weakness, peripheral neuropathy. GI: nausea/vomiting, diarrhea. Avoid strenuous exercise for 4 wks after rx.
Iodoquinol (Yodoxin) (650 mg) $1.09	Adults: 650mg po tid, children: 40mg/kg per day div tid.	Rarely causes nausea, abdominal cramps, rash, acne. Contraindicated if iodine intolerance.
Metronidazole/Ornidazole (Tiberal)	Side-effects similar for all. See *metronidazole in Table 10A*	See *Table 10C, page 91*
Paromomycin (Humatin)	Up to 750mg qid.	Drug is aminoglycoside similar to neomycin; if absorbed due to concomitant inflammatory bowel
Aminosidine in U.K.	250mg caps $3.57	disease can result in oto/nephrotoxicity. Doses >3 gm assoc. with nausea, abdominal cramps, diarrhea.
Quinacrineᵛˢ˒ᵉ (**Atabrine, Mepacrine**)	No longer available in U.S. 2 pharmacies will compare as a service: (1) Panorama Pharmacies, 800-247-9767 Connecticut 203-785-6816; (2) California 800-247-9767	Contraindicated for pts with history of psychosis or psoriasis. Yellow staining of skin. Dizziness, headache, vomiting, toxic psychosis (1.5%), hemolytic anemia, leukopenia, thrombocytopenia, urticaria, rash, fever, minor disulfiram-like reactions.
Antiprotozoan Drugs		
Tinidazole (Tindamax)	500mg tabs, with food. Regimen varies with indication. Cost: 500mg tab $4.56	Chemical structure similar to metronidazole but better tolerated. Seizures/peripheral neuropathy reported. **Adverse effects:** Metallic taste 4-6%, nausea 3-5%, anorexia 2-3%.
Extraintestinal Parasites		
Antimony compoundsᴬᵁˢ Stibogluconate sodium (Pentostam) from CDC or Meglumine antimoniate (Glucantime— French tradenames)	Dilute in 120ml of D₅W and infuse over 2hr. Ideally, monitor EKG.	Fatigue, myalgia, N/V and diarrhea common. ALT/AST ↑s, ↑ amylase and lipase occur. **NOTE: Reversible T wave changes in 30-60%. Risk of QTc prolongation.**
Atovaquone (Mepron) Ref. AAC 46:1163, 2002	Suspension: 1tsp (750 mg) po bid 750mg/5mL. Cost: 210mL $821	No. pts stopping rx due to side-effects was 9%, rash 22%, GI 20%, headache 16%, insomnia 10%, fever 14%
Atovaquone and proguanil (Malarone) For prophylaxis of P. falciparum; little data on P. vivax	**Prophylaxis:** 1 tab po (250mg + 100mg) q24h with food **Treatment:** 4 tabs po (1000mg + 400mg) once daily with food x 3 days Adult tab: 250/100mg. Peds tab 62.5/25mg. Peds dosage: footnote 1 page 97 Cost: 250/100mg tab $5.33	Adverse effects in rx trials: Adults—abd. pain 17%, N/V 12%, headache 10%, dizziness 5% Rx stopped in 1%. Asymptomatic mild ↑ in ALT/AST. Children—cough, headache, anorexia, vomiting, abd. pain. See *drug interactions, Table 22.* Safe in G6PD-deficient pts. Can crush tabs for children and give with milk or other liquid nutrients. Renal insufficiency: contraindicated if CrCl <30 mL per min.
Benznidazoleᴬᵁˢ (**Rochagan**, Roche, Brazil)	7.5mg/Kg per day po	Photosensitivity in 50% of pts. GI: abdominal pain, nausea/vomiting/anorexia. CNS: disorientation, insomnia, twitching/seizures, paresthesias, polyneuritis
Chloroquine phosphate (Aralen)	Dose varies—see *Malaria Prophylaxis and Rx, pages 124-125.* 500mg tabs $6.04	Minor: anorexia/nausea/vomiting, headache, dizziness, blurred vision, pruritus in dark-skinned pts. Major: protracted rx in rheumatoid arthritis can lead to retinopathy. Can exacerbate psoriasis. Can block response to rabies vaccine. Contraindicated in pts with epilepsy.

* See page 2 for abbreviations. All dosage recommendations are for adults (unless otherwise indicated) and assume normal renal function.

TABLE 13B (2)

CLASS, AGENT, GENERIC NAME (TRADE NAME)	USUAL ADULT DOSAGE (Cost)	ADVERSE REACTIONS/COMMENTS
Antiprotozoan Drugs/Extraintestinal Parasites (continued)		
Dapsone Ref.: CID 27:191, 1998	100mg po q24h 100mg tabs $0.20	Usually tolerated by pts with rash after TMP-SMX. Adverse effects: nausea/vomiting, rash, oral lesions (CID 18:630, 1994). Methemoglobinemia (usually asymptomatic); if > 10–15%, stop drug. Hemolytic anemia if G6PD deficient. Sulfone syndrome: fever, rash, hemolytic anemia, atypical lymphocytes, and liver injury (West J Med 156:303, 1992).
Eflornithine[NUS] (Ornidyl)	Approved in US for trypanosome infections but not market-ed. Hoechst Marion Roussel, (800) 552-3656.	Diarrhea in ½ pts, vomiting, abdominal pain, anemia/leukopenia in ⅓ pts, seizures, alopecia, jaundice, ↓ hearing.
Fumagillin	Eyedrops + po. Drug not avail. Call 800-547-1392.	Adverse events: Neutropenia & thrombocytopenia
Mefloquine (Lariam)	One 250mg tab/wk for malaria prophylaxis; for rx, 1250mg x 1 or 750mg & then 500mg in 6–8hrs. 250mg tab $12.40. In US: 250mg tab = 228mg base; outside US = 250mg tab = 250mg base	Side-effects in roughly 3%. Minor: headache, irritability, insomnia, weakness, diarrhea. Toxic psychosis, seizures can occur. Teratogenic—do not use in pregnancy. Do not use with quinine, quinidine, or halofantrine. Rare. Prolonged QT interval and toxic epidermal necrolysis (Ln 349:101, 1997). Not used for self-rx due to neuropsychiatric side-effects.
Melarsoprol (CDC) (Mel B, Arsobal) (Manufactured in France)	See Trypanosomiasis for adult dose. Peds dose: 0.36mg/kg IV, then gradual ↑ to 3.6mg/kg q1–5 days for total of 3–10 doses.	Post-rx encephalopathy (10%) with 50% mortality overall: risk of death 2° to rx 4–8%. Prednisolone 1 mg per kg per day po may ↓ encephalopathy. Other: Heart damage, albuminuria, abdominal pain, vomiting, peripheral neuropathy, Herxheimer-like reaction, pruritus.
Miltefosine[NUS] (Zentaris, Impavido)	100–150mg (approx 2.25mg/kg per day) po x 28 days Cutaneous leishmaniasis 2.25mg/kg po q24h x 6wk	Contact Astra Medica, Ger. **Pregnancy—No**, teratogenic. Side-effects vary: kala-azar pts, vomiting in up to 40%, diarrhea in 17%, mild to moderate in severity—may resolve in <1 day.
Nifurtimox (Lampit) (CDC) (Manufactured in Germany by Bayer)	8–10mg/kg per day po div. 4 x per day	Side-effects in 40–70% of pts. GI: abdominal pain, nausea/vomiting. CNS: polyneuritis (1/3), disorientation, insomnia, twitching, seizures. Skin rash. Hemolysis with G6PD deficiency.
Nitazoxanide (Alinia)	Adults: 500mg po q12h. Children 4–11: 200mg susp. po q12h. Take with food. 500mg tabs $13.02	Abdominal pain 7.8%, diarrhea 2.1%. Rev.: CID 40:1173, 2005; Expert Opin Pharmacother 7:953, 2006
Pentamidine (NebuPent)	300mg via aerosol q month. Also used IM. 300mg $98.75 + admin. costs	Hypotension, hypocalcemia, hypoglycemia followed by hyperglycemia, pancreatitis. Neutropenia (15%), thrombocytopenia. Nephrotoxicity. Others: nausea/vomiting, ↑ liver tests, rash.
Primaquine phosphate	26.3 mg (= 15mg base) $1.03	In G6PD def pts, can cause hemolytic anemia, esp. African, Asian peoples. Methemoglobinemia. Nausea/abdominal pain if on fasting. CID 39:1336, 2004.
Pyrimethamine (Daraprim, Malocide) Also combined with sulfadoxine as **Fansidar** (25–500 mg) $4.13	100mg po, then 25mg/day. 25mg $0.58 Cost of folinic acid (leucovorin) 5mg $2.36	Major problem is hematologic: megaloblastic anemia, ↓ WBC, ↓ platelets. Can give 5 mg folinic acid per day to ↓ bone marrow depression and not interfere with antitoxoplasmosis effect. If high-dose pyrimethamine, ↑ folinic acid to 10–50mg/day. Pyrimethamine + sulfadiazine can cause mental changes due to carnitine deficiency (AJM 95:112, 1993). Other: Rash, vomiting, diarrhea, xerostomia
Quinacrine[NUS]	For giardiasis: 100mg po tid x 5 days Peds dose: 2mg/kg po tid (max. 300mg/day) x 5 days	Compounded by Med. Carter Pharm., New Haven, CT. (203) 688-8816 or Panorama Compound. Pharm., Van Nuys, CA. (800) 247-9767
Quinidine gluconate	Loading dose of 10mg (equiv to 6.2mg of quinidine base) kg IV over 1–2hr, then constant infusion of 0.02mg of quinidine gluconate / kg per minute.	Adverse reactions of quinidine/quinine similar: (1) IV bolus injection can cause fatal hypotension, (2) hyperinsulinemic hypoglycemia, (3) ↓ rate of infusion of IV quinidine if QT interval *> 25% of baseline, (4) reduce dose 30–50% after day 3 due to ↓ renal clearance and ↓ vol. of distribution.
Quinine sulfate (300mg salt = 250mg base)	For malaria: 100mg po tid x 5 days or chloro-quine-resistant falciparum malaria: 650mg po tid x 3 days, then tetracycline 250mg po qid x 7 days 325mg $0.16 325 & 650mg tabs. No IV prep. in US. Oral rx of chloro-quine-resistant falciparum malaria 650mg po tid x 3 days, then tetracycline 250mg po qid x 7 days	Cinchonism, tinnitus, headache, nausea, abdominal pain, blurred vision. Rarely: blood dyscrasias, drug fever, asthma, hypoglycemia. Transient blindness in <1% of 500 pts (AnIM 136:339, 2002). Contraindicated if G6PD deficiency.

* See page 2 for abbreviations. All dosage recommendations are for adults (unless otherwise indicated) and assume normal renal/renal function.

TABLE 13B (3)

CLASS, AGENT, GENERIC NAME (TRADE NAME)	USUAL ADULT DOSAGE (Cost)	ADVERSE REACTIONS/COMMENTS
Antiprotozoan Drugs/Extraintestinal Parasites *(continued)*		
Spiramycin (Rovamycin) (*JAC* 42:572; 1998)	Up to 3-4gm/day. Not available in U.S. Can try FDA. (301) 827-2335.	GI and allergic reactions have occurred. Not available in U.S.
Sulfadiazine	1-1.5gm po q6h. 500mg $0.34	*See Table 10C, page 93, for sulfonamide side-effects*
Sulfadoxine & pyrimethamine combination (Fansidar)	Contains 500mg sulfadoxine & 25mg pyrimethamine One tab $4.13	Very long mean half-life of both drugs: Sulfadoxine 169hrs, pyrimethamine 111hrs allows weekly dosage. Do not use in pregnancy. Fatalities reported due to Stevens-Johnson syndrome and toxic epidermal necrolysis. Renal excretion—use with caution in pts with renal impairment.
DRUGS USED TO TREAT NEMATODES, TREMATODES, AND CESTODES		
Bithionol (CDC)	Adults & children: 30-40mg/kg (to max. of 2gm/day) po every other day x 10-15 doses	Photosensitivity, skin reactions, urticaria, GI upset
Diethylcarbamazine (Hetrazan) (CDC)	Used to treat filariasis. Licensed (Lederle) but not available in US	Headache, dizziness, nausea, fever. Host may experience inflammatory reaction to death of adult worms: fever, urticaria, asthma, GI upset (Mazzotti reaction).
Ivermectin (Stromectol, Mectizan)	Strongyloidiasis dose: 200mcg/kg x 1 dose po Onchocerciasis: 150mcg/kg x 1 po Scabies: 200 mcg/kg po x 1 3mg tabs $5.44	Mild side-effects: fever, pruritus, rash. In rx of onchocerciasis, can see tender lymphadenopathy, headache, bone/joint pain. Can cause Mazzotti reaction (see above).
Mebendazole (Vermox)	Doses vary with indication. 100mg tab $13.23	Rarely causes abdominal pain, nausea, diarrhea. Contraindicated in pregnancy & children <2yrs old.
Oxamniquine (Vansil)[NUS]	For S. mansoni. Some experts suggest 40-60mg/kg over 2-3 days in all of Africa	Rarely, dizziness, drowsiness, neuropsychiatric symptoms, GI upset. EKG/EEG changes. Orange/red urine
Praziquantel (Biltricide)	Doses vary with parasite, see Table 13A. 600 mg $11.90	Mild: dizziness/drowsiness, N/V, rash, fever. Only contraindication is ocular cysticercosis. Metabolism induced by anticonvulsants and steroids: can negate effect with cimetidine 400mg po tid
Pyrantel pamoate (over-the-counter as Reese's Pinworm Medicine)	Oral suspension. Dose for all ages: 11mg/kg (to max. of 1gm) x 1 dose	Rare GI upset, headache, dizziness, rash
Suramin (Germanin) (CDC)	For early trypanosomiasis. Drug powder mixed to 10% solution with 5mL water and used within 30 min	Does not cross blood-brain barrier; no effect on CNS infection. Side-effects: vomiting, pruritus, urticaria, fever, paresthesias, albuminuria (discontinue drug if casts appear). Do not use if renal/liver disease present. Deaths from vascular collapse reported.
Thiabendazole (Mintezol)	Take after meals. Dose varies with parasite; see Table 12A. 500mg $1.25	Nausea/vomiting, headache, dizziness. Rarely: liver damage, ↓ BP, angioneurotic edema, Stevens-Johnson syndrome. May ↓ mental alertness.

* See page 2 for abbreviations. All dosage recommendations are for adults (unless otherwise indicated) and assume normal renal function.

TABLE 14A – ANTIVIRAL THERAPY (NON-HIV)*

VIRUS/DISEASE	DRUG/DOSAGE	SIDE EFFECTS/COMMENTS
Adenovirus: Cause of RTIs including fatal pneumonia in children esp. <2 yrs old & 60% mortality in transplant pts (CID 43:331, 2006). **Findings include:** fever, ↑ liver enzymes, leukopenia, thrombocytopenia, diarrhea, pneumonia, & hemorrhagic cystitis.	In severe cases especially HSCT or pneumonia: **Cidofovir** • 5mg/kg q 2 wks, then q2 wks + **probenecid** 1.25gm/M given 3hrs before cidofovir and 3 & 9 hrs after infusion • Or 1 mg/kg 3x/wk. • Or intravesical cidofovir (5mg/kg in 100 ml saline instilled into bladder) successful Rx of adenovirus hemorrhagic cystitis (CID 40:199, 2005)	Successful in 3/8 immunosuppressed children (CID 38:45, 2004) & 8 of 10 children with HSCT (CID 41: 1812, 2005). ↓ in virus load predicted response to cidofovir
Coronavirus—SARS-CoV (Severe Acute Respiratory Distress Syn.) (see comment) A new coronavirus, isolated Spring 2003 (NEJM 348:1953 & 1967, 2003) emerged from China & spread from Hong Kong to 32 countries. Effective infection control guidelines likely responsible for controlling the epidemic. Only 4 mini-outbreaks in 2004, 3/4 from research labs testing live virus (Science 304:1097, 2004); none reported in 2005 (7/05)	Therapy remains predominantly supportive care. Therapy tried or under evaluation (see Comments): **Ribavirin**—ineffective. Interferon alfa ± steroids—small case series. Peglyated IFN-a effective in monkeys. Value of corticosteroids alone unclear. Inhaled nitric oxide improved oxygenation & improved chest x-ray (CID 39:1531, 2004).	Other coronaviruses (HCoV-229E, OC43, NL63, etc.) implicated as cause of croup, asthma exacerbations, & other RTIs in children (CID 40:1721, 2005; JID 191:492, 2005). May be associated with Kawasaki disease (JID 191:499, 2005).
Enterovirus—Meningitis: most common cause of aseptic meningitis. PCR on CSF valuable for early dx (Scand J Inf Dis 34:359, 2002) but sensitivity only 2 days of symptoms. PCR on feces pos. in 12/13 specimens, 5–16 days after clinical onset (CID 40:982, 2005)	**No rx currently recommended;** however, **pleconaril** (VP 63843) still under investigation. [For compassionate use call Viropharma (610) 458-7300, ext. 6297 (Donna Kolbush, RN)]	No clinical benefit demonstrated in double-blind placebo-controlled study in 21 infants with enteroviral aseptic meningitis (PIDJ 22:335, 2003).
Hemorrhagic Fever Virus Infections: For excellent reviews, see Med Lab Observer, May 2005, p. 16, www.mlo-online.com and LnID 4:487, 2004		
Congo-Crimean Hemorrhagic Fever (HF) (CID 39:284, 2004) Tickborne; symptoms include NV, fever, headache, myalgias, & stupor (1/3). Signs: conjunctival injection, hepatomegaly, petechiae (1/3). Lab: ↓ WBC, ↑ ALT, AST, LDH & CPK (100%).	Oral **ribavirin**, **30mg/kg** as initial loading dose, & 15mg/kg q6h x 4 days & then 7.5mg/kg x 6 days (WHO recommendation) (see Comment)	3/3 healthcare workers in Pakistan had complete recovery (Ln 346:472, 1995) & 61/69 (89%) with confirmed CCHF survived with ribavirin in Iran (CID 36:1613, 2003)
Ebola/Marburg HF (Central Africa) Severe outbreak of Ebola in Angola 308 cases with 277 deaths by 5/2005 (NEJM 352:2155, 2005) (JID 196 S.5.331, 2006). Major epidemic of Marburg 1998–2000 in Congo & 2004+ in Angola (NEJM355:866, 2006)	No effective antiviral rx (J Virol 77: 9733, 2003).	Intense inflammatory response within 4 days after infection may control viral proliferation & result in asymptomatic infection (Ln 355:2210, 2000). Can infect gorillas & chimps that come in contact with other dead animal carcasses (Science 303:387, 2004). Bats also suspected (LnID 5:331, 2005)
With pulmonary syndrome: Hantavirus pulmonary syndrome, "sin nombre virus"	No benefit from ribavirin has been demonstrated (CID 39:1307, 2004).	Acute onset of fever, headache, myalgias, non-productive cough, thrombocytopenia and non-cardiogenic pulmonary edema with respiratory insufficiency following exposure to rodents.
With renal syndrome: Lassa, Venezuelan, Korean, HF, Sabia, Argentinian HF, Bolivian HF, Junin, Machupo	**Ribavirin** IV 2 gm loading dose, then 1 gm q6h times 4 days, then 0.5 gm q8h times 6 days (See Comment: Congo-Crimean HF)	Toxicity low, hemolysis reported but recovery when treatment stopped. No significant changes in platelets, hepatic or renal function. Effective in Lassa and in 2 cases of Bolivian HF (CID 24:718, 1997). No data on others. See CID 5:1254, 2003, for management of contacts.

* See page 2 for abbreviations. NOTE: All dosage recommendations are for adults (unless otherwise indicated) and assume normal renal function.
Costs from 2006 DRUG TOPICS RED BOOK, Medical Economics. Price is average wholesale price (AWP).

TABLE 14A (2)

VIRUS/DISEASE	DRUG/DOSAGE	SIDE EFFECTS/COMMENTS
Hemorrhagic Fever Virus Infections (continued)		
Dengue and dengue hemorrhagic fever (DHF) http://www.cdc.gov/ncidod/dvbid/dengue/dengue-hcp.htm Think dengue in traveler to tropics or subtypes (incubation period usually 4-7 days) with fever, bleeding, thrombocytopenia, or hemoconcentration with shock. Dx by viral isolation or serology serum to CDC (telephone 787-706-2399).	**No data on antiviral rx.** Fluid replacement with careful hemodynamic monitoring critical. Rx of **DHF** with colloids effective: 6% hydroxyethyl starch preferred in 1 study (NEJM 353:9, 2005)	Of 77 cases dx at CDC (2001-2004), recent (2-wk) travel to Caribbean island 30%, Asia 17%, Central America 15% (MMWR 54:556, June 10, 2005). 5 pts with severe **DHF** given dengue antibody-neg gamma globulin 500 mg per kg IV for 3-5 days; rapid ↑ in platelet counts (CID 36:1623, 2003).
West Nile virus (see AnIM 104:545, 2004) A flavivirus transmitted by mosquitoes, blood transfusions, transplanted organs (NEJM 348:2196, 2003; CID 38:1257, 2004), & breast-feeding (MMWR 51:877, 2002). Birds (>200 species) are main host with man & horses incidental hosts. WNV epidemic continues unabated in the US in 2006	**No proven rx to date.** 2 clinical trials in progress: (1) Interferon alfa-N3 (CID 40:764, 2005). See www.nyhq.org/posting/nahal.html (2) IVIG from Israel with high titer antibody West Nile (JID 188:5, 2003; Transpl Inf Dis 4:160, 2003). Contact NIH, 301-496-7453, see www.clinicaltrials.gov/show/NCT00068055.	Usually nonspecific febrile disease but 1/150 cases develops meningoen-cephalitis, aseptic meningitis or polio-like paralysis (AnIM 104:545, 2004; JCI 113: 1102, 2004). Long-term sequelae (neuromuscular weakness & psychiatric) common (CID 43:723, 2006). Dx by ↑ IgM in serum & CSF or ↑↑ PCR (contact State Health Dept./CDC). Blood supply now tested in U.S.; ↑ serum lipase in 11/17 cases (NEJM 352:420, 2005).
Yellow fever	**No data on antiviral therapy**	Reemergence in Africa & S. Amer. due to urbanization of susceptible population (Lancet Inf 5:604, 2005). Vaccination effective. (JAMA 276:1157,1996)
Chikungunya fever: A self-limited arbovirus illness spread by Aedes mosquito that has caused a massive epidemic in countries near the Indian ocean in 2004-6 with hundreds of thousands of cases	**No antiviral therapy**	Clinical presentation: high fever, severe myalgias & headache, macular papular rash with occ thrombocytopenia. Rarely hemorrhagic complications. Dx by increase in IgM.
Hepatitis Viral Infections		
Hepatitis A (Ln 351:1643, 1998)	No therapy recommended. If within 2 wks of exposure, IVIG 0.02 mL or kg IM times 1 protective.	Vaccine recommendations in Table 20. Coverage of only 50% in states that recommend Hep A vaccination (MMWR 54:141, 2005). 40% of pts with chronic Hep C who developed superinfection with Hep A developed fulminant hepatic failure (NEJM 338:286, 1998)
Hepatitis B **Acute**	No therapy recommended	Most common cause of death from acute hepatitis in Italy (Dig Liver Dis 35:404, 2003). Screen for HIV.
Chronic **HBeAg+:** Consider rx if ↑ ALT/AST (1) Symptomatic if ↑ ALT/AST (2) HBeAg positive (3) HBV DNA plasma "viral load" > 10⁴ or 20,000 copies/mL; if >10⁴-<10⁵ copies/mL, no rx unless active inflammation/ fibrosis on biopsy, then 200ml telbivudine. <10⁴, no rx. (continued on next page)	Data on treatment changing rapidly. 6 approved options now approved & available—no consensus on initial rx (see Clin/Gastro/Hepat 4:936, 2006). • **Adefovir** (ADF) 10 mg po q24h. For HBeAg (+), treat 12mo & recheck HBeAg. For HBeAg (-), rx min. 6mo after seroconversion or indefinitely. If previous LAV treatment or known YMDD mutation, use 1mg q24h. If previous LAV mutation, use 1mg q24h. Treat 1yr or min. 6mo after seroconversion OR • **Entecavir** (ENT) 0.5mg po fasting q24h. If previous LAV treatment or seroconversion OR	**Specific drug comments** (side-effects & cost in Table 14B) • **ADV:** Preferred rx. YMDD mutant strains & ENT resistant strains but resistance to ADV may reach 15% min. toxicity at baseline but should ↓ resistance. Clin improvement. Histologic improvement in many. Superior to LAV in 2 large trials (HBVeAg+, and -Ag -) NEJM 354:10 & 1011, 2006). Resistance rare but was 7.4% at 1/2yr in LAM-resistant pts and 6% pre-existing LAM(1R) at baseline. • **ENT:** Min. toxicity. Active vs. YMDD LAV mutants & ADV-resistant strains. (continued on next page)

* See page 2 for abbreviations. NOTE: All dosage recommendations are for adults (unless otherwise indicated) and assume normal renal function. Costs from 2006 Drug Topics Red Book, Medical Economics. Price is average wholesale price (AWP).

TABLE 14A (3)

VIRUS/DISEASE	DRUG/DOSAGE	SIDE EFFECTS/COMMENTS
Hepatitis Viral Infections/Hepatitis B/Chronic *(continued)*	*(continued from previous page)*	*(continued from previous page)*
(continued from previous page) **Goal of rx:** ↓ liver inflammation, stop progression of cirrhosis & prevent hepatocellular carcinoma. If all drugs listed, ideal response: ↓ plasma HB DNA to <20,000 copies/ml; Normal ALT/AST; HBsAg to anti-HBs; HBeAg to anti-HBe.	• Another option: (**Tenofovir** 300mg) + **entricitabine** 200mg) as **Truvada**[aB34] + 1 tab po q24h looks promising, but don't use alone in HIV co-infected patients OR 1x/wk times at least 1 year OR • **Interferon alfa-2a** 180 mcg subcut. OR **PEG IFN alfa-2b** 1.5mcg/kg 1x/wk times at least 1 year OR • **Interferon alfa-2b** 10 million units 3x/wk or 5 million units q24h subcut. for 16–24 wks. Don't use IFNs in cirrhosis or decompensated liver diseases—hepatitis flares common & associated with further decompensation OR	• **Truvada** not yet approved for this indication but highly effective with low resistance potential. • **Interferon:** PEG IFN 2x more effective than standard IFN (*J Viral Hep* 10:298, 2003) & ?effective than LAV for HBeAg(–) pts. (*NEJM 351:1206, 2004*). Genotypes A & B respond better (40–50%) than C & D (25–30%). • **LAV:** Some still start with LAV and switch when YMDD emerges. Cheapest therapy and minimal toxicity. YMDD mutants less virulent than wild type. Sustained viral response (SVR) if initial ALT >2x normal is 65% at 3 yrs (*J Viral Hep 9:208, 2002*).
HBeAg: Rx indefinitely, consult specialist! **Refs:** *NEJM 350:1118, 2004; Clin Gastro & Hep 2:87, 2004; NEJM 354:10, 2006.* Prevention of re-infection after liver transplant for Hepatitis	**Lamivudine** (LAV) 100 mg po q24h x 12mo or until HBsAg seroconversion. If hepatitis flare or persistent HBeAg(+), continue rx. **Refs:** *NEJM 351:1521, 2004*), switch to ENT or ADF. Don't use for first-line rx in cirrhotic; ? clinical breakthrough with resistance & hepatitis flares. **Lamivudine** 100 mg po q24h from 4 wks pre-transplant to 12 wks post-transplant OR **Adefovir** 10mg po q24h	**Combination:** *NEJM 352:26, 2005; AnIM 142:240, 2005*). May have role for LAV or ADF resistance in Pts with cirrhosis & in preventing resistance in HBeAg(–) pts. Effective in pts with LAV YMDD mutations. *Hepatology, Hpt 34:888 & 895, 2001.* Based on uncontrolled studies. *Hpt 30:222A, 1999; J Hpt 34:888 & 895, 2001.* Some add HBIG (*Hpt 28:585, 1998*).
Hepatitis C (up to 3% of world infected, 4 million in U.S., 36,000 new cases annually). Co-infection with HIV common—see Sanford Guide to HIV/AIDS Therapy, See *AnIM 136:747, 2002.* www.va.gov/hepatitis; www.hepnet.com/hepc.html		
Acute Usually asymptomatic. (>75%). Can detect by PCR within 13 days; antibody in 36+ days.(*JID 189:3, 2004; CID 40:951, 2005*) **Chronic:** www.va.gov/hepatitis; *Sem Liver Dis 23(Suppl 1):35, 2003; AASLD/IDSA Guidelines: Hpt 39:1147, 2004*	Follow plasma HCV viral load by PCR: If clear within 3–4 mos. no treatment. If persists: PEG IFN ± ribavirin as below, albeit controversial (*NEJM 345:1091, 2002*) **Treat if:** persistent elevated ALT/AST, + HCV RNA plasma viral load, fibrosis &/or inflam on biopsy.	
Genotypes 1 *AnIM 140:346, 2004*	**PEG IFN** Either alfa-2a (Pegasys) 180mcg subcut 1x/wk **OR** **Alfa-2b** (PEG-INTRON) 1.5mcg/kg subcut 1x/wk **Monitor response by quantification:**	In U.S., 90% due to genotype 1. Sustained viral response (SVR) of genotype 1 42–51%, (SVR of genotype 2 or 3 76–82%. Avoid alcohol—accelerates HCV disease. HIV accelerates HCV disease. See *Table 14B for drug adverse events & cost. Interferon alfa can cause serious depression.* Ribavirin is teratogenic & has dose-related hematologic toxicity. For drugs in development, see *Hepatol Res, July 12, 2005.* For genotypes 2 & 3, some use standard IFN, results similar & ↓ cost.
	+ Ribavirin 400mg po bid **Weight** **Ribavirin Dose** <75 kg 400mg am & 600mg pm >75 kg 600mg am & 600mg pm **Action** <1 log → Discontinue therapy <2 log↓ Discontinue therapy >2 log↓ or undetectable Treat 48 wks	
	HCV RNA **Result** **Action** After 4 wks rx: Undetectable >2 log↓ or undetectable After 12 wks rx: <2 log↓ Discontinue therapy	
Genotype 2 or 3	**PEG IFN alfa-2a or 2b**—dose as for types 1 & 4 above **+ Ribavirin** 400 mg po (*NEJM 352:2609, 2005*) **Quant. HCV RNA** **Result** **Action** After 4 wks rx: >1 log↓ Treat 12 wks, if relapse Treat 24 wks	Some would treat 24wks for high titer Genotype 3.
For prevention of acute and chronic infection, see Table 15D, page 169		

TABLE 14A (4)

VIRUS/DISEASE	DRUG/DOSAGE	SIDE EFFECTS/COMMENTS
Herpesvirus Infections (see review: CID 26:541, 1998)		
Cytomegalovirus (CMV) Marked ↓ in CMV infections & death from CMV with Highly Active Antiretroviral Rx: there is a progressive ↓ in CMV DNA & most pts actually become neg. after a median time of 13mos (AIDS 13:1203 & 1497, 1999; AIDS 14:582, 2004; EJCMID 23:550, 2004). Initial rx for CMV infections should include optimization of HAART	Primary prophylaxis not generally recommended; preemptive rx in pts with ↑ CMV DNA titers in plasma & CD4 <100/mm³, associated with 3.1-fold & each log₁₀ associated with 3.1-fold ↑ in dis-ease (JCI 101:497, 1998; CID 28:758, 1999).	Risk for developing CMV disease correlates with quantity of CMV DNA in plasma. (+DNA=↑ 3.4-fold & each log₁₀ associated with 3.1-fold ↑ in disease (JCI 101:497, 1998; CID 28:758, 1999).
	Primary prophylaxis not recommended. CMV titers in plasma & CD4 <100/mm³. Recommended by some. **valganciclovir** 900mg po q24h (CID 32: 783, 2001). Authors rec. primary prophylaxis (se dc if response to HAART CD4 >100 for 6mos. (MMWR 53:98, 2004).	
Colitis, Esophagitis Dx best by biopsy of ulcer base/edge (Clin Gastro Hepatol 2:564, 2004)	**Ganciclovir** as with retinitis except induction period extended for 3-6wks. Responses less predictable than for retinitis (AJM 98:169, 1994). **Foscarnet** 90mg/kg q12h effective in 9/10 pts (AAC 41:1226, 1997). **Valganciclovir also likely effective.** Switch to oral valganciclovir when po tolerated & when symptoms not severe enough to interfere with absorption.	No agreement as with retinitis; may not be necessary except after relapse (AJM 98:169, 1994). **Foscarnet** 90mg/kg q12h effective in 9/10 pts (AAC 41:1226, 1997). Disease may develop while taking ganciclovir as suppressive rx.
CMV of the nervous system: Encephalitis & ventriculitis. [See Herpes 11(Suppl 12):954, 2004] Lumbosacral polyradiculopathy	**Ganciclovir** as with retinitis. Consider combination of ganciclovir & foscarnet, esp. if prior CMV rx used. Switch to valganciclovir when possible. Suppression continued until CD4 remains >100/mm³ for 6mos.	About 50% will respond (CID 20:747, 1995), survival ↑ (5.4wks to 14.6wks) (CID 27:345, 1988).
Mononeuritis multiplex	Not defined	Due to vasculitis & may not be responsive to antiviral rx (AnNeurol 29:139, 1991).
	Ganciclovir/valganciclovir as with retinitis	11/16 pts showed initial improvement with either ganciclovir or foscarnet but disease eventually progressed despite maintenance (CID 23:76, 1996). In BMT recipients, serial measure of pp65 antigen was useful in establishing early dx of CMV interstitial pneumonia with good results if GCV was initiated within 6 days of antigen positivity (Bone Marrow Transplant 26:413, 2000). For preemptive therapy, see Table 10.
CMV pneumonia—seen predominantly in transplants (esp. bone marrow), **rare in HIV** pts only when histologic evidence present in AIDS pts & other pathogens not identified.	**Ganciclovir** 5mg/kg IV q12h x14-21d, then **valganciclovir** 900mg po q24h **OR** **Foscarnet** 60mg/kg IV q8h or 90mg/kg IV q12h x14-21d, then 90-120mg/kg IV q24h	
CMV retinitis (most common in AIDS) Still the most common cause of blindness in AIDS patients with <50mm³ CD4 counts. 19/30 pts (63%) with inactive CMV retinitis who responded to HAART (↑ of ≥60 CD4 cells/ml) developed immune recovery vitreitis (vision ↓ & floaters with posterior segment inflammation —vitreitis, papillitis & macular changes) an average of 43 wks after rx started (JID 179: 697, 1999). Another report noted corticosteroid rx ↓ inflammatory reaction of immune recovery vitreitis without reactivation of CMV retinitis, either periocular corticosteroids or short course of systemic steroid.	**For immediate sight-threatening lesions:** **Ganciclovir intraocular implant** & **valganciclovir** 900mg po q24h **For peripheral lesions:** **Valganciclovir** 900mg po q12h x14-21d, then 900mg po q24h	Differential dx: HIV retinopathy, herpes simplex retinitis (Arch Ophthal 114: 834, 1996), varicella-zoster retinitis (rare, hard to diagnose). **Valganciclovir** po equal to GCV in induction of remission: 7/71 progressed on Val & 7/70 on GCV during 1ˢᵗ 4wks & 72% of Val & 77% of GCV-treated pts had satisfactory responses to induction rx. Adverse events were similar (NEJM 346:1119, 2002).
	Cidofovir 5mg/kg IV q1wk x2wks, then 5mg/kg every other wk; each dose should be administered with IV saline hydration & oral probenecid **OR** Repeated intravitreal injections with **fomivirsen** (for relapses only, not as initial therapy).	Cannot use GCV ocular implant alone as approx. 50% risk of CMV retinitis in other eye at 6 mos. & 31% risk visceral disease. Risk w/ systemic rx but when contralateral retinitis does occur, ganciclovir-resistant mutation often present (JID 189:611, 2004). **Concurrent systemic rx recommended!** Response to fomivirsen similar to other therapies (med. time to progression 267–403days). Because of unique mode of action, fomivirsen may have a role if isolates become resistant to other therapies. *(continued on next page)*

---

* See page 2 for abbreviations. NOTE: All dosage recommendations are for adults (unless otherwise indicated) and assume normal renal function.
Costs from 2005 DRUG TOPICS RED BOOK, Medical Economics. Price is average wholesale price (AWP).

TABLE 14A (5)

VIRUS/DISEASE	DRUG/DOSAGE	SIDE EFFECTS/COMMENTS
		(continued from previous page)
	Suppression, 1[*]: Chronic maintenance therapy (secondary prophylaxis): **Valganciclovir** 900mg po q24h OR **foscarnet** 90-120mg/kg IV q24h. Maintenance can be discontinued if CD4 >100/mm³ x6mos.	Retinal detachments 50–60% within 1 yr of dx of retinitis. In 271 AIDS pts with CMV retinitis, both 2° eye involvement & retinal detachment markedly ↓ with HAART but only if good CD4 cell response: 2° eye involvement: 0.02/person yr with CD4 >200 vs 0.34 with <50/mm³ retinal detachment 0.02/person yr for CD4 >200 vs 0.30 with <50/mm³ *(Ophtha 111:2232, 2004)*. Equal efficacy of IV GCV & FOS. GCV avoids nephrotoxicity of FOS; FOS avoids bone marrow suppression of GCV. Although bone marrow toxicity may be similar to ganciclovir. **Oral valganciclovir should replace both.** Reports indicate success of combination rx with GCV at 1/2 dose 5mg/kg/day q24h & FOS up to 125mg/kg/day for GCV-resistant isolates in solid organ transplants *(CID 34:1337, 2002)*. Hypomagnesemia common complication.
	Suppression, 2[*]: Chronic maintenance therapy: **Cidofovir** 5mg/kg IV every other week with **probenecid** 2gm po 3hrs before the dose followed by 1gm po 2hrs after then dose, & 1 gm po 8hrs after the dose (total of 4 gm); OR **fomivirsen** 1 vial (330 mg) injected into the vitreous, then repeated every 2–4 wks.	Potential emergence of resistant CMV. 27.5% pts treated 9mos developed CMV isolates resistant to GCV *(JID 177:770, 1998)*, hence may be reason for clinical failure. DC in a great advantage since IV-related complications are common: 1.2/person²/yr with mortality rate of 5.8% *(AIDS 12:2321, 1999)*. Valganciclovir 900mg q24h has similar efficacy (17% progressed over 1 year) & toxicity profile as IV ganciclovir but with fewer IV-related events *(J AIDS 30:392, 2002)*. There is also a significant ↓ in cost with oral vs IV rx *(J AIDS 36:972, 2004)*.

CMV in transplant patients: The prevention and management of CMV infections in transplant pts is beyond the scope of this Guide. Use of valganciclovir to prevent infections in CMV seronegative recipients who receive organs from a seropositive donor & in seropositive receivers has been highly effective *(Ln 365:2105, 2005)*. Others evaluate CMV antigenemia post-transplant *(Transplant 79:85, 2005)*.

EBV—Mononucleosis *(Ln D:3:131, 2003)*	**No treatment.** Corticosteroids for tonsillar obstruction or CNS complications.	*(See JAC 56:277, 2005 for current status of drugs in development.)*
HHV-6—implicated as cause of roseola (exanthem subitum) & other febrile diseases of childhood *(NEJM 352:768, 2005)*. Reactivation in 47% of 110 U.S. HSCT pts assoc. with delayed monocytes & platelet engraftment *(CID 40:932, 2005)*. Recognized in assoc. with meningoencephalitis in immunocompromised adults. Dx made by pos. PCR in CSF, ↑ viral copies in response to **ganciclovir** *(CID 40:890 & 894, 2005)*. Foscarnet rx improved thrombotic microangiopathy *(Am J Hematol 76:156, 2004)*.		
HHV-7—ubiquitous virus (>90% of the population is infected by age 5 yrs). No relationship to human disease. Infects CD4 lymphocytes like CD4 lymphocytes via CD4 receptor; transmitted via saliva		
HHV-8—The agent of Kaposi's sarcoma, Castleman's disease, & body cavity lymphoma	**No antiviral treatment.** Effective anti-HIV rx may help.	Localized lesions: radiotherapy, laser surgery or intralesional chemotherapy. Systemic: chemotherapy, Castleman's disease responded to ganciclovir *(Blood 103:1632, 2004)* & valganciclovir *(JID 2006)*. Valganciclovir reduced HHV-8 replication in saliva by 79% vs placebo *(IDSA 2005, Abst 0066)*.
Herpes simplex virus (HSV Types 1 & 2) *(See Ln 357:1513, 2001 & CID Suppl 39:S237, 2004 for rx HSV in HIV-infected persons)*		
Bell's palsy may be caused by H. zoster, Lyme disease, HHV-6) *(CID 30:529, 2000)*	**Either Acyclovir** 400 mg 5x/day for 10 days] with or without [**prednisone po** [30mg (tid or 1mg/kg daily dose given tid) x 5 days, then taper to 5mg bid and dc after total of 10 days)] **or no rx.**	Pts with symptoms <3 days had faster recovery & less neural degeneration when rx with acyclovir + prednisone compared to prednisone alone *(Am Otol/Rhinol/Laryngol 105:371, 1996)*, another study was inconclusive. Valacyclovir also effective in one study *(AnnOto/Rhinol/Laryngol 112:197, 2003)*. More data needed *(Cochrane Database Syst Rev CD001869, 2004)*. Surgical decompression within 14 days of symptoms controversial *(NEJM 352:416, 2005)*. It caused by VZV, acyclovir may help *(PIDJ 21:615, 2002)*.

*See page 2 for abbreviations. NOTE: All dosage recommendations are for adults (unless otherwise indicated) and assume normal renal function.
Costs from 2006 Drug Topics Red Book, Medical Economics. Price is average wholesale price (AWP).

TABLE 14A (6)

VIRUS/DISEASE	DRUG/DOSAGE	SIDE EFFECTS/COMMENTS
Herpesvirus infections/Herpes Simplex Virus (HSV Types 1 & 2) *(continued)*		
Encephalitis *(Excellent reviews: CID 35: 254, 2002; UK experience (EID 9:234, 2003; Eur J Neurol 12:331, 2005)*	**Acyclovir** IV 10mg/kg IV (infuse over 1 hr) q8h x 14–21 days. Up to 20mg/kg q8h in children <12 yrs	HSV-1 is most common cause of sporadic encephalitis. Survival & recovery from neurological sequelae are related to mental status at time of initiation of rx. **Early dx and rx imperative.** Mortality rate reduced from >70% to 19% with acyclovir rx. PCR analysis of CSF for HSV-1 DNA is 100% sensitive & 75–98% sensitive. 8/33 (25%) CSF samples drawn before day 3 were neg. by PCR; neg. PCR assoc. with ↓ protein & <10 WBC per mm³ in CSF (CID 36:1335, 2003). All were + after 3 days. Relapse after successful rx reported in 7/27 (27%) children. Relapse was associated with a lower total dose of initial acyclovir rx (285 ± 82 mg per kg in relapse group vs. 462 ± 149 mg per kg., p <0.03) (CID 30:185, 2000; Neuropediatrics 35:371, 2004)
Genital, immunocompetent: Emerging problem in adolescents (Sem in Ped Int Dis 16:224, 2005). ACOG guidelines for management Ob Gyn 104:1111, 2004. Recommendations from International Herpes Management Forum, Herpes 12:15, 2005. See **Sexually Transmitted Treatment Guidelines 2006: www.cdc.gov/std/treatment/2006/genital-ulcers, MMWR Recomm Rep. 2006 Aug 4:55 (RR-11):1–94.**		
Primary (initial episode) See excellent reviews: NEJM 350:1970, 2004 & AnIM 137:257, 2002 or CDC 2002 Guidelines	**Acyclovir** (Zovirax or generic) 400 mg po tid x 7–10 days (FDA-approved dosage is 200 mg po 5 times per day x 10 days). (NB $150 per course; G $35 per course.) **OR** **Valacyclovir** (Valtrex) 1000 mg po bid x 10 days ($99 per course). **OR** **Famciclovir** (Famvir) 250 mg po tid x 7–10 days (not FDA-approved for this indication) ($97–139 per course)	All effective with few differences. Choice can be made on basis of cost & convenience. Trend is to ↓ duration of rx. The 2-day course of acyclovir was equivalent to 5 days, duration of episode & lesions 4.4 days (CID 34:958, 2002). Famciclovir 125 bid effective (CID 41:1097, 2005). Famciclovir 1 gm bid x 1 day was effective (CID 42:8, 2006)
Episodic recurrences	**Acyclovir** 400 mg po tid **x 5 days** or 800 mg po tid **x 2 days** or **famciclovir** 1000 mg bid **x 1 day** or **valacyclovir** 500 mg po bid **x 3 days**	An ester of acyclovir, which is well absorbed, bioavailability 3–5 times greater than acyclovir. Found to be **equal to acyclovir** (See Trans Dis 24:481, 1997). Metabolized to penciclovir, which is active component. Side effects and activity similar to acyclovir. Famciclovir 250 mg po tid found to be **equal to acyclovir** 200 mg 5 times per day.
Chronic suppression *(JAMA 280:928, 1998; JID 178:603, 1998) Decision to rx arbitrary, but rx sig. improves quality of life over 1 yr (Sex Trans Infect 75:398, 1999).*	**Suppressive rx reduces the frequency of genital herpes recurrences by 70–80% among pts who have frequent recurrences (i.e., >6 recurrences per yr) & many report no symptomatic outbreaks** (NEJM 51:RR-6, 2002). **Acyclovir** 400 mg po bid (cost/yr ↓ $562), or **famciclovir** 250 mg po bid (cost per yr $2969), **or valacyclovir** 1 gm po q24h ($3268 per yr.) for pts with <9 recurrences per yr. use 500 mg po q24h ($1825 per yr). May use 1 gm po q24h if breakthrough at lower dose.	All effective HSV-2 shedding between episodes of active disease. Vala = acyclovir in 69 immunocompetent pts. Vala x risk of transmission by 48% vs placebo in double-blind crossover study (JID 190:1374, 2004). Vala ↓ risk of transmission by 48% vs placebo (NEJM 350:11 & 67, 2004). Drug resistance unlikely to develop with 1 use. After 20 yrs of use in immunocompetent pts v. Control 327, 2005). However, in immunocompetent BMT) 6–7% HSV are resistant (CID 38:S248, 2004). Suppressive rx could also ↓ HIV transmission (JID 191:5107, 2005). Since 2/3 of pts demonstrate ↓ in recurrences between yrs 1 & 5, daily suppressive rx should be reassessed periodically, and after 3–5 yrs, episodic rx may become more practical (AnIM 131:14, 1999). Rarely failure of suppression in immunocompetent could indicate resistant virus (JID 192:156, 2005; CID 41:320, 2005)

TABLE 14A (7)

VIRUS/DISEASE	DRUG/DOSAGE	SIDE EFFECTS/COMMENTS
Herpesvirus Infections/Herpes Simplex Virus (HSV Types 1 & 2)/Genital, immunocompetent *(continued)*		
Gingivostomatitis, primary (children)	**Acyclovir** 15 mg/kg po 5x/day x 7 days	Efficacy demonstrated in randomized double-blind placebo-controlled trial *(BMJ 314:1800, 1997)*.
Kerato-conjunctivitis and recurrent epithelial keratitis	**Trifluridine** (Viroptic), 1 drop 1% solution q2h (max. 9 drops per day) for max. of 21 days (see *Table 1, page 12*)	In controlled trials, response % > idoxuridine. Suppressive rx with acyclovir (400 mg bid) reduced recurrences of ocular HSV from 32% to 19% over 12-month period *(NEJM 339:300, 1998)*.
Mollaret's recurrent "aseptic" meningitis (usually HSV-2) *(Ln 363:1772, 2004)*	No controlled trials of antiviral rx & resolves spontaneously. In severe cases, IV or po acyclovir or valacyclovir or famciclovir recommended	Pos. PCR for HSV in CSF confirms dx *(EJCMID 23:560, 2004)*. Daily suppression rx might ↓ frequency of recurrence but no clinical trials.
Mucocutaneous		
Oral labial, "fever blisters": [[star]] *(CDC STD Guidelines 2006, CID 43:347, 2006)*	Start rx with prodrome symptoms (tingling/burning) before lesions show.	
Normal host: *AnPharmacotherapy 38:705, 2004; JAC 53:703, 2004*	**Oral:**	Penciclovir *(J Derm Treat 13:67, 2002; JAMA 277:1374, 1997; AAC 46: 2848, 2002)*. Docosanol *(J Am Acad Derm 45:222, 2001)*. Oral acyclovir 5% cream *(AAC 46:2238, 2002)*. Oral famciclovir *(JID 179:303, 1999)*. Topical fluocinonide (0.05% Lidex gel) q8h times 5 days in combination with famciclovir ↓ lesion size and pain when compared to famciclovir alone *(JID 181:1906, 2000)*.
	Drug — **Dose** — **Cost**	
	Valacyclovir — 2 gm q12h x 1 day — $36	
	Famciclovir — 500 mg po bid x 7 days — $123	
	Acyclovir^NUS — 400 mg po 5x per day (q4h while awake) x 5 days — $19 (generic)	
	Topical:	
	Penciclovir 1% cream — q2h during day x 4 days — $25	
	Docosanol 10% cream² — 5x/day until healed — $14	
	Acyclovir 5% cream¹ — 6x/day (q3h) x 7 days — $37 per 2 gm / $86 per 5 gm	
	¹ FDA approved only HIV; ² Approved for immunocompromised	
	See *Table 1, page 24*	
Herpes Whitlow		
Oral labial or genital: Immunocompromised (includes pts with AIDS) and critically ill pts in ICU setting/large necrotic ulcers in perineum or face. (See Comment)	**Acyclovir** 5 mg per kg IV (infused over 1 hr) q8h times 7 days (250 mg per M² or 400 mg/M² po 5 times per day times 14-21 days (see Comment if suspect acyclovir-resistant) **OR Famciclovir** [in HIV-infected, 500 mg po bid for 7 days for recurrent episodes of genital herpes **OR Valacyclovir** [in HIV-infected, 500 mg po bid for 5-10 days for recurrent episodes of genital herpes or 500 mg po bid for chronic suppressive rx].	Acyclovir-resistant HSV occurs, esp. in large ulcers. Most will respond to IV **foscarnet**, but recur after drug discontinued [median 6 weeks *(NEJM 325:551, 1991)*]. Suppressive rx with valaciclovir (500 mg po bid) reduced viral shedding and clinical recurrences (total days with lesions 18% vs 5%) in HIV-infected pts *(AnIM 128:21, 1998)*, similar to findings with acyclovir & valacyclovir 500 mg po bid [at 6 mos. 65% of vala-rx were recurrence-free vs 26% of placebo-rx *(JID 188:1009, 2003)*]. Cidofovir (topical) has been used with moderate success *(JID 176:892, 1997)*.
Episodic/Recurrent Genital: HIV/AIDS *(CDC STD Guidelines 2006, CID 43:347, 2006)*	**Acyclovir** 400 mg po 3x a day for 5-10 d or **Famciclovir** 500 mg po bid for 5-10 days or **Valacyclovir** 1 gm po bid x 5-10 days	
Daily suppression:	**Acyclovir** 400-800 mg po 2-3x a day or **Famciclovir** 500 mg po 2x a day or **Valacyclovir** 500 mg po 2x a day	
Perinatal (genital in pregnancy at delivery)	In ≥25% HSV reactivated in last mo of preg. Infant exposure to primary lesion 50% risk, recurrent lesion 4%, 50% mortality in infected neonates. If visible genital lesion, deliver by **C-sec.** regardless of duration of membrane rupture. If no lesions/symptoms, vaginal delivery. Routine HSV cultures no longer rec. **Acyclovir** useful in dose of 10mg/kg (20mg/kg if premature) q8h x 10-21 days if recurrent *(PIID 14:827, 1995; NEJM 337:509, 1997)*.	

* See *page 2* for abbreviations. NOTE: All dosage recommendations are for adults (unless otherwise indicated) and assume normal renal function.
Costs from *2006 Drug TOPICS Red Book, Medical Economics*. Price is average wholesale price (AWP).

TABLE 14A (8)

VIRUS/DISEASE	DRUG/DOSAGE	SIDE EFFECTS/COMMENTS
Herpesvirus infections (continued)		
Monkey bite (Herpes B virus) *CID 35:1191, 2002*	**Postexposure prophylaxis:** Valacyclovir 1 gm po q8h times 14 days or acyclovir 800 mg po 5 times per day times 14 days. **Treatment of disease:** (1) CNS symptoms absent: Acyclovir 12.5-15 mg per kg IV q8h or ganciclovir 5 mg per kg IV q12h. (2) CNS symptoms present: Ganciclovir 5 mg per kg IV q12h.	Fatal human cases of myelitis and hemorrhagic encephalitis have been reported following bites, scratches, or eye inoculation of saliva from monkeys. Initial sx include fever, headache, myalgias and diffuse adenopathy. Incubation period of 2-14 days (*EID 9:246, 2003*)
Herpes Varicella-Zoster Virus (VZV) **Varicella:** Vaccination has markedly ↓ incidence of varicella & morbidity (*NEJM 352:450, 2005 including incidence & severity of post herpetic neuralgia (NEJM 353:2377, 2005)*). Our understanding of the disease still undeveloped (*COID 18:235, 2005*).		
Normal host (chickenpox) Child (2-12 years)	Rx not recommended by Amer Acad of Peds. Oral acyclovir rec for healthy persons at ↑ risk for moderate to severe varicella, ie, >12yrs of age, chronic cutaneous or pulmonary diseases, chronic salicylate rx (↑ risk of Reye syndrome), use **acyclovir 20mg/kg** po qid x 5 days (start within 24 hrs of rash).	Acyclovir slowed development and ↓ number of new lesions; duration of disease ↓ in children receiving acyclovir: 7.6 vs 9.0 days (*PIDJ 21:739, 2002*). Oral dose of acyclovir in children should not exceed 80 mg per kg per day or 3200 mg per day
Adolescents, young adults	**Acyclovir** 800mg po 5x/day x 5-7 days (start within 24 hrs of rash) or **valacyclovir**[AHFS] 1000mg po 3x/day x 5 days). **Famciclovir**[AHFS] 500 mg po 3x/day probably effective but data lacking (*AnIM 130:922, 1999*).	↓ duration of fever, time to healing, and symptoms (*AnIM 117:358, 1992*).
Pneumonia or chickenpox in 3rd trimester of pregnancy	**Acyclovir** 800 mg po 5 times per day or 10 mg per kg IV q8h times 5 days. Risks and benefits to fetus and mother still unknown. Many experts recommend rx, especially in 3rd trimester. Some would use VZIG (varicella-zoster immune globulin).	Varicella pneumonia severe in pregnancy (41% mortality, *Ob Gyn 25:734, 1965*) and acyclovir ↓ incidence and severity (*JID 185:422, 2002*). If varicella-susceptible mother exposed and respiratory symptoms develop within 10 days after exposure, start acyclovir (*CCTD 13:123, 1993*). Acyclovir is pregnancy category B, no evidence of ↑ birth defects (*MMWR 42:806, 1993*). Disseminated 1° varicella infection reported during infliximab rx of rheumatoid arthritis (*J Rheum 31:2517, 2004*).
Immunocompromised host	**Acyclovir** 10-12 mg per kg IV (infused over 1 hr) q8h times 7 days	Continuous infusion of high-dose acyclovir (2 mg per kg per hr) successful in 1 pt with severe hemorrhagic varicella (*NEJM 336:732, 1997*). Mortality high (43%) in AIDS pts (*Int J Inf Dis 6:6, 2002*)
Prevention—Post-exposure prophylaxis Varicella was the leading cause of vaccine-preventable deaths in children in the US (*MMWR 47:365, 1998*). Now markedly reduced with vaccine, but still deaths in unvaccinated (*MMWR 54:272, 2005*).	**CDC Recommendations for Prevention:** Since <5% of cases of varicella occur in adults >20 yrs of age, the CDC recommends a more aggressive approach in this age group: **1st, varicella-zoster immune globulin** (VZIG) 125units/10 kg (22 lbs) body weight IM up to a max. of 625 units; minimum dose is 125 units) is recommended for post-exposure prophylaxis in susceptible persons at greater risk for complications (immunocompromised such as HIV, malignancies, pregnancy, and steroid rx) as soon as possible after exposure (<96 hrs). If varicella develops, initiate rx quickly (<24 hrs of rash) with **acyclovir** as below. Some would rx presumptively with acyclovir in high-risk pts. **2nd,** susceptible adults should be vaccinated. Check antibody in adults with negative or uncertain hx of varicella (10-30% will be Ab-neg) and vaccinate those who are Ab-neg. **3rd** susceptible children should receive vaccination. Recommended routinely before age 12-18 mos. but OK at any age	

* See page 2 for abbreviations. NOTE: All dosage recommendations are for adults (unless otherwise indicated) and assume normal renal function.
Costs from 2006 DRUG TOPICS RED BOOK, Medical Economics. Price is average wholesale price (AWP)

TABLE 14A (9)

VIRUS/DISEASE	DRUG/DOSAGE	SIDE EFFECTS/COMMENTS
Herpesvirus Infections/Herpes Varicella-Zoster Virus (VZV) (continued)		
Herpes zoster (shingles) (See NEJM 342:635, 2000; 347:340, 2002) **Normal host** Effective rx most evident in pts >50 yrs. Rx *of post-herpetic neuralgia*, see p. 143 *and* 151 *below*.	**NOTE: Trials showing benefit of rx: only in pts treated within 3 days of onset of rash** **Valacyclovir** 1000 mg po tid times 7 days (adjust dose for renal failure) **OR** **Famciclovir** 500 mg tid x 7 days. Adjust for renal failure (see table 17) **OR**	Valacyclovir ↓ post-herpetic neuralgia more rapidly than acyclovir in pts >50 yrs of age: median duration of zoster-associated pain was 38 days with valacyclovir and 51 days on acyclovir (AAC 39:1546, 1995). Toxicity of both drugs similar (Arch Fam Med 9:863, 2000). Time to healing more rapid. Reduced post-herpetic neuralgia (PHN) vs placebo in pts >50 yr of age: duration of PHN with famciclovir 63 days, placebo 163 days. Famciclovir similar to acyclovir in reduction of acute pain and PHN (J Micro Immunol Inf 37:75, 2004).
New vaccine ↓ herpes zoster & post-herpetic neuralgia (NEJM 352:2271, 2005; JAMA 292:157, 2006).	**Acyclovir** 800 mg po 5 times per day times 7–10 days **Prednisone** 30 mg bid days 1–7, 15 mg bid days 8–14 and 7.5 mg bid days 15–21 also recommended by some authorities in pts >50 yrs of age (NEJM 335:32, 1996)] and especially when pt has large number of lesions (>21) and/or severe pain at presentation (JID 179:9, 1999)	A meta-analysis of 4 placebo-controlled trials (691 pts) demonstrated that acyclovir accelerated by approx. 2-fold pain resolution by all measures employed and reduced post-herpetic neuralgia at 3 & 6 mos (CID 22:341, 1996)]. ↓ med. time to resolution of pain 41 days vs 101 days in those >50 yrs. Prednisone added to acyclovir improved quality of life measurements (↓ acute pain, sleep, and return to normal activity) (AnIM 125:376, 1996). In post-herpetic neuralgia, controlled trials demonstrated effectiveness of gabapentin, the lidocaine patch (5%), & opioid analgesic in controlling pain (Days: 64:937, 2004; J Clin Virol 29:248, 2004). Nortriptyline & amitriptyline are equally effective but nortriptyline is better tolerated (CID 36:877, 2003). Role of antiviral drugs in rx of PHN unproven (Neurol 64:21, 2005) but 8 of 15 pt improved with IV acyclovir 10 mg/kg q 8 hrs x 14 days followed by oral valacyclovir 1 gm 3x a day for 1 month (Arch Neur 63:940, 2006).
Immunocompromised host Not severe	**Acyclovir** 800 mg po 5 times per day times 7 days. **Options: Famciclovir** 750 mg po q24h or 500 mg bid or 250 mg 3 times per day times 7 days **OR valacyclovir** 1000 mg po tid times 7 days, though both are not FDA-approved for this indication]	If progression, switch to IV
Severe: >1 dermatome, trigeminal nerve or disseminated	**Acyclovir** 10–12 mg per kg IV (infusion over 1 hr) q8h times 7–14 days. In older pts, ↓ to 7.5 mg per kg. If nephrotoxicity and pt improving, ↓ to 5 mg per kg q8h.	A common manifestation of immune reconstitution following HAART in HIV-infected children (J All Clin Immun 113:742, 2004). Rx must be begun within 72 hrs. Acyclovir-resistant VZV occurs in HIV+ pts previously treated with acyclovir. Foscarnet (40 mg per kg IV q8h for 14–26 days) successful in 4/5 pts but 2 relapsed in 7 and 14 days (AnIM 115:19, 1997).

---

* See page 2 for abbreviations. NOTE: All dosage recommendations are for adults (unless otherwise indicated) and assume normal renal function.
Costs from 2006 DRUG TOPICS RED BOOK, Medical Economics. Price is average wholesale price (AWP).

TABLE 14A (10)

VIRUS/DISEASE	DRUG/DOSAGE	SIDE EFFECTS/COMMENTS
Influenza (A & B) **Suspect or proven acute disease** Rapid flu tests available. Antiviral rx most-effective if given within first 48 hrs of onset of typical symptoms during influenza season. **Pathogenic avian influenza** (H5N1) emerged in poultry (mainly chickens & ducks) in *East & Southeast Asia*. From Dec. 1, 2003 to August 30, 2006, 246 laboratory confirmed cases reported in 10 countries with 144 deaths (see *www.cdc.gov/flu/ avian*). Human-to-human transmission reported (*NEJM 352:333, 2005*); most have had direct contact with poultry (*NEJM 350:1179, 2004*). One human cluster of 8 cases reported from Sumatra island with 6 deaths. According to WHO, mortality highest in young age 10-19 (73%) vs 50% overall and associated with high viral load and cytokine storm (*Nature Medicine Sept. 2006*). Human isolates are resistant to amantadine/rimantadine. Oseltamivir rx recommended if avian H5N1 suspected (*MMWR 53:97, 2004*). ↑ dose & duration of oseltamivir necessary for maximum effect in mouse model (*JID 192:665, 2005; Nature 456:418, 2005*). **Prevention**. See *MMWR 54:RR-8:1, 2005*	**If fever & cough; known community influenza activity; and 1st 48 hrs of illness, consider:** **For Influenza A & B: also avian (H5N1):** **Oseltamivir** 75 mg po bid times 5 days (also approved for rx of children age 1-12 yrs, dose 2 mg per kg up to a total of 75 mg bid times 5 days) or **Zanamivir** 2 inhalations (2 times 5 mg) bid times 5 days **Prevention of influenza A & B:** give vaccine and/or ≥13 yrs age, consider **oseltamivir** 75 mg po q24h for duration of peak influenza in community or for outbreak control in high-risk populations (*CID 39:459, 2004*). (Consider for similar populations as immunization recommendations.)	Pts with COPD or asthma, **potential risk of bronchospasm with zanamivir**. All ↓ duration of symptoms by approx. 50% (1-2 days) if given within 30-36 hrs after onset of symptoms. Benefit influenced by duration of sx before rx. Oseltamivir rx within 12 hrs after fever onset ↓ total median illness duration by 74.6 hrs (*JAC 51:123, 2003*). ↓ risk of pneumonia & hospitalization (*Curr Med Res Opin 21:761, 2005*). **Disturbing report** of oseltamivir-resistant virus detected after 4 days of rx (*Ln 364: 733 & 759, 2004*). In another study of 298 rx cases of adults & children, two oseltamivir-resistant viruses found (*JID 189:440, 2004*). Concern about postinfluenza complications including community-acquired MRSA pneumonia (*CID 40:1693, 2005*). Rimantadine and amantadine no longer recommended by the CDC because of high level resistance emerging since 2005.
Measles While measles in the US is at the lowest rates ever (.55/100,00) much higher rates reported in developing countries	No therapy or **vitamin A**	Immunization contraindicated if hypersensitivity to hen's eggs. Both amantadine and rimantadine are about 60-90% effective against influenza A. Both oseltamivir and zanamivir reported efficacious (82 & 84% respectively) in clinical trials (*JAMA 285: 748, 2001; JID 186:1582, 2002*). In families, rx of index case as well as contact cases was more effective than rx index case alone (p <0.01) (*JID 189:440, 2004*).
Children	No rx or **ribavirin** IV (i) (0.20-35 mg per kg per day times 7 days	↓ severity of measles in one study (*NEJM 323:160, 1990*), not in others.
Adults		Vitamin A↓ severity of illness in adults (*CID 20:454, 1994*). ↓ severity of illness in adults (*CID 20:454, 1994*).
Metapneumovirus (HMPV) A paramyxovirus isolated from pts of all ages, with mild bronchiolitis/bronchospasm to pneumonia (*PIDJ 23:S215, 2004*). Can cause lethal pneumonia in HSCT pts (*Ann Intern Med 144:344, 2006*).	No proven antiviral therapy	Human metapneumovirus isolated from 6.2% of children with respiratory infections (*JID 190:20, 2004*). 12% of children with lower respiratory infections (*NEJM 350:443, 2004*) & 21% of hospitalized children with RSV (*PIDJ 23:436, 2004; JID 190:27, 2004*). Dual infection with RSV assoc. with severe bronchiolitis (*JID 191:382, 2005*).
Monkey pox (orthopox virus) (see *LnID 4:17, 2004*) In 2003, 72 pts contracted from contact with ill prairie dogs. Source likely imported Gambian giant rats (*MMWR 42:642, 2003*).	**No proven antiviral therapy.** Cidofovir is active in vitro & in mouse model (*AAC 46:1329, 2002; Antiviral Res 57:13, 2003*)	Incubation period of 12 days, then fever, headache, cough, adenopathy, & a vesicular papular rash that pustulates, umbilicates, & crusts on the head, trunk, & extremities. Transmission in healthcare setting rare (*CID 40:789, 2005*).

* See page 2 for abbreviations. NOTE: All dosage recommendations are for adults (unless otherwise indicated) and assume normal renal function.
Costs from 2006 Drug Topics Red Book, MedicalEconomics. Price is average wholesale price (AWP)

TABLE 14A (11)

VIRUS/DISEASE	DRUG/DOSAGE	SIDE EFFECTS/COMMENTS
Norovirus (Nowalk-like virus, or NLV) Caused 93% of outbreaks of non-bacterial gastroenteritis reported to CDC 1997–2000. Transmission by contaminated food, fecal-oral, contaminated surfaces, or fomites.	No antiviral therapy. Replete volume.	Sudden onset of nausea, vomiting, & watery diarrhea lasting 12–60 hours. Ethanol-based hand rubs effective against norovirus (*J Hosp Inf* 60:144, 2005).
Papillomaviruses. 81.7% of 60 adolescent females infected over 2.2 yrs (*JID* 191:182, 2005). Therapies unsatisfactory with limited efficacy, high recurrence rates & ↑ side-effects (*JAC* 53:137, 2004) **Vaccine against HPV 16/18 highly effective & safe in preventing HPV infection & preventing cervical lesions. (*Lancet* 367; 1247, 2006) Use should become routine!**		2005; *CID* 41:1742, 2005; *CID* 41:1765, 2005).
Anogenital Warts: Condyloma acuminatum (HPV types 6 & 11 most common but types 16 & 18 most likely premalignant.) (See *Med Lett* 43:1, 2001; *CID* 28:S37, 1999.) [NOTE: Results of Pap smear should be available prior to rx; **avoid rx in pregnant women**) NOTE: Recurrences common after all treatments Warts occurred within 36 mos. after infection with HPV-16/18 in 64% (*JID* 191:731, 2005)	**Podofilox** (Condylox) 2x/day app with cotton swab for 3 days followed by 4 days without rx; repeat cycle 4–6 x as necessary] **OR** [25% **podo-phyllin** in tincture of benzoin (Podocon-25) apply 1x/wk up to 6wk, allow to air dry—1–4 hr) If no regression after 4 wks, use alt rx. **interferon alfa-2b** (Intron A), **alfa-n3** (Alferon N): 1 million units (0.1 mL) into lesion 3 times per week times 3 weeks. Intralesional injection of skin test antigens (mumps, candida or trichophyton) with or without interferon alfa-2b	**Podofilox:** Local reactions—pain, burning, inflammation in 50%. No systemic effects. Efficacy in penile warts 74% vs placebo 8%. Recurrences 55% vs 100% with placebo. (Podocon-25 15 mL, $32.40, Condylox 3.5 mL, $56.64.) Condylox Warts recur in 1/3 with either agent within 1" month after rx. Painful; dilute to 10 million units per 1 mL. Other concentrations are hypertonic (*CID* 28:S37, 1999). Use when other rx fails, esp. in AIDS. More effective than placebo in ↑ warts. IFN alfa-2b did not ↑ response rate & given alone, not better than saline placebo in one 235-pt randomized single-blind placebo-controlled trial (*AJDerm* 141:589, 2005). An in vitro positive monocyte proliferation assay to antigen predicted resolution of wart
	Imiquimod (5% cream): Apply 3 times per week prior to sleep, remove 6–10 hrs later when awake. Continue until cleared or max. 16 wks.	Clearance rates of warts in immunocompetent: at 8 wks 50%, 16 wks 72% with follow-up to 16wk or until warts cleared. 3x/wk overnight x 16 wks (*AIDS* 12:F27, 1998). Less effective in immunosuppressed pts: Benefit in 5/12 pts who completed 24-month course (*Brit J Derm* 152:122, 2005). Cost of 1–4 wks rx: $108–432. [Imiquimod: Local reactions—mild erythema 60%, erosion 30%.
Skin papillomas	**Topical α-lactalbumin** (from human milk) applied 1x/day for 3 wks	↓ lesion size & recurrence vs placebo (p <0.001) (*NEJM* 350:2663, 2004). Further studies warranted.
Parvo B19 Virus (Erythrovirus B19). See *NEJM* 350:586, 2004 Uncomplicated or self-limited acute arthritis. May be chronic in children.	No treatment recommended	Bone marrow shows selective erythrocyte maturation arrest with giant pronormoblasts. IgM antibody for diagnosis. Parvo B19 also associated with respiratory distress syndrome (*CID* 27:900, 1998) and myocarditis/myocardiopathy (*CID* 28:1343, 1999). One 16-year-old boy with chronic infection (fatigue, fever, rash) responded to high dose IVIG (*PIDJ* 24:272, 2005).
Acute profound anemia: in utero, in hemolytic anemia, in HIV and in solid organ transplant & HSCT. (*CID* 43:40, 2006)	**IVIG** 0.4gm/kg IV q24h × 5 days in immune def. states with severe anemia has been reported successful.	IVIG contains anti-parvo B19 antibody. Longterm remission reported (*Transpl Inf Dis* 7:30, 2005). In pts with pre-existing hemolytic anemia, parvo B19-induced bone marrow arrest can result in sudden severe anemia.
Papovavirus/Polyomavirus **Progressive multifocal leukoencephalopathy** (PML/JC virus) Pts with advanced HIV disease or organ trans-plant. Requested in pts receiving natalizumab, a monoclonal antibody against α4 integrins (*NEJM* 353:362, & 369, 2005)	See *SANFORD GUIDE TO HIV/AIDS THERAPY.* **HAART** ↑ survival (545 days vs 60 days, p < 0.0001) and either improved (50%) or stabilized (50%) neurological deficits in 12 pts (*AIDS* 12: 2467, 1999). Others less optimistic (*CID* 28: 1152, 1999). integrins for Crohn's disease (1) & MS (2)	Cytarabine of no value in controlled trial (*NEJM* 338:1345, 1998). Camptothecin, a human topoisomerase I inhibitor, was administered to a single pt with slowing of progression (*Ln* 349:1366, 1997). Use of cidofovir controversial (*Clin Micro Rev* 16:569, 2003; *J Infect Neurol* 19:35, 2004; *J Neurol Sci* 213:29, 2004). DC immunosuppression in transplant pts resulted in successful outcome (*Am J Transpl* 5:1151, 2005).

* See page 2 for abbreviations. *NOTE: All dosage recommendations are for adults (unless otherwise indicated) and assume normal renal function.*
Costs from 2006 DRUG TOPICS RED BOOK, Medical Economics. Price is average wholesale price (AWP).

TABLE 14A (12)

VIRUS/DISEASE	DRUG/DOSAGE	SIDE EFFECTS/COMMENTS
Polyomavirus-associated nephropathy Due to BK virus, post renal transplant		Possible rx for cidofovir (*CID* 36:1111, 2003)
Rabies [see *table 20F*, pages 182–183; see Mayo Clin Proc 79:671, 2004; MMWR 54:RR-3:1, 2005, CDC Guidelines for Prevention and Control 2006, MMWR/55/RR-5,2006]		
Rabid dog accounts for 50,000 deaths worldwide. Most cases in the U.S. are cryptic, i.e., no documented evidence of bite or contact with a rabid animal (*CID* 35:738, 2003). 70% assoc. with 2 rare bat species (*EID* 9:151, 2003). An organ donor infected. 4 recipients (2 kidneys, liver & artery) who all died of rabies avg. 13 days after transplant (*NEJM* 352:1103, 2005).	**Mortality↑100% with only survivors those who receive rabies vaccine before the onset of illness/symptoms** (*CID* 36:61, 2003). A 15-year-old female who developed rabies 1 month post-bat bite but survived after drug induction of coma (+ vme rx for 7 days; did not receive immunoprophylaxis (*NEJM* 352:2508, 2005).	Corticosteroids ↑ mortality rate and ↓ incubation time in mice. Therapies that have failed after symptoms develop: include rabies vaccine, rabies immunoglobulin, rabies virus neutralizing antibody, ribavirin, alfa interferon, & ketamine.
Respiratory Syncytial Virus Major cause of morbidity in neonates/infants. In adults, RSV accounted for 10.6% of hospitalizations for pneumonia, 11.4% for COPD, 7.2% for asthma, 5.4% for CHF in pts >65 yrs of age (*NEJM* 352:1749, 2005). RSV caused 11% of clinically important respiratory illnesses in military recruits (*CID* 41:311, 2005).	Rapid dx by antigen detection on nasopharyngeal wash. **No rx proven to ↑ survival.** Various combinations of ribavirin, RSV-IVIG & palliclumab have been used; see Comments (*PIDJ* 23:707, 2004; *Pharmacotherapy* 24:932, 2004; *Ped Drugs* 6:177, 2004).	Ribavirin reported to ↓ fever and other symptoms and signs. However, in controlled studies, ribavirin had no beneficial effect (*J Ped* 126: 422, 1996; *AJRCCM* 160:829, 1999). Still recommended by some authorities for immunocompromised children (*PIDJ* 19:253, 2000) & still controversial (*PIDJ* 22:589, 2003).
Prevention (1) Children <24 mos. old with bronchopulmonary dysplasia (BPD) requiring supplemental O₂ (<26 wks gestation) and <6 mos. old at start of RSV season (2) Perhaps premature infants	**RSV immune globulin intravenous** (RSV-IVIG) 100 mg per kg IV once monthly Nov. through April (for northern hemisphere) 1ˢᵗ week of life for premature. Perhaps up to 60 months of age for pts with BPD — **OR** **Palivizumab** 15 mg per kg I.M. q month Nov–April as above (*Scand J Inf Dis* 33:323, 2001). Cost: \$500–5000/yr.	RSV-IVIG very expensive—estimated cost per infusion \$1175. See consensus opinion for details: *Ped Int Dis J* 15:1059, 1996. See *Ln* 354:847, 1999 for updated review. Palivizumab reduced hospitalization due to RSV in 1500 premature infants & children with chronic lung disease from 10.6% to 4.8% (*Pediatrics* 102:531, 1998). Expensive but often recommended, but in 2003, approx. 100,000 infants received drug annually in U.S. (*PIDJ* 23:1051, 2004).
Rhinovirus (Colds) See *Ln* 361:51, 2003 Found in 1/2 of children with community-acquired pneumonia, role in pathogenesis unclear (*CID* 39:681, 2004). Antiviral Kleenex may reduce spread (*Med Lett* 47:3, 2005).	No antiviral rx indicated (*Ped Ann* 34:53, 2005). Symptomatic rx: • ipratropium bromide nasal (2 sprays per nostril tid) • clemastine 1.34 mg 1–2 tab po bid-tid (OTC)	Six relief (ipratropium nasal spray + sneezing and sneezing vs placebo (*AnIM* 125:89, 1996). Clemastine (an antihistamine) ↓ sneezing, rhinorrhea but associated with dry nose, mouth & throat in 6–19% (*CID* 22:656, 1996). Zinc lozenges were ineffective (*JID* 31:1202, 2000). Oral **pleconaril** given within 24 hrs of onset reduced duration (1 day) & severity of "cold symptoms" in DBPCT (*n* <.001) (*CID* 36:1523, 2003). A combination of intranasal interferon alfa-2b, oral chlorpheniramine & ibuprofen + symptom score by 33–73% vs placebo when started 24 hrs after intranasal rhinovirus (*JID* 186:147, 2002). Echinacea didn't work (*CID* 38:1367, 2004 & 40:807, 2005)—put it to rest!
Rotavirus Leading recognized cause of diarrhea-related illness among infants and children worldwide and kills 2 million children annually.	No antiviral rx available; oral hydration life-saving. In one study, **Nitazoxanide 7.5 mg/kg 2x/d x3 days** reduced duration of illness from 75 to 31 hrs in Egyptian children. Impact on rotavirus or other parameters not measured. (*Lancet* 368:124, 2006). Too early to recommend routine use (*Lancet* 368:100, 2004)	Two live-attenuated vaccines highly effective (85 and 98%) and safe in preventing rotavirus diarrhea and hospitalization (*NEJM* 354, 1 & 23, 2006)
SARS-CoV: See page 134		
Smallpox (*NEJM* 346/1300, 2002) **Contact vaccinia** (*JAMA* 288:1901, 2002)	Smallpox vaccine (if within 4 days of exposure) + cidofovir (dosage uncertain (dosage uncertain) (AWP)). From vaccination: Progressive vaccinia—vaccinia immune globulin may be of benefit. To obtain immune globulin, contact CDC: 770-488-7100. (*CID* 39:759, 776 & 819, 2004)	
West Nile virus: See page 135		

* See page 2 for abbreviations; NOTE: All dosage recommendations are for adults (unless otherwise indicated) and assume normal renal function. Costs from 2006 DRUG TOPICS RED BOOK, Medica Economics. Price is average wholesale price (AWP).

TABLE 14B – ANTIVIRAL DRUGS (OTHER THAN RETROVIRAL)

DRUG NAME(S) GENERIC (TRADE)	DOSAGE/ROUTE/COST*	COMMENTS/ADVERSE EFFECTS
CMV (See SANFORD GUIDE TO HIV/AIDS THERAPY)		
Cidofovir (Vistide)	5 mg per kg IV q week times 2, then q2 weeks. (375 mg **$888**) Probenecid and IV prehydration with normal saline and oral probenecid **must be used with each cidofovir infusion** (see pkg insert for details). Renal function (serum creatinine and urine protein) must be monitored prior to each dose (see pkg insert for details).	**Adverse effects: Nephrotoxicity:** dose-dependent proximal tubular injury (Fanconi-like syndrome): proteinuria, glycosuria, bicarbonaturia, phosphaturia, polyuria (nephrogenic diabetic insipidus. Ln 350:413, 1997). ↑ creatinine. Concomitant saline prehydration, probenecid, extended dosing intervals allowed use. 25% of pts on IV cidofovir due to nephrotoxicity. Other toxicities: nausea 48%, fever 31%, alopecia 16%, myalgia 16%, proberecid hypersensitivity 16%, neutropenia 29%. No effect on hematocrit, platelets, LFTs. **Comment:** Recommended dosage, frequency or infusion rate must not be exceeded. Dose must be reduced or discontinued if changes in renal function occur during rx. For ↑ of 0.3-0.4 mg per dL in serum creatinine, reduce dose ↓ from 5 to 3 mg per kg; discontinue cidofovir if ↑ of 0.5 mg per dL above baseline or 3+ proteinuria develops (for 2+ proteinuria, observe pts carefully and consider discontinuation).
Foscarnet (Foscavir)	90 mg per kg IV q12h (induction) 90 mg per kg q24h (maintenance) Dosage adjust with renal dysfunction (see Table 17) (6 gm $70)	**Adverse effects: Major clinical toxicity is renal impairment (1/3 of patients)**—↑ creatinine, proteinuria, nephrogenic diabetes insipidus. ↓ K+, ↓ Ca++, ↓ Mg++ (↓Ca++) Toxicity (↓ with other nephrotoxic drugs (ampho B, aminoglycosides or pentamidine (especially severe ↓ Ca++)). Adequate hydration may ↓ toxicity. Other: headache, mild (10%), fatigue (100%), nausea (80%), fever (25%). CNS: seizures. Hematol: ↓ WBC, ↓ Hgb. Hepatic: liver function tests ↑. Neurop: Penile ulcers.
Ganciclovir (Cytovene)	IV 5 mg per kg q12h times 14 days (induction) 5 mg per kg q24h or 6 mg per kg 5 times per wk (maintenance) Dosage adjust with renal dysfunction (see Table 17) (500 mg IV $47)	**Adverse effects:** Absolute neutrophil count dropped below 500 per mm³ in 15%, thrombocytopenia 21%, anemia 6%. Fever 48%, GI 50%: nausea, vomiting, diarrhea, abdominal pain 19%, rash 10%. Retinal detachment 11% (relationship to ganciclovir?). Confusion, headache, psychiatric disturbances and seizures. Neutropenia may respond to granulocyte colony stimulating factor (G-CSF or GM-CSF). Severe myelosuppression may be ↑ with coadministration of zidovudine or azathioprine. 32% dc/interrupted rx, principally for neutropenia.
	Oral: 1.0 gm tid with food (fatty meal) (500 mg cap $9.60)	Hematologic: less frequent than with IV. Granulocytopenia 18%, anemia 12%, thrombocytopenia 6%. GI, also sense as with IV. Retinal detachment 8%.
Ganciclovir (Vitrasert)	Intraocular implant (~ $5000 per device + cost of surgery.)	**Adverse effects:** Late retinal detachment (7/30 eyes). Does not prevent CMV retinitis in good eye or visceral dissemination. **Comment:** Replacement every 6 months recommended.
Valganciclovir (Valcyte)	900 mg (two 450 mg tabs) po bid times 21 days for induction. followed by 900 mg po q24h. Take with food. (450 mg cap $33.30, ~ $2,000 for 60 caps)	A prodrug of ganciclovir with better bioavailability. 60% with food **Adverse effects:** Similar to ganciclovir.
Herpesvirus (non-CMV) Acyclovir (Zovirax) or generic	Doses: see Table 14A 400 mg tab G $0.30–0.70 (to $110–200/yr for chronic suppression) 800 mg tab G $0.97 200 mg cap G $0.60 Suspension 200 mg per 5 mL $137 Ointment 5% 15 gm $109	**po:** Generally well-tolerated with occ. diarrhea, vertigo, arthralgia. Less frequent rash, fatigue, insomnia, fever, menstrual abnormalities, acne, sore throat. Uncommon: lymphadenopathy. hallucinations, delirium, seizures, coma **IV:** Phlebitis, caustic with vesicular lesions with IV infiltration. CNS (1%): lethargy, tremors, confusion, hallucinations, delirium, seizures, coma (CID 21:435, 1995). Improve 1–2 weeks after rx stopped. Renal (5%): ↑ creatinine, hematuria. With high doses may crystallize in renal tubules → obstructive uropathy (rapid infusion, dehydration, renal insufficiency and ↑ dose ↑ risk). Adequate pre-hydration may prevent such nephrotoxicity. Hepatic: ↑ ALT, AST. Uncommon: neutropenia (CID 20: 1557, 1995), rash, diaphoresis, hypotension, headache, nausea

---

* See page 2 for abbreviations. NOTE: All dosage recommendations are for adults (unless otherwise indicated) and assume normal renal function.
Costs from 2006 DRUG TOPICS RED BOOK, Medical Economics. Price is average wholesale price (AWP).

TABLE 14B (2)

DRUG NAME(S) GENERIC (TRADE)	DOSAGE/ROUTE/COST*	COMMENTS/ADVERSE EFFECTS
Herpesvirus (non-CMV) *(continued)*		
Famciclovir (Famvir)	250 mg cap $4.70 500 mg cap $9.33	Metabolized to penciclovir. **Adverse effects:** similar to acyclovir, included headache, nausea, diarrhea, and dizziness but incidence did not differ from placebo *(JAMA 276:47, 1996)*. May be taken without regard to meals. Dose should be reduced for CrCl < 60 mL per min *(see package insert & Table 14A, page 136 & Table 17, page 174)*.
Penciclovir (Denavir)	Topical ¼% cream 1.5 gm $31	Apply to area of recurrence of herpes labialis with start of sx, then q2h while awake times 4 days. Well tolerated.
Trifluridine (Viroptic)	1 drop 1% solution q2h (max. 9 drops per day) for max. of 21 days (7.5 mL 1% solution $111)	Mild burning (5%), palpebral edema (3%), punctate keratopathy, stromal edema.
Valacyclovir (Valtrex)	500 mg cap $3.50, 1000mg caplet (capsule-shaped tablet)	An ester pro-drug of acyclovir that is well-absorbed, bioavailability 3-5 times greater than acyclovir. **Adverse effects** similar to acyclovir *(see JID 186:540, 2002)*. Thrombotic thrombocytopenic purpura/hemolytic uremic syndrome reported in pts with advanced HIV disease and transplant recipients participating in clinical trials at doses of 8 gm per day.
Hepatitis		
Adefovir dipivoxil (Hepsera)	10 mg po q24h (with normal CrCl); see *Table 17A if renal impairment* Cost $20/ea = $596 per month	Adefovir dipivoxil is a prodrug of adefovir. It is an acyclic nucleotide analog with activity against hepatitis B [early on 0.2, 0.5 mM (IC₅₀). See Table 5 for Cmax & T½. Active against YMDD mutant strains, ENT resistant strains, and HepB virus immunoglobulin mutants. Primarily renal excretion—adjust dose. No food interactions. Remarkably low side effects. No nephrotoxicity at 10 mg per day. Monitor renal function. esp. with pts with pre-existing or other risks for renal impairment. Lactic acidosis reported with nucleoside analogs, esp. in women. Pregnancy Category C. Hepatitis may exacerbate after nx dc: 6-25% of pts developed ALT ↑ 10 times normal when nx dc; usually responds to re-treatment or self-limited.]
Entecavir (Baraclude)	0.5 mg po q24h, 1 mg if refractory to lamivudine 1 mg per day ($714.60 per month) (0.5 = $23.70ea = $710/mo)	A nucleoside analog active against HBV including lamivudine-resistant mutants. Minimal adverse effects reported: headache, fatigue, dizziness, & nausea reported in 22% of pts. Potential for lactic acidosis but not reported to date. Adjust dosage in renal impairment *(see Table 17, page 174)*.
Interferon alfa-2a (Roferon-A), alfa-2b Intron-A)	3 million units: (Roferon $45, Intron $49; Infergen 9 mcg $74)	A pocketbook drug in renal impairment has appeared. **Adverse effects:** Flu-like symptoms in up to ½ of pts *(J Clin Psych 64:708, 2003)* (depression, anxiety, 73%, headache 71%, GI: anorexia 46%, diarrhea 29%, CNS: dizziness 21%. Rash 18%, later profound fatigue & psychiatric symptoms in up to ½ of pts *(J Clin Psych 64:708, 2003)* (depression, anxiety, emotional lability and agitation), alopecia, ↑ TSH, autoimmune thyroid disorders with hypo- or hyperthyroidism 0.2%. Serum sickness reported *(J Rheum 32:329, 2005)*. Hematol ↓ WBC 49%, ↓ Hgb 27%, ↓ platelets 35%. Consider prophylactic antidepressant in pts with history. Acute reversible hearing loss and/or tinnitus in up to 1/3 *(Ln 343:1134, 1994)*. Optic neuropathy (retinal hemorrhage, cotton wool spots, ↓ in color vision) reported *(AIDS 18:1805, 2004)*. Cryoglobulinemia assoc. with HCV usually responds to IFN nx but exacerbations with vasculitis also reported with nx *(Clin Rheum, e30, June 2005)*. Side-effects ↑ with ↑ doses and dose reduction necessary in up to 46% receiving chronic nx for HBV.
PEG interferon alfa-2b (PEG-Intron)	0.5-1.5 mcg per kg subcut. q wk (120 mcg) $414)	
Pegylated-40k interferon alfa-2a (Pegasys)	180 mcg subcut. q wk times 48 wks (180 mcg) $429)	Attachment of IFN to polyethylene glycol (PEG) prolongs half-life and allows weekly dosing. Better efficacy data with similar adverse effects profile compared to regular formulation.
Lamivudine (3TC) (Epivir-HBV)	**Adverse effects:** See *Table 14D, page 157.* NOTE: 100 mg po q24h times 1 yr for hepatitis B. (100 mg tab) $7, or $205 per month	

* See page 2 for abbreviations. NOTE: All dosage recommendations are for adults (unless otherwise indicated) and assume normal/renal function.
Costs from 2006 DRUG TOPICS RED BOOK, Medical Economics. Price are average wholesale price (AWP).

TABLE 14B (3)

DRUG NAME(S) GENERIC (TRADE)	DOSAGE/ROUTE/COST*	COMMENTS/ADVERSE EFFECTS
Hepatitis (continued)		
Ribavirin–Interferon alfa-2b combination pack (Rebetron) or **PEG IFN + ribavirin in combination**	Combination kit contains 2 wk. supply of IFN and 42, 70, or 84 caps of 200 mg ribavirin. **Dose:** IFN 3 million units subcut. 3 times per wk AND ribavirin 400 mg p.o. a.m. + 600 mg p.o. q.p.m. (<75 kg BW) or 600 mg p.o. a.m. (>75 kg). Rebetron (1000 mg per day ribavirin dose pack). Cost \$650 per 24 wk course). **Ribavirin:** Hgb: <10 ↓ to 200 mg a.m. & 200 mg p.m. <8.5 DC **Interferon** No change DC	**Ribavirin:** Hemolytic anemia common but usually responds to ↓ ribavirin dosage (see package insert). Ribavirin plasma level correlates with degree of efficacy against HBV but also with efficacy against HBV (see package insert). 1 Japanese study suggests levels between 3000 to 3500 ng per mL 8 wks after initiating rx optimal (Intervirol 48:138, 2005). Erythropoietin (Epoetin alfa) effective in ↑ Hgb levels & quality of life while allowing adequate dosage of ribavirin to be maintained (Pharmacother 25:862, 2005). Pure red cell aplasia 2° to anti-erythropoietin antibodies reported (Am J Gastro 100:1415, 2005). **Since ribavirin is teratogenic, drug must not be used during pregnancy or within 6 months of pregnancy.** Also should not be used in pts with endstage renal failure, severe heart disease, or hemoglobinopathies. ARDS reported (Chest 124:406, 2003).
	Interferon WBC <1500 ↓ to 1.5 million units subcut. 3 times per wk <1000 No change DC Abs. PMNs <750 ↓ to 1.5 million units subcut. 3 times per wk <500 DC Platelets: <50,000 ↓ to 1.5 million units subcut. 3 times per wk <25,000 DC	**Interferon alfa: Severe psychiatric effects, esp. depression, most common (23–36%) reason for discontinuation of rx. Suicidal behavior reported.** Preemptive rx with antidepressants effective in 1 open-label study (J Hpt 42:793, 2005). Hyper- & hypothyroidism, alopecia (30%) including reversible alopecia universalis (J Chemother 17:212, 2005), & pulmonary disease reported (Mayo Clin Proc 74:367, 1999). Uncommon side-effects include exacerbation of psoriasis (Chemotherapy 51:167, 2005) & other rheumatological conditions (Rheumatol 44:1016, 2005), sexual dysfunction with ↑ testosterone levels (J Endo 186:545, 2005), risk of lipoatrophy 2° to mitochondrial toxicity when administered with nucleoside analogs to HIV-HBV co-infected pts (Antivir Ther 10:557, 2005), & sarcoidosis (AtDerm 141:865, 2005).
Ribavirin (Rebetol)	Use with pegylated interferons (alfa-2a & 2b) for treatment of hepatitis C. Available as 200 mg capsules. Dose: <75 kg BW = 2 caps in a.m. & 3 caps in p.m.; >75 kg BW 3 caps in a.m. & 3 caps in p.m. Cost: 200 mg \$10.60	Side-effects as above, esp. hemolytic anemia (during 1st 1–2 wks of rx) with hemoglobin ↓ of 3–4 gm. Should not be used with CrCl <50 mL per min & cautiously with cardiac disease.
Influenza A **Amantadine (Symmetrel)** or **Rimantadine (Flumadine)**	**Currently not recommended by the CDC for Influenza A because of high level resistance found in 2005 isolates!** Amantadine and rimantadine doses are the same (rimantadine approved only for prophylaxis in children, not treatment). Amantadine 100 mg bid, >65 y.o., 100 mg q24h. (G: 100 mg cap \$0.50, 100 mg 10 mL soln. \$1.80. Rimantadine 100 mg tab/syrup \$2	**Side-effects/toxicity:** CNS (nervousness, anxiety, difficulty concentrating, and lightheadedness). Symptoms occurred in 6% on amantadine vs 14% on rimantadine. They usually ↓ after 1st week and disappear when drug DC. GI (nausea, anorexia). Some serious side-effects—delirium, hallucinations, and seizures—are associated with high plasma drug levels resulting from renal insufficiency, esp. in older pts with prior seizure disorders, or psychiatric disorders. In pts with impaired renal function, dosage of both drugs should be reduced (amantadine: creatinine clearance <50 mL per min, rimantadine: CrCl <10 mL per min); see package inserts (Clin Ther 26:76; Curr Eye Res 11).
Influenza A and B—For both drugs, initiate within 48 hrs of symptom onset **Zanamivir (Relenza)** For pts ≥12 yrs of age	2 inhalations (2 times 5 mg) bid times 5 days. Powder is inhaled using specially designed breath-activated device. Each medication-containing blister contains 5 mg of zanamivir. \$60 per course	Active by inhalation against neuraminidase of both Influenza A and B and inhibits release of virus from epithelial cells of respiratory tract. Approx. 4–17% of inhaled dose absorbed into plasma. Excreted by kidney but with low absorption, dose reduction not necessary in renal impairment. Minimal side-effects: <3% cough, sinusitis, diarrhea, nausea and vomiting. **Reports of respiratory adverse events in pts with or without h/o airway disease, should be avoided in pts with respiratory disease.**

* See page 2 for abbreviations. NOTE: All dosage recommendations are for adults (unless otherwise indicated) and assume normal renal function.
Costs from 2006 Drug Topics Red Book, Medical Economics. Price is average wholesale price (AWP).

TABLE 14B (4)

DRUG NAME(S) GENERIC (TRADE)	DOSAGE/ROUTE/COST*	COMMENTS/ADVERSE EFFECTS
Oseltamivir (Tamiflu)	75 mg po bid for treatment (pediatric suspension [12 mg per mL] approved for treatment, not prevention, in children age 1–12 at dose of 2 mg per kg (up to 75 mg total) bid times 5 days) For prevention: 75 mg po q24h for duration of peak of flu epidemic. $73 per 5 day course	Well absorbed (80% bioavailable) from GI tract as ethyl ester of active compound GS-4071. T½ 6–10 hrs; excreted unchanged by kidney. Adverse effects in 15% include diarrhea 1.6%, nausea 0.5%, vomiting, headache (*J Am Ger Soc* 50:608, 2002). Nausea ↓ with food. Also available as 12 mg per mL oral suspension.
Respiratory Syncytial Virus (RSV) and other		
Palivizumab (Synagis) (See *Med Lett* 41:1, 1999) Used only for prevention of RSV infection in high-risk children *Pediatrics* 102:1211 (1998)	15 mg per kg IM q month 100 mg vial (for 1 injection) $1646	A monoclonal antibody directed against the F glycoprotein on surface of virus; side-effects are nominal, occ. ↑ ALT (*JID* 176:1215, 1997).
Ribavirin (Virazole)	1.1 gm per day (6 gm vial for inhalation $1700)	**Ribavirin side-effects:** Anemia, rash, conjunctivitis. Read package insert. Avoid procedures that lead to drug precipitation in ventilator tubing with subsequent dysfunction. Significant teratogenicity in animals. **Contraindicated in pregnant women and partners.** Pregnant health care workers should avoid direct care of pts receiving aerosolized ribavirin.
RSV-IV Immunoglobulin (IG) (RespiGam)	100 mg per kg IV q month (50 mL $1–87)	RespiGam side-effects rare but include fatal anaphylaxis, pruritus, rash, wheezing, fever, joint pain.
Warts (See *CID* 28:S37, 1999)		
Interferon alfa-2b or alfa-n3	Apply 1 million units into lesion	Interferon alfa-2b 3 million units per 0.5 mL, interferon alfa-n3 5 million units per 1 mL. Cost $10
Podofilox (Condylox)	3.5 mL for topical application: $130	**Side-effects:** Local reactions—pain, burning, inflammation in 50%. No systemic effects.
Imiquimod (Aldara)	Cream applied 3 times per week to maximum of 16 wks. 250 mg packets $16	Mild erythema, erosions, itching and burning

* See page 2 for abbreviations. NOTE: All dosage recommendations are for adults (unless otherwise indicated) and assume normal renal function. Costs from 2006 Drug Topics Red Book, Medical Economics. Price is average wholesale price (AWP).

Table 14C – ESTIMATED IN VIVO ACTIVITY OF ANTIVIRAL AGENTS AGAINST TREATABLE PATHOGENIC VIRUSES

Virus	ANTIVIRAL AGENT													
	Acyclovir	Amantadine	Adefovir Entecavir Lamivudine	Cidofovir	Famciclovir	Foscarnet	Ganciclovir	αInterferon Or PEG INF	Oseltamivir	Ribavirin	Rimantidine	Valacyclovir	Valganciclovir	Zanamivir
Adenovirus	·	·	·	+	·	·	±	·	·	·	·	·	±	·
BK virus	·	·	·	+	·	·	·	·	·	·	·	·	·	·
Cytomegalovirus	±	·	·	+++	±	+++	+++	·	·	·	·	±	+++	·
Hepatitis B	·	·	+++	·	·	·	·	+++	·	±	·	·	·	·
Hepatitis C	·	·	·	·	·	·	·	+++*	·	+++*	·	·	·	·
Herpes simplex virus	+++	·	·	++	+++	++	++	·	·	·	·	+++	·	·
Influenza A Influenza B	·	±**	·	·	·	·	·	·	+++	·	±**	·	·	+++
Respiratory Syncytial Virus	·	·	·	·	·	·	·	·	·	+	·	·	·	·
Varicella-zoster virus	++	·	·	+	++	++	+	·	·	·	·	++	+	·

* 1st line rx = an IFN + Ribavirin   ** not CDC recommended

- = no activity; ± = possible activity; + = active, 3rd line therapy (least active clinically)
++ = Active, 2nd line therapy (less active clinically); +++ = Active, 1st line therapy (usually active clinically)

TABLE 14D – ANTIRETROVIRAL THERAPY IN TREATMENT-NAIVE ADULTS

(See the 2006 SANFORD GUIDE TO HIV/AIDS THERAPY, Table 6, for additional information regarding treatment and complications of antiretroviral agents)

In 2006, guidelines and recommendations for the treatment of individuals infected with HIV-1 were updated. DHHS guidelines for treatment of infected adults and adolescents and recommendations for ART in pregnant women, guidelines for the use of antiretroviral therapy (ARV) in pediatrics were updated in late 2005 (all documents are available online at www.aidsinfo.nih.gov. New treatment recommendations by the International AIDS Society–USA Panel were also published (*JAMA* 296:827, 2006). Since the previous edition of this guide, a new formulation and protease inhibitor were approved in the US by FDA. Whenever starting antiretroviral therapy, **resistance testing** should be performed to help guide choice of agents Note that **immune reconstitution syndromes** may result from initiation of antiretroviral therapy, and may require medical intervention. For additional explanation and other acceptable alternatives relating to these tables, see www.aidsinfo.nih.gov.

A. When to start therapy? (www.aidsinfo.nih.gov)

HIV Symptoms	CD4 cells per mcL	Start Treatment	Comment
Yes	Any	Yes	
No	<200	Yes	
No	200–350	Offer (see Comment)	Risk for progression to AIDS also depends on viral load; consider on individual basis
No	>350	No (see Comment)	Maybe if CD4 decreasing rapidly and/or viral load >100,000 copies per mL

• **Acute retroviral syndrome**—See page 152, section C

B. Suggested Initial Therapy Regimens for Untreated Chronic HIV Infection *(For pregnancy, see below and Table 6 of the Sanford Guide to HIV/AIDS Therapy, 2006)*

Regimen	Pill strength (mg)	Usual Daily Regimen (oral)	No. pills per day	Cost/month (Avg. Wholesale Price)	Comment (See also Individual agents)
1. Preferred Regimens					
a. (Tenofovir + Emtricitabine)+ Efavirenz	(300) + (200) + 600	(Combination—Truvada 1 tab q24h) + 1 tab q24h at bedtime, empty stomach.	2	$1207	Good efficacy; low pill burden. The three drugs are available in a single pill as Atripla (see information for individual agents). Tenofovir: reports of renal toxicity (*CID* 42:283, 2006). Avoid efavirenz in pregnancy or in women who might become pregnant (**Pregnancy Category D**).
OR					
(Emtricitabine/tenofovir/efavirenz	(300+200+ 600)	(Combination—Atripla 1 tab q24h) at bedtime, empty stomach.	1	$1222	48-week analysis of ongoing trial reported superior viral suppression, CD4 ↑, and AEs of emtricitabine/tenofovir/efavirenz over 3TC/ZDV/efavirenz in rx-naive pts (*NEJM* 354:251, 2006)
b. (Zidovudine + Lamivudine)+ Efavirenz	(300) + (150) + 600	(Combination—Combivir 1 tab bid) + 1 tab q24h at bedtime, empty stomach	3	$1198	Good efficacy; low pill burden; low AE profile. **If rx stopped, do efavirenz 1–2 wks before NRTIs** (for explanation, see page 154). Avoid efavirenz in pregnancy or in women who might become pregnant (**Pregnancy Category D**). Food may ↑ serum efavirenz concentration, which can lead to ↑ adverse events.
c. (Zidovudine + Lamivudine) + Lopinavir/Ritonavir	(300) + (150) + 200/50	2 tabs bid without regard to food (Combination—Combivir 1 tab bid)	6	$1483	Good wirlogic efficacy and durable effect. Tolerable AEs. Alternative regimen: lopinavir/ritonavir can be given as 4 tabs once daily in combinations for rx-naive pts
d. (Zidovudine + Lamivudine) + Atazanavir + Ritonavir	(300) + (150) + 300 + 100	1 cap q24h + (Combination—Combivir 1 tab bid)	4	$1765	Lower potential for lipid derangement by (unboosted) atazanavir than w/other PIs. May ↑ PR interval & bilirubin. Acid-lowering agents can markedly ↓ absorption, avoid with PPIs & give 2hr before or 10h after H2-blockers. Alternative regimen: atazanavir (400 mg q24h with food without ritonavir) can be given in combo for rx-naive pts.
e. (Zidovudine + Lamivudine) + Fosamprenavir + Ritonavir	(300) + (150) + 100	1 cap q24h, both with food (Combination—Combivir 1 tab bid) + 1 tab bid fed or fasting + 1 tab bid fed or fasting +	6	$2021	Can take with food without ritonavir. GI symptoms. Contains sulfa moiety. Alternative regimens: once-daily fosamprenavir/ritonavir or fosamprenavir without ritonavir can be used in combinations for rx-naive pts (see label for doses)

TABLE 14D (2)

Regimen	Dosage	Directions	No.	Cost	Comments
2. Alternative Regimens (for additional alternatives, see Comments sections above and www.aidsinfo.nih.gov)					
a. Didanosine EC + Lamivudine + Efavirenz	400 + 300 + 600	1 cap q24h at bedtime, fasting + 1 tab q24h + 1 tab q24h at bedtime, empty stomach. **Didanosine dosage shown for ≥60 kg.**	3	$1159	Low pill burden. Efficacy & durability under study. Potential didanosine AEs (pancreatitis, peripheral neuritis). Avoid efavirenz in pregnancy or in women who might become pregnant (**Pregnancy Category D**). Food may ↑ serum efavirenz concentration, which can lead to ↑ adverse events. Can substitute emtricitabine 200 mg po q24h for lamivudine 300 mg po q24h.
b. (Abacavir + Lamivudine) + Efavirenz	(600 + 300) + 600	(**Combination—Epzicom** 1 tab q24h without regard to food) + 1 tab q24h at bedtime, empty stomach	2	$1256	Low pill burden. **However, note risk of abacavir hypersensitivity reaction.** Avoid efavirenz in pregnancy or in women who might become pregnant (**Pregnancy Category D**). Food may ↑ serum efavirenz concentration, which can lead to ↑ adverse events.
3. Triple nucleoside or nucleoside/nucleotide regimen: Due to inferior virologic activity, use only when preferred or alternative regimen not possible.					
a. (Zidovudine + Lamivudine) + Abacavir	(300 + 150) + 300	(**Combination—Trizivir** 1 tab bid)	2	$1219	Reduced efficacy as compared to preferred & alternative regimens. Potentially serious **abacavir hypersensitivity reaction** (See comments for individual agents)
4. During pregnancy. Expert consultation mandatory. Timing of rx initiation & drug choice must be individualized. Viral resistance testing should be strongly considered. Longterm effects of agents unknown. Certain drugs hazardous or contraindicated (see SANFORD GUIDE TO HIV/AIDS THERAPY, Table 17). See www.aidsinfo.nih.gov for additional information & alternative rx options, and (see SANFORD GUIDE TO HIV/AIDS THERAPY, Table 8A) for regimens to prevent mother-child transmission.					
a. (Zidovudine + Lamivudine) + Nevirapine	(300 + 150) + 200	(**Combination—Combivir** 1 tab bid) + 1 tab bid fed or fasting [after 14-day lead-in period of 1 tab q24h]	4	$1160	See nevirapine Black Box warnings (page 155)—among others, ↑ risk of **potentially fatal hepatotoxicity** in women with CD4 >250. Avoid in this group unless benefits clearly > risks; monitor intensively if drug must be used.
b. (Zidovudine + Lamivudine)+ Nelfinavir	(300 + 150) + 625	(**Combination—Combivir** 1 tab bid) + 2 tabs bid, with food	6	$445	Nelfinavir-assoc diarrhea in 20%. Nelfinavir contraindicated w/ drugs highly dependent on CYP3A4 elimination where ↑ levels may cause life-threatening toxicity. Time to loss of virological response shorter than that of lopinavir/ritonavir. (NEJM 346:2039, 2002).
c. (Zidovudine + Lamivudine) + Lopinavir/Ritonavir	(300 + 150) + 200/50	(**Combination—Combivir** 1 tab bid) + 2 tabs bid without regard to food	6	$483	Optimum dose in 3rd trimester unknown. May need TDM as ↑ dose of Lop/Rit may be required. For Lopinavir/Ritonavir once daily dosing not recommended.
Alternative regimen (DHHS 2006)					
a. (Zidovudine + Lamivudine) + Saquinavir + Ritonavir	(300 + 150) + 500 + 100	(**Combination—Combivir** 1 tab bid) + 2 tabs bid + 1 cap bid (both within 2 h after a meal)	8	$2060	Use saquinavir tabs only in combination with ritonavir. Certain drugs metabolized by CYP3A4 are contraindicated with saquinavir/ritonavir. (DHHS recommendations based on www.aidsinfo.nih.gov). Saquinavir softgel caps, which are no longer available, plus ritonavir.
C. Suggested Regimen for Acute Primary HIV Infection (see Comment)					
(Zidovudine + Lamivudine) + Efavirenz	(300 + 150) + 600	(**Combination—Combivir** 1 tab bid) + 1 tab q24h at bedtime, empty stomach. Food may ↑ serum efavirenz concentration, which can lead to ↑ adverse events.	3	$1198	Benefits of rx acute HIV infection uncertain; treatment is considered optional, and best undertaken in research setting. Perform resistance testing. Optimal duration of rx unknown. (See www.aidsinfo.nih.gov). Avoid efavirenz in pregnancy or in women who might become pregnant (**Pregnancy Category D**).
D. Some Antiretroviral Therapies Should NOT Be Offered, see 2006 SANFORD GUIDE TO HIV/AIDS THERAPY, Table 6, for details					

TABLE 14D (3)

E. Selected Characteristics of Antiretroviral Drugs
1. Selected Characteristics of Nucleoside or Nucleotide Reverse Transcriptase Inhibitors (NRTIs)
   All agents have Black Box warning: Risk of lactic acidosis/hepatic steatosis. Also, labels note risk of fat redistribution/accumulation with ARV rx. For combos, see comments for component agents.

Generic/Trade Name	Pharmaceutical Prep. (Avg. Wholesale Price)	Usual Adult Dosage & Food Effect	Absorbed, %, po	Serum T½, hrs	Intracellular T½, hrs	Elimination	Major Adverse Events/Comments (See Table 14E)
Abacavir (ABC, Ziagen)	300mg tabs or 20mg per mL oral solution ($466 per month)	300 mg po bid or 600 mg po q24h. Food OK	83	1.5	20	Liver metab/renal excretion of metabolites 82%. Alcohol ↑ AUC.	**Hypersensitivity reaction:** fever, rash, N/V, malaise, diarrhea, abdominal pain, respiratory symptoms. (Severe reactions may be ↑ with 600 mg dose). **Do not rechallenge!** Report to 800-270-0425.
Abacavir/ lamivudine/ zidovudine (Trizivir)	Film-coated tabs: ABC 300mg + 3TC 150mg + ZDV 300mg ($1219 per month)	1 tab po bid (not recommended for wt <40 kg or CrCl <50 mL per min or impaired hepatic function)	(See individual components)			(See Comments for individual components) **Note: Black Box warnings** for ABC hypersensitivity reaction & others. Should only be used for regimens intended to include these 3 agents. **Black Box warning**—limited data for VL >100,000 copies per mL	
Didanosine (ddI; Videx, Videx EC) (Ru EC) ↓ Concomitant: Potential ↑ toxicity & ↓ efficacy if used with tenofovir (see AIDS Reader 15:403, 2005)	125, 200, 250, 400 enteric-coated caps 100, 167, 250, 375 per packet for oral solution; ($332 per month Videx EC) ($1122 per month). (Tablets discontinued in US in 2006)	≥60 kg: Usually 400 mg enteric-coated po q24h. 1 hr before or 2 hrs after meal. **Do not crush.** <60 kg: 250 mg EC po q24h. Food ↓ levels See Comment	30–40	1.6	25–40	Renal excretion. 50%	**Pancreatitis,** peripheral neuropathy, diarrhea, lactic acidosis & hepatic steatosis (rare but life-threatening, esp. combined with stavudine in pregnancy). Retinal, optic nerve changes reported. **If ddI + TDF is used, ↓dose from 400 mg to 250 mg EC q24h for ≥60 kg; for <60 kg, use 200 mg EC for adults (<60 kg). This combination is generally avoided but, if needed, monitor for ↑ toxicity & possible ↓ efficacy; combination may result in ↓CD4.**
Emtricitabine (FTC, Emtriva)	200mg caps; 10mg per mL solution ($306 per month)	200 mg po q24h. Food OK	93	Approx. 10	39	Renal excretion 86%, minor biotransformation; 14% excretion in feces	Well tolerated: headache, nausea, vomiting & diarrhea occasionally, skin rash rare. Skin hyperpigmentation. Differs only slightly in structure from lamivudine (5-fluoro substitution). **Exacerbation of Hep B reported after stopping FTC**
Emtricitabine/ tenofovir disoproxil fumarate (Truvada)	Film-coated tabs: FTC 200mg + TDF 300mg ($799 per month)	1 tab po q24h for CrCl ≥50 mL per min. Food OK	92/25	10/17	—	Primarily renal/renal	See Comments for individual agents Black Box warning—not indicated for rx of Hep B. Exacerbation after stopping.
Emtricitabine/ tenofovir/ efavirenz (Atripla)	Film-coated tabs: FTC 200 mg + TDF 300 mg + efavirenz 600 mg ($1279 per month)	1 tab po q24h on an empty stomach, preferably at bedtime. Do not use if CrCl <50 mL/min	(See individual components)				See Comments for individual components **Exacerbation of hepB** reported for individual components; not indicated for rx of hepB. **Pregnancy Category D**—may cause fetal harm. Avoid in preg. in women who might become preg.)
Lamivudine (3TC; Epivir)	150, 300 mg tabs; 10 mg per mL oral solution ($347 per month)	150 mg po bid or 300 mg po q24h. Food OK	86	5–7	18	Renal excretion, minimal metabolism	**Use HIV dose, not Hep B dose.** Usually well-tolerated. **Risk of exacerbation of Hep B after stopping 3TC**
Lamivudine/ abacavir (Epzicom)	Film-coated tabs: 3TC 300 mg + abacavir 600 mg ($777 per month)	1 tab po q24h. Food OK. Not recommended for CrCl <50 mL per min or impaired hepatic function	86/86	5–7/1.5	—	Primarily renal/ metabolism	See Comments for individual agents. Note abacavir **hypersensitivity Black Box warnings** (severe reactions may be more frequent with 600mg dose).

TABLE 14D (4)

E. Selected Characteristics of Antiretroviral Drugs/1.

Generic/Trade Name	Pharmaceutical Prep. (Avg. Wholesale Price)	Usual Adult Dosage & Food Effect	Absorbed, % po	Serum T½, hrs	Intracellular T½, hrs	Elimination	Major Adverse Events/Comments (See Table 14E)
		Selected Characteristics of Nucleoside or Nucleotide Reverse Transcriptase Inhibitors (NRTIs) (continued)					
Lamivudine/zidovudine (Combivir)	Film-coated tabs: 3TC 150 mg + ZDV 300 mg ($719 per month)	1 tab bid. Not rec: for ClCr <50 mL per min or impaired hepatic function. Food OK	86/64	5–7/0.5–3		Primarily renal/ metabolism with renal excretion of glucuronide	See Comments for individual agents. See Black Box warning—exacerbation of Hep B in pts stopping 3TC
Stavudine (d4T; Zerit)	15, 20, 30, 40 mg capsules; 1 mg per mL oral solution ($370/mo 40 mg caps)	≥60 kg: 40 mg po bid; <60 kg: 30 mg po bid. Food OK.	86	1.2–1.6	3.5	Renal excretion, 40%	**Highest incidence of lactic acidosis of all NRTIs** (See Comments for individual agents.) Pancreatitis. Peripheral neuropathy. High incidence of lipoatrophy, hyperlipidemia.
Tenofovir disoproxil fumarate (TDF; Viread)—a nucleotide **Black Box warning**—Not indicated for treatment of Hep B; exacerbations of Hep B reported after stopping tenofovir.	300 mg tabs ($500 per month)	ClCr ≥50 mL, per min: 300 mg po q24h. Food OK; high-fat meal ↑ absorption	39 (with food); 25 (fasted)	17	>60	Renal excretion 70–80%	Headache, N/V. Cases of renal dysfunction reported: avoid concomitant nephrotoxic agents. Must adjust dose of ddI (↓) if used concomitantly (see ddI Comments box). Atazanavir & lopinavir/ritonavir ↑ tenofovir concentrations: monitor for adverse effects.
Zalcitabine (ddC; Hivid)	0.375, 0.75 tabs (To be discontinued by end of 2006)	0.75 mg po q8h. Food OK	85	2	3	Renal excretion, 70%	**Peripheral neuropathy:** stomatitis, rarely life-threatening lactic acidosis, pancreatitis
Zidovudine (ZDV, AZT; Retrovir)	100 mg caps, 300 mg tabs; 10 mg per mL IV solution, 10 mg per mL oral syrup ($387 per month)	300 mg po q12h. Food OK	60	1.1	11	Metabolized to glucuronide & excreted in urine	**Bone marrow suppression.** GI intolerance, headache, insomnia, malaise, myopathy

2. Selected Characteristics of Non-Nucleoside Reverse Transcriptase Inhibitors (NNRTIs)

Generic/Trade Name	Pharmaceutical Prep. (Avg. Wholesale Price)	Usual Adult Dosage & Food Effect	Absorbed, % po	Serum T½, hrs	Elimination	Major Adverse Events/Comments (See Table 14E)
Delavirdine (Rescriptor)	100, 200 mg tabs ($316 per month)	400 mg po q8h. Food OK	85	5.8	Cytochrome P450 (3A inhibition), 51% excreted in urine (<5% unchanged), 44% in feces	Rash severe enough to stop drug in 4.3%. ↑ AST/ALT, headaches. Not recommended.
Efavirenz (Sustiva) **Pregnancy Category D—may cause fetal harm**—avoid in preg women or those who might become preg (Note: No single method of contraception is 100% reliable)	50, 100, 200 mg capsules; 600 mg tablet ($479 per month)	600 mg po q24h at bedtime, without food. Food may ↑ serum conc., which can lead to ↑ in risk of adverse events.	42	40–55 See Comment	Cytochrome P450 (3A mixed inducer/inhibitor), 14–34% of dose excreted in urine as glucuronidated metabolites, 16–61% in feces	Rash severe enough to d/c use of drug in 1.7%. High frequency of diverse CNS AEs: somnolence, dreams, confusion, agitation. Serious psychiatric symptoms. False-pos. cannabinoid screen. Very long T½: if efavirenz to be discontinued, stop efavirenz ~2 wks before stopping companion drugs. Otherwise, risk of developing efavirenz resistance, as after 1–2 days only efavirenz in blood and/or tissue. Some authorities add a PI to NRTI backbone to bridge this period after efavirenz is discontinued (CID 42:401, 2006).

TABLE 14D (5)

(See Table 14E)

Generic/Trade Name	Pharmaceutical Prep. (Avg. Wholesale Price)	Usual Adult Dosage & Food Effect	Absorbed, %, po	Serum T½, hrs	Elimination	Major Adverse Events/Comments (See Table 14E)
E. Selected Characteristics of Antiretroviral Drugs / 2. Selected Characteristics of Non-Nucleoside Reverse Transcriptase Inhibitors (NNRTIs) *(continued)*						
Nevirapine (Viramune) **Black Box warning —** fatal **hepatotoxicity**, esp. vulnerable, Women with CD4 >250 including preg women. Avoid in this group unless benefits clearly > risks (see www.fda.gov/cder/drug/advisory/nevirapine.htm)	200 mg tabs: 50 mg per 5 mL oral suspension ($442 per month)	200 mg po q24h for 14 days then 200 mg po bid (see Comments & Black Box warning) Food OK	>90	25–30	Cytochrome P450 (3A4, 2B6) inducer 80% of dose excreted in urine as glucuronidated metabolites, 10% in feces	If used, intensive monitoring advised. Men with CD4 >400 also at ↑ risk. Rash severe enough to stop drug in 7%, **severe or life-threatening skin reactions** in 2%. Do not restart if any suspicion of such reactions. 2-week dose escalation period may ↓ skin reactions. As with efavirenz, in because of long T½, consider continuing companion agents for several days if nevirapine is discontinued.
3. Selected Characteristics of Protease Inhibitors (PIs).						
All PIs: Glucose metabolism: new diabetes mellitus or deterioration of glucose control; hyperlipidemia; hypertriglyceridemia or hypercholesterolemia. Exercise caution re: potential drug interactions. QTc prolongation has been seen in a few pts taking PIs; some PIs can cause hemophilia bleeding; fat redistribution; possible hemophilia bleeding. Some PIs can block HERG channels in vitro (*Lancet 365:682, 2005*).						
Atazanavir (Reyataz)	100, 150, 200, 300 mg capsules ($857 per month)	400mg po q24h with food (exception is atazanavir 300mg po q24h + ritonavir 100mg po q24h in combo with efavirenz 600mg po q24h) or TDF 300mg po q24h). Take with food 2hrs pre or 1hr post buffered ddI. Ritonavir-boosted dose also rec for ARV-tx-experienced pts.	Good oral bioavailability, food enhances bioavailability & pharmacokinetic variability. Absorption ↓ by antacids, H₂-blockers, proton pump inhibitors.	Approx. 7	Cytochrome P450 (3A4, 1A2 & 2C9 inhibitor); UGT1A1 inhibitor, 13% excreted in urine (7% unchanged), 79% excreted in feces (20% unchanged)	No ↑ lipids in available studies. Asymptomatic unconjugated hyperbilirubinemia common, especially likely in Gilbert syndrome (*IJID 192:1381, 2005*). Headache in 1% for nucleoside reverse transcription system disease or with drugs that ↑ block. **Prolongation of PR interval** / rare cases of **2° or 3° (1st degree AV block) block.** Caution in pre-existing conduction system disease or with drugs that ↑ block. **Efavirenz & tenofovir** ↓ **atazanavir exposure: use atazanavir/ritonavir regimen; also, atazanavir** ↑ **tenofovir concentrations—watch for adverse events.**
Darunavir (Prezista)	300 mg tablet ($731 per month)	600 mg darunavir (2 tabs) + 100 mg ritonavir) po bid, with food	82% absorbed (taken with ritonavir)	Approx. 15 hr (with ritonavir)	Metabolized by CYP3A and is a CYP 3A inhibitor	Contains sulfa moiety. Rash, nausea, headaches seen. Co-admin of certain drugs cleared by CYP3A is contraind (see label). Use with caution in pts with hepatic dysfunction. May cause hormonal contraception failure.
Fosamprenavir (Lexiva)	700 mg tablet ($659 per month if with ritonavir)	1400mg (two 700 mg tabs) po bid OR 1400mg [1400mg fosamprenavir (2 tabs)] + ritonavir 200mg] po q24h OR [700mg fosamprenavir (1 tab) + ritonavir 100mg] po bid	Bioavailability not established. Food OK	7.7	Hydrolyzed to amprenavir, then Cytochrome P450 (3A4 substrate, inhibitor, inducer)	Amprenavir prodrug. *(See amprenavir adverse events, **Table 14E**.)* (2) Potential for serious drug interactions. Rash, including Stevens-Johnson syndrome. Once-daily regimen (1) not recommended for PI-experienced pts, (2) additional ritonavir needed if given with efavirenz (see label). Boosted twice-daily regimen is recommended for PI-experienced pts.
Indinavir (Crixivan)	100, 200, 333, 400 mg capsules ($385 per month if with ritonavir) Store in original container with desiccant	Two 400mg caps (800mg) po q8h w/o food or w/ light meal. Can take with water or skim milk; e.g. Videx. [If taken w/ ritonavir (e.g. 800mg ritonavir + 100mg ritonavir po bid, no food restrict)]	65	1.2–2	Cytochrome P450 (3A4 inhibitor)	Maintain hydration. **Nephrolithiasis**, nausea, inconsequential ↑ of indirect bilirubin, ↑ AST/ALT, headache, asthenia, blurred vision, metallic taste, hemolysis, ↑ urine WBC >100 per mm³ in up to 30% with assoc. nephritis/medullary calcification, cortical atrophy.

TABLE 14D (6)

Generic/Trade Name	Pharmaceutical Prep. (Avg. Wholesale Price)	Usual Adult Dosage & Food Effect	Absorbed, %, po	Serum T½, hrs	Elimination	Major Adverse Events/Comments (See Table 14E)
E. Selected Characteristics of Antiretroviral Drugs [3. Selected Characteristics of Protease Inhibitors (PIs) *(continued)*]						
Lopinavir + ritonavir (Kaletra)	200 mg lopinavir + 50 mg ritonavir tablets. Tabs do not need refrigeration. Oral solution: (80 mg lopinavir + 20 mg ritonavir) per mL. ($764 per month)	Two tabs (400mg lopinavir + 100mg ritonavir)—po bid. ↑ dose may be needed in non-rx-naive pts when used w/ efavirenz, nevirapine, amprenavir (or unboosted fosamprenavir (tabs)). *(See Table 22B & C & label for specific agents)*	No food effect with tablets. *(Previous capsule formulation required food.)*	5–6	Cytochrome P450 (3A4 inhibitor)	Nausea, vomiting, diarrhea, ↑ AST/ ALT, pancreatitis. Oral solution 42% alcohol. Lopinavir + ritonavir can be taken as single daily dose of 4 tabs (total 800 mg lopinavir + 200 mg ritonavir), except in rx-experienced pts or those taking concomitant efavirenz, nevirapine, amprenavir, or nelfinavir.
Nelfinavir (Viracept)	625, 250 mg tabs: 50 mg per gm oral powder ($726 per month)	Two, 625 mg tabs (1250 mg) po bid, with food	20–80 Food ↑ exposure & ↓ variability	3.5–5	Cytochrome P450 3A4	Diarrhea. Coadministration of drugs with life-threatening toxicities & which are cleared by CYP34A is contraindicated.
Ritonavir (Norvir)	100 mg capsules. 600 mg per 7.5 mL solution. Refrigerate caps but not solution. Room temperature times 1 mo. ($10.72 per capsule)	Full dose (**not recommended**): 6 caps (600mg) po bid, with food. Escalate to full dose: 300mg bid times 2 days; 400mg bid times 3 days; 500mg bid times 7 days; then full dose. *(See Comment)*	Food ↑ absorption	3–5	Cytochrome P450 Potent 3A4 & 2D6 inhibitor	**With rare exceptions, used only to enhance pharmacokinetics of other PIs, using lower ritonavir doses.** Nausea/vomiting/diarrhea, extremity & circumoral paresthesias; hepatitis, pancreatitis, taste perversion, ↑CPK & uric acid. **Black Box warning**—potentially fatal drug interactions—see Table 22A. *Table 22C, pg 184–191*
Saquinavir (Invirase—hard gel caps or tabs) + ritonavir	200 mg caps, 500 mg film-coated tabs. ($719 per month)	(5 caps saquinavir (1000 mg) + 1 cap ritonavir (100 mg)) po bid with food OR (2 tabs saquinavir (1000 mg)) + 1 cap ritonavir (100 mg) po bid with food	Erratic, 4 (saquinavir alone)	1–2	Cytochrome P450 (3A4 inhibitor)	Nausea, diarrhea, headache. ↑ AST/ALT. Avoid rifampin with saquinavir + ritonavir: ↑ hepatitis risk (www.fda.gov/cder/drug/new.html, accessed 2/26/05). **Black Box warning**—Invirase to be used only with ritonavir
Tipranavir (Aptivus) For rx-experienced pts or PI-resistant strains	250 mg capsules. Refrigerate unopened bottles. Use opened bottles within 2 months. ($1073 per month)	(500 mg (two 250 mg caps) + ritonavir 200 mg) po bid, with food	Absorption low, but with ritonavir most of drug is eliminated in feces. ↑ with high fat meal. ↓ with Al+++ & Mg++ antacids	5.5–6	Cytochrome 3A4, but with ritonavir most of drug is eliminated in feces	Contains sulfa moiety. **Black Box warning—reports of fatal & nonfatal intracranial hemorrhage, hepatitis, fatal & nonfatal hepatic failure.** Use cautiously in pts with liver disease, esp. Hep B or C; contraindicated in Child-Pugh class B-C. Monitor LFTs. Coadministration of certain drugs contraindicated (see *Drug-Drug Interactions, Table 22*)
4. Selected Characteristics of Fusion Inhibitors						
Enfuvirtide (T20, Fuzeon)	Single-use vials of 90 mg per mL when reconstituted. Vials should be stored at room temperature. Reconstituted vials can be refrigerated for 24 hrs only. ($2223 per month)	90 mg (1 mL) subcut. bid. Rotate injection sites, avoiding those currently inflamed.	84	3.8	Catabolism to its constituent amino acids with subsequent recycling of amino acids in the body pool. Elim pathway(s) have not been performed in humans. Does not inhibit CYP3A4, CYP2D6, CYP1A2, CYP2C19 or CYP2E1 substrates.	Local injection site reactions 98%; 4% discontinue. Erythema/induration reports—~80%. HYpersensitivity reactions reported (fever, rash, chills, N/V ↑BP &/or ↑ALT/AST)—do not restart if it occurs. Incl background regimens: peripheral neuropathy 8.9%, insomnia 11.3%, ↓ appetite 6.3%, myalgia 5%, lymphadenopathy 2.3%, eosinophilia ~10%, ↑ incidence of bacterial pneumonia. Adverse effects offers little benefit to a failing regimen (*NEJM* 348:2249, 2003).

TABLE 14E– ANTIRETROVIRAL DRUGS AND ADVERSE EFFECTS
(www.aidsinfo.nih.gov— May 2006)

ADVERSE EFFECTS

DRUG NAME(S): GENERIC (TRADE)	ADVERSE EFFECTS
Nucleoside Reverse Transcriptase Inhibitors (NRTI) [Black Box warning for all nucleoside/nucleotide RTIs: lactic acidosis/hepatic steatosis, potentially fatal. Also carry Warnings that fat redistribution has been observed]	
Abacavir (Ziagen)	**Most common:** Headache 7-13%, nausea 7-19%, diarrhea 7%, malaise 7-12% **Most significant: Black Box warning—Hypersensitivity reaction** in 8% with malaise, fever, GI upset, rash, lethargy, & respiratory symptoms most commonly reported; myalgia, arthralgia, edema, paresthesia less commonly reported. Appears to be assoc with presence of HLA-B*5701 allele (CID 43:99, 2006). Severe hypersensitivity reaction may be more common with once-daily dosing. **Rechallenge contraindicated; may be life-threatening.**
Didanosine (ddl) (Videx)	**Most common:** Diarrhea 28%, nausea 6%, rash 9%, headache 7%, fever 12%, hyperuricemia 2% **Most significant: Pancreatitis 1-9%. Black Box warning—Cases of fatal and nonfatal pancreatitis** have occurred in pts receiving ddl, especially when used in combination with d4T or d4T + hydroxyurea. Fatal lactic acidosis in pregnancy with ddl + d4T Peripheral neuropathy in 20%, 12% required dose reduction. Rarely, retinal changes
Emtricitabine (FTC, Emtriva)	**Most common:** Headache, diarrhea, nausea, rash, skin hyperpigmentation **Most significant:** Anti-HBV rx may be warranted if FTC stopped. **exacerbation of hepatitis B on stopping drug; monitor clinical/labs for several months after stopping.**
Lamivudine (3TC) (Epivir)	Well tolerated. Headache 35%, nausea 33%, diarrhea 18%, abdominal pain 9%, insomnia 11% (all in combination with ZDV). Pancreatitis more common in pediatrics (15%). **Black Box warning: Lactic acidosis and hepatic steatosis in pregnant women receiving d4T + ddl. Fatal lactic acidosis/labs for several months after stopping.** Anti-HBV rx may be warranted. Make sure to use HIV dosage, not Hep B dosage. **exacerbation of hepatitis B on stopping drug; monitor clinical/labs for several months after stopping.** HBC rx may be warranted if 3TC stopped
Stavudine (d4T) (Zerit)	**Most common:** Diarrhea, nausea, vomiting, headache **Most significant: Peripheral neuropathy** 15-20%. Pancreatitis 1%. Appears to produce lactic acidosis more commonly than other NRTIs. **Black Box warning—Fatal & nonfatal pancreatitis with d4T + ddl ± hydroxyurea. Fatal lactic acidosis in pregnant women receiving d4T + ddl.** Motor weakness in the setting of lactic acidosis (rare) mimicking the clinical presentation of Guillain-Barré syndrome (including respiratory failure) (rare).
Zalcitabine (ddC) (Hivid)	**Most common:** Oral ulcers 3%, rash 3% Nausea 50%, anorexia 20%, vomiting 17%, **headache 62%.** Also reported: asthenia, insomnia, myalgias, fever. **Peripheral neuropathy** <1%. Severe continuous pain, slowly reversible when ddC is discontinued, ↑ risk with diabetes mellitus. **Black Box warning—Pancreatitis** <1% and **Hepatic failure in pts with Hep B.**
Zidovudine (ZDV, AZT) (Retrovir)	**Most common:** Nausea 50%, anorexia 20%, vomiting 17%, **headache 62%.** Also reported: asthenia, insomnia, myalgias, fever. Macrocytosis expected with all dosage regimens. **Most significant: Black Box warning—hematologic toxicity, myopathy, Anemia** (<8 gm, 1%), **granulocytopenia** (<750, 1.8%). Anemia may respond to epoetin alfa if endogenous serum erythropoietin levels are <500 milli-International Units per ml.
Nucleotide Reverse Transcriptase Inhibitor (NRTI) [Black Box warning for all nucleoside/nucleotide RTIs: lactic acidosis/hepatic steatosis, potentially fatal. Also carry Warnings that fat redistribution has been observed]	
Tenofovir (TDF) (Viread)	**Most common:** Diarrhea 11%, nausea 8%, vomiting 5% (generally well tolerated) **Most significant: Black Box Warning—Severe exacerbations of hepatitis B reported in pts who stop tenofovir.** Not indicated to treat Hep B. Monitor carefully if drug is stopped, and HBV rx may be warranted if TDF stopped. Possible ↑ bone demineralization. Reports of Fanconi syndrome & renal injury induced by tenofovir (CID 37:e174, 2003; JAIDS 35:269, 2004). Modest decline in Ccr with TDF may be greater than with NRTIs (CID 40:1194, 2005)
Non-Nucleoside Reverse Transcriptase Inhibitors (NNRTI)	
Delavirdine (Rescriptor)	**Most common:** Nausea, diarrhea, vomiting, headache **Most significant: Skin rash** has occurred in 18%, can continue or restart during therapy in most cases. Stevens-Johnson syndrome and erythema multiforme have been reported rarely. ↑ in liver enzymes **pregnancy category D—may cause fetal harm**, avoid in pregnant women or those who might become pregnant (see 2006 SANFORD GUIDE TO HIV/AIDS THERAPY, Table 8).
Efavirenz (Sustiva)	**Most common: CNS side-effects 52%;** symptoms include dizziness, insomnia, somnolence, impaired concentration, psychiatric sx, and abnormal dreams, symptoms are worse after 1st or 2nd dose and improve over 2-4 weeks; discontinuation rate 2.6%. Rash 26%, improves with oral antihistamines; discontinuation rate 1.7%. Can cause false-positive urine test results for cannabinoid with CEDIA DAU multi-level THC assay. **Most significant:** Serious neuropsychiatric symptoms, including severe depression, ↑ suicidal ideation 0.7%. Elevation in liver enzymes. **Teratogenicity reported in primates.** **pregnancy category D—may cause fetal harm,** avoid in pregnant women or those who might become pregnant (see 2006 SANFORD GUIDE TO HIV/AIDS THERAPY, Table 8). NOTE: No single method of contraception is 100% reliable. Contraindicated with certain drugs metabolized by CYP3A4

TABLE 14E (2)

DRUG NAME(S): GENERIC (TRADE)	ADVERSE EFFECTS (continued)
Non-Nucleoside Reverse Transcriptase Inhibitors (NNRTI)	
Nevirapine (Viramune)	**Most significant: Rash 37%:** occurs during 1st 6 wks of therapy. Follow recommendations for 14-day lead-in period to ↓ risk of rash (see *Table 14D*). Women experience 7-fold ↑ in risk of severe rash (*CID* 32:124, 2001). 50% resolve with 2wks of dc drug and 80% by 1mo. 6.7% discontinuation rate. **Black Box warning—Severe life-threatening skin reactions reported:** Stevens-Johnson syndrome, toxic epidermal necrolysis, & hypersensitivity reaction 7-fold ↑ in severe rash with nevirapine & systemic symptoms (*AnIM* 133:192, 2001). **Black Box warning—Severe life-threatening hepatotoxicity:** esp. within 18 wks, some fatal. ↑ risk of rash, drug rash with eosinophilia & systemic symptoms (DRESS syndrome). **Severe symptomatic hepatotoxicity reported:** 2/3 during first 12wks of rx. Pts with pre-existing ↑ in ALT &/or history of chronic Hep B or C, susceptible (*AnIM* 35:182, 2002). Women with CD4 >250, inc. preg women, at ↑ risk. Avoid in this group unless no other option. Men with CD4 >400 also at ↑ risk. Monitor pts intensively (clinical & LFTs), esp. during first 12wks of rx. If clinical hepatotoxicity, severe skin or hypersensitivity reactions occur, dc drug, & never rechallenge.
Protease inhibitors (PI)	Abnormalities in glucose metabolism, dyslipidemias, fat redistribution syndromes are potential problems. Pts taking PI may be at ↑ risk for developing osteopenia/osteoporosis. Spontaneous bleeding episodes reported in HIV+ pts with hemophilia being treated with PI. Rheumatoid complications have been reported with use of Pts *Ann Rheum Dis* 61:82, 2002). **Caution for all PIs**—Coadministration with certain drugs dependent on CYP3A for elimination &/or which ↑ levels can cause serious toxicity may be contraindicated.
Amprenavir (Agenerase)	**Most common:** Nausea 43-74%, vomiting 24-34%, diarrhea 39-60%, paresthesias 26-31%. ↑ ALT/AST. Contains sulfa moiety. **Most significant:** Skin rash 28%. Most maculopapular of mild-mod intensity, some with pruritus. Severe/life-threatening rash, inc. Stevens-Johnson syndrome, in 1%. Rash onset 7-73d, median 11d. **Black Box warning**—potential propylene glycol toxicity with oral solution. Do not use in preg, children <4y, renal/hepatic failure, with disulfiram or metronidazole.
Atazanavir (Reyataz)	**Most common:** Asymptomatic unconjugated hyperbilirubinemia in up to 60% of pts, jaundice in 7-9%, especially in Gilbert syndrome (*JID* 192:1381, 2005). Moderate to severe events. Diarrhea 1-3%, nausea 6-14%, abdominal pain 4%, headache 6%, rash 5-7%. **Most significant:** ↑ PR interval (1st degree AV block; rarely 2nd AV block). Acute interstitial nephritis and ureteral calculi (*AIDS* 20:2131, 2006).
Darunavir (Prezista)	**Most common:** With background regimens, headache 15%, nausea 18%, diarrhea 20%, ↑ amylase 17%. Rash in 7% of treated, 0.3% discontinuation. **Most significant:** Stevens-Johnson syndrome, erythema multiforme. May cause failure of hormonal contraceptives. Use caution in pts with hepatic dysfunction.
Fosamprenavir (Lexiva)	**Most common:** Skin rash 20-30% (moderate or worse in 3-8%), nausea, headache, diarrhea. **Most significant:** Rarely Stevens-Johnson syndrome, hemolytic anemia. Pro-drug of amprenavir. Contains sulfa moiety.
Indinavir (Crixivan)	**Most common:** ↑ in indirect bilirubin 10-15% (≥2.5 mg per dL), with overt jaundice more likely in those with Gilbert syndrome (*JID* 192:1381, 2005). Nausea 12%, vomiting 4%, diarrhea 5%. Paronychia reported (*CID* 32:140, 2001). **Black Box warning:** Nephrolithiasis in 12% of adults. ↑ In pedis. Prevent (minimize) by good hydration (≥48oz. water/day) (*AAC* 42:332, 1998). Tubulointerstitial nephritis/renal cortical atrophy reported in assoc with asympt ↑ urine WBC. Severe hepatitis reported (*Ln* 349:924, 1997). Hemolytic anemia reported.
Lopinavir/Ritonavir (Kaletra)	**Most common: GI: diarrhea** 14-24%, nausea 2-16%, lipid abnormalities in up to 20-40%. More diarrhea with q24h dosing. **Most significant:** Pancreatitis, inflammatory edema of the legs. For diarrhea: Oat bran tabs, calcium, or oral anti-diarrheal agents (e.g. loperamide, diphenoxylate/atropine sulfate).
Nelfinavir (Viracept)	**Most common:** Mild-moderate **diarrhea** 20%. For diarrhea, use Imodium. **Most significant:** Potential for drug interactions
Ritonavir (Norvir)	**Most common: Diarrhea,** abdominal discomfort, nausea, headache. **Black Box Warning—**Invirase & Fortovase are not bioequivalent. (NOTE: Fortovase discontinued in 2006.) **Use Invirase only with ritonavir.** **Most serious: Black Box warnings—**associated with fatal/non-fatal hemorrhage (can inhibit platelet aggregation in vitro); caution in those with bleeding risk. Associated with hepatitis & fatal hepatic failure. Risk of hepatotoxicity↑ in Hep B or Hep C co-infection. Potential for major drug interactions.
Saquinavir (Invirase, hard cap, tablet)	**Most common:** Nausea & vomiting, diarrhea, abdominal pain. Rash in 8-14%, more common in women, & 33% in women taking ethinyl estradiol. Major lipid effects. Circumoral paresthesias 5-6%. ↑ dose >100mg q12h assoc. with ↑ GI side-effects & ↑ in lipid abnormalities. With rare exceptions, used in low doses to enhance levels of other antiretrovirals because of ↑ toxicity/interactions with full-dose ritonavir.
Tipranavir (Aptivus)	**Most common:** Nausea & vomiting, **diarrhea,** abdominal pain. Rash in 8-14%, more common in women, & 33% in women taking ethinyl estradiol. Major lipid effects. **Black Box Warnings**—associated with fatal/non-fatal intracranial hemorrhage (can inhibit platelet aggregation in vitro); caution in those with bleeding risk. Associated with hepatitis & fatal hepatic failure. Risk of hepatotoxicity↑ in Hep B or Hep C co-infection. Potential for major drug interactions.
Fusion Inhibitor	
Enfuvirtide (T20, Fuzeon)	**Most common:** local injection site reactions (98% at least 1 local [ISR, 4% dc because of ISR), hypersensitivity reactions <1% (rash, fever, nausea & vomiting, chills, rigors, hypotension, & ↑ serum liver transaminases); can occur with re-exposure. **Most significant:** ↑ rate of bacterial pneumonia (6.7 pneumonia events per 100 pt yrs).

TABLE 15A – ANTIMICROBIAL PROPHYLAXIS FOR SELECTED BACTERIAL INFECTIONS*

CLASS OF ETIOLOGIC AGENT/DISEASE/CONDITION	PROPHYLAXIS: AGENT/DOSE/ROUTE/DURATION [CDC Guidelines, MMWR 51(RR-11):1, 2002]	COMMENTS
Group B streptococcal disease (GBS), neonatal: Approaches to management [CDC Guidelines, MMWR 51(RR-11):1, 2002]:		
Pregnant women—intrapartum antimicrobial prophylaxis procedures:	**Prophylactic regimens during labor:**	Careful observation of signs & symptoms. 95% of infants with early-onset GBS disease
1. Rx during labor if GBS at 35–37 wks gestation (unless other indications for prophylaxis exist. GBS bacteriuria during this pregnancy or previously delivered infant with invasive GBS disease; even then cultures may be useful for susceptibility testing). Use transport medium; GBS survive at room temp. up to 96 hrs. **Rx during labor if swab culture positive.**	**All women:** Ampicillin 2 gm IV (load) then 1 gm IV q4h, or Penicillin G 5 million units IV (load) then 2.5 million units IV q4h. **Pen-allergic: Pts not at high risk for anaphylaxis: Cefazolin** 2 gm IV initial dose, then 1 gm IV q8h. **Pts at high risk for anaphylaxis:** GBS susceptible to clinda & erythro. **Clindamycin** 900 mg IV q8h or **erythromycin** 500 mg IV q6h. Vancomycin for pts at high risk for anaphylaxis and when alternative to clindamycin or erythromycin needed (e.g., GBS-resistant or unknown susceptibility).	will show clinical signs of infection during the 1st 24 hrs whether mother received intrapartum antibiotics or not (Pediatrics 106:244, 2000). For gestational age <35 wks or intrapartum antibiotics <4 hrs, lab evaluation (CBC, diff, blood culture) & ≥48 hr observation recommended. See algorithm, MMWR 51(RR-11):1, 2002.
2. Rx during labor if previously delivered infant with invasive GBS infection, or if any GBS bacteriuria this pregnancy (MMWR 53:506, 2004).		**Comment:** Universal screening has resulted in continued declines in early-onset GBS disease (MMWR 54:1205, 2005).
3. Rx if GBS status unknown but if any of the following are present: (a) delivery at <37 wks gestation [see MMWR 51(RR-11):1, 2002 algorithm for threatened preterm delivery], or (b) duration of ruptured membranes ≥18 hrs, or (c) intrapartum temp. ≥100.4°F [≥38.0°C].		
Neonate of mother given prophylaxis		
Preterm, premature rupture of the membranes in Group B strep-negative women	**(IV ampicillin 2 gm q6h + IV erythromycin 250 mg q6h) for 48 hr followed by (po amoxicillin 250 mg q8h + po erythromycin base 333 mg q8h times 5 days).** Decreases infant morbidity. (JAMA 278:989, 1997) (Note: May require additional antibiotics for therapy of specific existing infections)	Antibiotic rx reduced infant respiratory distress syndrome (50.6% to 40.8%, p = 0.03), necrotizing enterocolitis (5.8% to 2.3%, p = 0.03) and prolonged pregnancy (2.9 to 6.1 days, p < 0.001) vs placebo. In larger study (4809 children) po erythromycin to improved neonatal outcomes vs placebo (11.2% vs 14.4% for single births) but not co-AM-CL or both drugs in combination (both assoc. with ↑ necrotizing enterocolitis (Ln 357:979, 2001). (See ACOG discussion, Ob Gyn 102:875, 2003)
Post-splenectomy bacteremia. Likely agents: Pneumococci (4%), H. influenzae, meningococci, N. meningitidis. Babesia sp. and malaria, severe babesiosis, and Capnocytophaga spp.) Ref.: 2006 Red Book, 27th Ed., Amer Acad Pediatrics	**Immunizations:** Ensure admin. of pneumococcal vaccine, H. influenzae B, & quadrivalent meningococcal vaccines at recommended times. (see Table 20) In addition, asplenic children with sickle cell anemia, thalassemia, & perhaps others, daily antimicrobial prophylaxis until at least age 5—see Comments.	Antimicrobial prophylaxis until age 5: Amox 20mg/kg/day or Pen V-K 125 mg bid. Over age 5: Consider Pen V-K 250 mg bid for at least 1 yr in children post-splenectomy. Some suggest prophylaxis until at least age 18. Maintain immunizations plus self-administer AM-CL (with onset of any febrile illness while seeking physician assistance. Pen. allergy: TMP-SMX or clarithro are options, but resistance in S. pneumo may be significant in some areas, particularly among pen-resistant isolates.
Sexual Exposure		
Sexual assault survivor [likely agents and risks, see NEJM 332:234, 1995; MMWR 55(RR-11):1, 2006]	**(Ceftriaxone** 125 mg IM once) + **(metronidazole** 2 gm po single dose) + **(azithromycin** 1 gm po single dose) or **(doxycycline** 100 mg po bid times 7 days)** [MMWR 55(RR-11):1, 2006]**	Obtain expert advice re: forensic exam & specimens; pregnancy, physical trauma, psychological support. If decision is to proceed with spec. collection, at initial exam: Test for gonococci & chlamydia, wet mount for T. vaginalis (& culture vaginal swab). Serologic evaluation for syphilis, Hep B, HIV, others as appropriate. Initiate post-exposure protocols for HIV & hepatitis as appropriate (see). Follow-up exam for STD at 1–2 wks. Retest syphilis & HIV serology at 6, 12, 24 wks if negative earlier.
Sexual contacts, likely agents. N. gonorrhoeae, C. trachomatis	**(Ceftriaxone** 125 mg IM once) or **(cefixime** 400 mg po once)] for GC, plus **(doxycycline** 100 mg po times 7 days) or **azithromycin** 1 gm po once)]. for Chlamydia	Be sure to check for evidence incubating syphilis. Consider also T. vaginalis. Identify & rx contacts as appropriate to suspected STD [see MMWR 55(RR-11):1, 2006 for other etiologies & rx options].
Syphilis exposure	**Penicillin V** 125 mg po bid	Presumptive rx for exposure within 3 mos. as tests may be negative. See , page 21. Make effort to do syphilis
Sickle-cell disease. Likely agents: S. pneumoniae (see post-splenectomy, above) Ref.: 2006 Red Book, 27th Ed., Amer Acad Pediatrics	Children <5 yrs: **Penicillin V** 125 mg po bid ≥5 yrs: **Penicillin V** 250 mg po bid (Alternative in children: Amoxicillin 20 mg per kg per day)	Start prophylaxis by 2 mos. (Pediatrics 106:367, 2000). Age-appropriate vaccines, including pneumococcal, Hib, influenza, meningococcal. Treating infections, consider possibility of penicillin non-susceptible pneumococcus.

* See page 2 for abbreviations

TABLE 15B – SURGICAL ANTIBIOTIC PROPHYLAXIS IN ADULTS*
(EID 7:220, 2001; CID 38:1706, 2004; Am J Surg 189:395, 2005)

Surgical Procedures: To be optimally effective, **antibiotics must be started in the interval: 2 hrs before time of surgical incision** (NEJM 326:281, 1992). For most procedures the number of doses needed for optimal coverage is not defined. Most authorities employ a single dose (Treat Guide Med Lett. 2:27, 2004) although FDA-approved product labelling is often for 2 or more doses. The surgical procedure lasts >3 hrs, additional intraoperative doses of rapidly eliminated drugs should be given at approx. 3-hr intervals. A recent consensus statement from the National Surgical Infection Prevention Project (CID 38:1706, 2004) advises antibiotic prophylaxis be started within 1 hr before incision (except vancomycin or fluoroquinolones begun within 2 hrs before surg); half-lives of the prophylactic agent, and for longest-procedures, not be continued beyond 24 hrs. In patients with normal renal function & not intolerant of these agents are for the most part those approved in FDA product labeling. For single-dose regimens, the dosage & route are the same. (See Table 15C for regimens to reduce risk of endocarditis.
General Comments: In some centers, ↑ resistance may render certain regimens (e.g., quinolones) unacceptable. Pharmacokinetic considerations suggest that typical prophylaxis dosing may yield suboptimal serum/tissue levels in pts with high BMI (see Surgery 136:738, 2004 for cefazolin; Eur J Clin Pharm 54:632, 1998 for vancomycin), although clinical implications uncertain.

TYPE OF SURGERY	PROPHYLAXIS	COMMENTS
Cardiovascular Surgery Antibiotic prophylaxis in cardiovascular surgery has been proven beneficial only in the following procedures. Reconstruction of abdominal aorta Procedures on the leg that involve a groin incision Any vascular procedure that inserts prosthesis/foreign body Lower extremity amputation for ischemia Cardiac surgery Perhaps permanent pacemakers (see Comment)	**Cefazolin** 1–2 gm IV as a single dose or q8h for 1–2 days, or **cefuroxime** 1.5 gm IV as a single dose or q12h for total of 6 doses or **vancomycin** 1 gm IV as single dose or q12h for 1–2 days. Consider **intranasal mupirocin**, evening before, day of surgery, & bid for 5 days post-op in pts with pos. nasal culture for S. aureus.	Single injection just before surgery probably as effective as multiple doses. Not recommended for cardiac catheterization or prosthetic heart valves, customarily given to stop prophylaxis either after removal of retrosternal drainage catheters or just a 2nd dose after coming off bypass. Vancomycin may be preferable in hospitals with ↑ frequency of MRSA or Gm-neg. bacilli, therefore would add cefazolin for groin incisions. Meta-analysis failed to demonstrate overall superiority of vancomycin over β-lactam prophylaxis for cardiac surgery (CID 38:1357, 2004). A meta-analysis of 7 placebo-controlled randomized studies of antibiotic prophylaxis for permanent pacemaker implantation, sig. ↓ in incidence of infection (Circulation 97:1796, 1998). Intranasal mupirocin ↓ sternal wound infections from S. aureus in 1850 pts; used historical controls (An Thor Surg 71:1572, 2001); in another trial, it reduced nosocomial S. aureus infections only in nasal carriers (NEJM 346:1871, 2002).
Gastric, Biliary and Colonic Surgery **Gastroduodenal/Biliary** Gastroduodenal, includes percutaneous endoscopic gastrostomy (high-risk only; see Comments) Biliary, includes laparoscopic cholecystectomy (high-risk only; see Comments) Endoscopic retrograde cholangiopancreato-graphy Not controversial: No benefit from single dose piperacillin in randomized placebo-controlled trial, AnIM 125:442, 1996 (see Comment)	**Cefazolin** or **cefoxitin** or **cefotetan** or **cefuroxime** 1.5 gm IV as a single dose (some give additional doses q12h for 2–3 days). In biliary surgery, cefazolin 1 gm & ceftizoxime 1 gm (± repeat dosing at 12 & 24 hrs) were equivalent (AAC 40:70, 1996). No rx without obstruction. If obstruction: **Cip** ofloxacin 500–750 mg po 2 hrs prior to procedure or **Ceftizoxime** 1.5 gm IV 1 hr prior to procedure and **Piperacillin** 4 gm IV 1 hr prior to procedure	**Gastroduodenal:** High-risk is marked obesity, obstruction, ↓ gastric acid or ↓ GI motility. **Biliary:** Cholecystectomy if: age >70, acute cholecystitis, common duct stones, jaundice or obstructive jaundice. With low-risk elective laparoscopic cholecystectomy, prophylaxis not needed (most would not use). **Oral CIP** as effective as cephalosporins in 2 studies & less expensive (CID 23:380, 1996). Most studies show that achieving adequate drainage will prevent sepsis and thus not benefit from prophylactic antibiotics. With inadequate drainage or suspected biliary obstruction: antibiotics may be of value. American Society for GI Endoscopy recommends use for known or suspected biliary obstruction. Biliary: cholangiocarcinoma if obstruction yet clinically evidence as prophylaxis either surgery. With cholangitis, treat as infection, not prophylaxis; Tc-CL3, 3.0 gm q6h IV or PIP-TZ 3.375 gm q6h or 4.5 gm q8h IV or AM-SB 3.0 gm q6h IV. Biliary high-risk: age >70, acute cholecystitis, non-functioning gallbladder, obstructive jaundice or common duct stones. Meta-analysis supports use in percutaneous endoscopic gastrostomy (Am J Gastro 95:3133, 2000).
Colorectal, Includes Appendectomy — Elective surgery — Emergency surgery or when parenteral rx needed	**Neomycin + erythromycin** po (see Comment for dose) or **Cefazolin** + **metronidazole** 0.5 gm IV (single dose) or **cefoxitin** or **cefotetan** 4 gm IV 1 hr prior to procedure	Elective colorectal prep: Pre-op day: (1) 10am 4L polyethylene glycol electrolyte solution (GoLYTELY) po over 2h, (2) clear liquid diet only, (3) 1pm, 2pm & 3pm: neomycin 1gm + erythromycin base 1gm po. As alternatives to (4) NG tube at midnight. Alternative have been less well studied: GoLYTELY 1–6pm, then neomycin 2gm po + metronidazole 2gm po at 7pm & 11pm. Oral regimen as effective as parenteral; parenteral is advantageous but often used (Am J Surg 189:395, 2005). For emergency colorectal surg, use parenteral. (CID 15 Suppl 1:S313, 1992). Ertapenem 1gm IV one hour pre-op approved for elective colorectal surg. Alternative is parenteral ampicillin-sulbactam (CID 43:322, 2006).

Ruptured Viscus: See Peritoneum/Peritonitis, Secondary, Table 1, page 42.

* See page 2 for abbreviations

TABLE 15B (2)

TYPE OF SURGERY	PROPHYLAXIS	COMMENTS
Head and Neck Surgery (Ann Otol Rhinol Laryngol 101 Suppl:16, 1992)		
Antimicrobial prophylaxis in head & neck surg appears efficacious only for procedures involving oral/pharyngeal mucosa (e.g., laryngeal or pharyngeal tumor) but even with high wound infection rate high when 1 o contaminated head & neck surg does not require prophylaxis. (Arch Otol HNS 23:447, 2007). Uncontaminated head & neck surg does not require prophylaxis.		
Neurosurgical Procedures [Prophylaxis not effective in + infection rate with intracranial pressure monitors in retrospective analysis of 215 pts (J Neurol Neurosurg Psych 69:381, 2000)]		
Clean, non-implant, e.g., craniotomy	**Cefazolin 1 gm IV x 1.** Alternative: **vanco 1 gm IV x 1.**	Reference: Ln 344:1547, 1994
Clean, contaminated (cross sinuses, or naso/oropharynx)	**Clindamycin 900 mg IV** (single dose)	British recommend amoxicillin-clavulanate 1.2 gm IV[A] or (cefuroxime 1.5 gm IV + metronidazole 0.5 gm) IV.
CSF shunt surgery. Meta-analysis suggests benefit (Cochrane Database (4) 2006)	**Cefazolin 1gm IV once.** Alternative: **vanco 1gm IV once.**	**Alternative: Vancomycin** 10 mg into cerebral ventricles + **gentamicin** 3 mg into cerebral ventricles (Ln 344:1547, 1994)
Obstetric/Gynecologic Surgery		
Vaginal or abdominal hysterectomy	**Cefazolin 1–2 gm** or **cefoxitin 1–2 gm** or **cefotetan 1–2 gm** or **cefuroxime 1.5 gm IV 30 min before surgery.**	1 study found cefotetan superior to cefazolin (CID 20:677, 1995). For prolonged procedures, doses can be repeated q4–8h for duration of procedure. Ampicillin-sulbactam is considered an acceptable alternative (CID43:322, 2006).
Cesarean section for premature rupture of membranes or active labor	**Cefazolin once, administer IV** as soon as umbilical cord clamped.	Prophylaxis decreases risk of endometritis/wound infection in elective as well as non-elective C-section; single dose regimen vs multiple dose regimens (Cochrane Database System Rev 2002, issue 3, & 1999, issue 1).
Abortion	1st trimester: aqueous **pen G 2 miU IV** or **doxycycline 300 mg po.** 2nd trimester: **Cefazolin 1 gm IV**	Meta-analysis showed benefit of antibiotic prophylaxis in all risk groups. One regimen was doxy 100 mg orally 1 hr before procedure, then 200 mg after procedure (Ob Gyn 87:884, 1996).
Orthopedic Surgery [Most pts with prosthetic joints do not need prophylaxis for routine dental procedures, but individual considerations prevail for high-risk procedures & prostheses (J Am Dental Assn 134:895, 2003; Med Lett 47:59, 2005)].		
Hip arthroplasty, spinal fusion	Same as cardiac	Customarily stopped after "Hemovac" removed. NSIPP workgroup recommends stopping prophylaxis within 24 hrs of surgery (CID 38:1706, 2004).
Total joint replacement (other than hip)	**Cefazolin 1–2 gm IV** pre-op (± 2nd dose) or **vancomycin 1 gm IV** or call to OR	Post-op: some would give no further rx (Med Lett 39:98, 1997). NSIPP workgroup recommends stopping prophylaxis within 24 hrs of surgery (CID 38:1706, 2004).
Open reduction of closed fracture with internal fixation	**Ceftriaxone 2 gm IV or IM once**	3.6% vs 8.3% (for placebo) infection found in Dutch trauma trial (Ln 347:1133, 1996).
Peritoneal Dialysis Catheter Placement	**Vancomycin** single 1000 mg dose 12 hrs prior to procedure	Effectively reduced peritonitis during 14 days post-placement in 221 pts. vanco 1%, cefazolin 7%, placebo 12% (p=0.02) (Am J Kidney Dis 36:1014, 2000).
Urologic Surgery/Procedures		
Antimicrobials not recommended in pts with sterile urine. Pts with pre-operative bacteriuria should be treated.	Recommended antibiotic to pts with pre-operative bacteriuria. **Cefazolin 1 gm IV q8h times 1–3 doses perioperatively, followed by oral antibiotics for 10 days.** Modify based on susceptibility test results.	
Transrectal prostate biopsy	**Ciprofloxacin 500 mg po 12 hrs prior to biopsy and repeated 12 hrs after 1st dose**	Bacteremia 7% with CIP vs 37% gentamicin (Urology 38:84, 1991; review in JAC 39:115, 1997). Levo 500 mg 30–60 min before procedure was effective in low-risk pts; additional doses were given for risk (J Urol 168:1021, 2002). ↑ Fluoroquinolone resistance in enteric gram-negatives is a concern.
Other		
Breast surgery, herniorrhaphy	**P Ceph 1,2,** dosage as Gynecologic Surgery, above	Meta-analysis did not show clear evidence of benefit from prophylaxis in elective inguinal hernia repair (Cochrane Database System Rev 2004, issue 4).

1 Gentamicin (12.5 mg per gm of acrylic bone cement) is released for at least 3 weeks. Usefulness not proven.

* See page 2 for abbreviations

TABLE 15C – ANTIMICROBIAL PROPHYLAXIS FOR THE PREVENTION OF BACTERIAL ENDOCARDITIS IN PATIENTS WITH UNDERLYING CARDIAC CONDITIONS*

[These are the Amer Heart Assoc recommendations (JAMA 277:1794, 1997). However, a population-based prospective case-controlled study brings into serious question whether dental procedures predispose to endocarditis & whether antibiotic prophylaxis is of any value (see AnIM 129:761, 1998; Brit Dent J 189:610, 2000). For new Brit Soc Antimicro Chemo guidelines, see JAC 57:1035, 2006]

ENDOCARDITIS PROPHYLAXIS RECOMMENDED	ENDOCARDITIS PROPHYLAXIS NOT RECOMMENDED
Cardiac conditions associated with endocarditis[1]	**Negligible-risk** (same as general population):
High-risk conditions:[1]	Atrial septal defect (secundum)
Prosthetic valves—bioprosthetic and homograft, as well as mechanical	Surgical repair of ASD, VSD, or PDA (beyond 6 months)
Previous bacterial endocarditis	Previous CABG; mitral prolapse without MR (see discussion JAMA 277:1794, 1997)
Complex cyanotic congenital heart disease, e.g.: single ventricle, transposition, tetralogy of Fallot	Physiologic, functional, or innocent heart murmurs
Surgically constructed systemic pulmonic shunts or conduits	Previous Kawasaki or rheumatic fever without valve dysfunction
Moderate-risk conditions:	Cardiac pacemakers (all) and implanted defibrillators
Most other congenital heart abnormalities or acquired valvular disease; hypertrophic cardiac myopathy; mitral prolapse with regurgitation	

ENDOCARDITIS PROPHYLAXIS RECOMMENDED	ENDOCARDITIS PROPHYLAXIS NOT RECOMMENDED
Dental and other procedures where prophylaxis is considered for patients with moderate- or high-risk cardiac conditions	
Dental: Extractions, periodontal procedures[1]	Dental: Filling cavities with local anesthetic
Implants, root canal, subgingival antibiotic fibers/strips	Placement of rubber dams, suture removal, orthodontic removal
Initial orthodontic bands (not brackets); intraligamentary local anesthetic	Orthodontic adjustments; dental x-rays
Cleaning of teeth/implants if bleeding anticipated	Shedding of primary teeth
Respiratory: T&A, surgery on respiratory mucosa, rigid bronchoscopy (BSC) guidelines (JAC 57:1035, 2006)	Respiratory: Intubation, flexible bronchoscopy[4] tympanostomy tube
GI: Sclerotherapy of esophageal varices; dilation of esophageal stricture, ERCP with biliary obstruction	Respiratory: Transesophageal cardiac echo[4]; EGD without biopsy[4]
GU: Prostate surgery; cystoscopy, urethral dilation	GU: Vaginal hysterectomy[4], vaginal delivery[4], C-section
	If uninfected, Foley catheter, uterine D&C, therapeutic abortion, tubal ligation, insert/remove IUD
	Other: Cardiac cath, balloon angioplasty; implanted pacemaker, defibrillators, coronary stents
	Skin biopsy, circumcision

Abbreviations: T&A = tonsillectomy/adenoidectomy, ERCP = endoscopic retrograde cholangiography, ASD/VSD = atrial septal defect/ventricular septal defect, PDA = patent ductus arteriosus, EGD = esophagogastroduodenoscopy, D&C = dilation and curettage.

PROPHYLACTIC REGIMENS FOR DENTAL, ORAL, RESPIRATORY TRACT, OR ESOPHAGEAL PROCEDURES

SITUATION	AGENT	REGIMEN[1]
Standard general prophylaxis	Amoxicillin	Adults 2 gm; children 50 mg per kg orally 1 hr before procedure
Unable to take oral medications	Ampicillin	Adults 2 gm IM or IV; children 50 mg per kg IM or IV within 30 min. before procedure
Allergic to penicillin	Clindamycin OR [Cephalexin[4] or cefadroxil[4]], OR Azithromycin or clarithromycin	Adults 600 mg; children 20 mg per kg orally 1 hr before procedure Adults 2 gm; children 50 mg per kg orally 1 hr before procedure. Adults 500 mg; children 15 mg per kg orally 1 hr before procedure
Allergic to penicillin and unable to take oral medications	Clindamycin OR Cefazolin[4]	Adults 600 mg, children 20 mg per kg IV within 30 min. before procedure Adults 1 gm; children 25 mg per kg IM or IV within 30 min. before procedure

[1] Some now recommend that for adults, prophylaxis prior to dental procedures should **only** be used for **extractions and gingival surgery** (including implant replacement) **and only for patients with prosthetic cardiac valves or previous endocarditis** (AnIM 129:829, 1998). If any of these 4 conditions exist = prophylactic antibiotics according to American Heart Association are recommended.
[2] Prophylaxis optional for high-risk patients.
[3] Total children's dose should not exceed adult dose.
[4] Cephalosporins should not be used in individuals with immediate-type hypersensitivity reaction (urticaria, angioedema, or anaphylaxis) to penicillins.

* See page 2 for abbreviations

TABLE 15C (2)
PROPHYLACTIC REGIMENS FOR GENITOURINARY/GASTROINTESTINAL (EXCLUDING ESOPHAGEAL) PROCEDURES

SITUATION	AGENT	REGIMEN
High-risk patients	Ampicillin + gentamicin	**Adults: ampicillin** 2 gm IM or IV + **gentamicin** 1.5 mg per kg (not to exceed 120 mg) within 30 min. of starting the procedure; 6 hr later, **ampicillin** 1 gm IM/IV or **amoxicillin** 1 gm orally. **Children: ampicillin** 50 mg per kg IM or IV (not to exceed 2 gm) + **gentamicin** 1.5 mg per kg IV/IM within 30 min. of starting the procedure; 6 hrs later, **ampicillin** 25 mg per kg IM/IV or **amoxicillin** 25 mg per kg orally
High-risk patients allergic to ampicillin or amoxicillin	Vancomycin + gentamicin	**Adults: vancomycin** 1 gm IV over 1–2 hrs + **gentamicin** 1.5 mg per kg IV/IM (not to exceed 120 mg); complete injection/infusion within 30 min. of starting the procedure. **Children: vancomycin** 20 mg per kg IV over 1–2 hrs + **gentamicin** 1.5 mg per kg IV/IM; complete injection/ infusion within 30 min. of starting the procedure
Moderate-risk patients	Amoxicillin or ampicillin	**Adults: amoxicillin** 2 gm orally 1 hr before procedure, or **ampicillin** 2 gm IM/IV within 30 min. of starting the procedure. **Children: amoxicillin** 50 mg per kg orally 1 hr before procedure, or **ampicillin** 50 mg per kg IM/IV within 30 min. of starting the procedure
Moderate-risk patients allergic to ampicillin or amoxicillin	Vancomycin	**Adults: vancomycin** 1 gm IV over 1–2 hrs; complete infusion within 30 min. of starting the procedure. **Children: vancomycin** 20 mg per kg IV over 1–2 hrs; complete infusion within 30 min. of starting the procedure

¹ Total children's dose should not exceed adult dose

TABLE 15D – MANAGEMENT OF EXPOSURE TO HIV-1 AND HEPATITIS*

OCCUPATIONAL EXPOSURE TO BLOOD, PENILE/VAGINAL SECRETIONS OR OTHER POTENTIALLY INFECTIOUS BODY FLUIDS OR TISSUES WITH RISK OF TRANSMISSION OF HEPATITIS B/C AND/OR HIV-1 (E.G., NEEDLESTICK INJURY)
[Adapted from MMWR 50(RR-11):1, 2001; NEJM 348:826, 2003 and MMWR 54(RR-9):1, 2005 (available at www.aidsinfo.nih.gov).]

Free medical consultation for occupational exposures, call (PEPline) 1-888-448-4911.

General steps in management:
1. Wash clean wounds/flush mucous membranes immediately (use of caustic agents or squeezing the wound is discouraged; data lacking regarding antiseptics).
2. Assess risk by doing the following: (a) Characterize exposure; (b) Determine/evaluate source of exposure by medical history, risk behavior, & testing for hepatitis B/C, HIV; (c) Evaluate and test exposed individual for hepatitis B/C & HIV.

Hepatitis B Exposure [Adapted from CDC recommendations: MMWR 50(RR-11), 2001]

Exposed Person	Exposure Source		
	HBs Ag+	HBs Ag–	Status Unknown
Unvaccinated	Give HBIG 0.06 per kg IM & initiate HB vaccine	Initiate HB vaccine	Initiate HB vaccine and if possible, check HBs Ag of source person. Consider HBIG if source high-risk.
Vaccinated (antibody status unknown)	Do anti-HBs on exposed person: If titer ≥10 milli-International units per mL, no rx If titer <10 milli-International units per mL, give HBIG + 1 dose HB vaccine!	No rx necessary	Do anti-HBs on exposed person: If titer ≥10 milli-International units per mL, no rx If titer <10 milli-International units per mL, give 1 dose of HB vaccine plus 1 dose HBIG (if source high-risk)

For known vaccine series responder (titer ≥10 milli-International units per mL), monitoring of levels or booster doses not currently recommended. Known non-responder (<10 milli-International units per mL) exposed to HBsAg+ source or suspected high-risk source—rx with HBIG & re-initiate vaccine series or give 2 doses HBIG 1 month apart. For non-responders after a 2⁰ vaccine series, 2 doses HBIG 1 month apart is preferred approach to new exposure [MMWR 40(RR-13):21, 2001].

! Follow-up to assess/address vaccine response and rx being series.

Hepatitis C Exposure
Determine the antibody to hepatitis C for both exposed person and, if possible, exposure source. If source +, follow-up HCV testing advised. **No recommended prophylaxis:** immune serum globulin (not effective). Monitor for early infection, as therapy may ↓ risk of progression to chronic hepatitis. See page 136 and discussion in Clin Micro Rev 16:546, 2003.

* See page 2 for abbreviations

TABLE 15D (2)

HIV: Occupational exposure management

- The decision to initiate post-exposure prophylaxis (PEP) for HIV is a clinical judgment that should be made in concert with the exposed healthcare worker (HCW). It is based on:
  1. Likelihood of the source patient having HIV infection: ↑ with history of high-risk activity—injection drug use, sexual activity with known HIV+ person, unprotected sex with multiple partners (either hetero- or homosexual), receipt of blood products 1978–1985. ↑ with clinical signs suggestive of acute HIV (unexplained wasting, night sweats, thrush, seborrheic dermatitis, etc.).
  2. Remember, the vast majority of persons are **not** infected with HIV (1,000 women infected with HIV in larger U.S. cities) and likelihood of infection is low if not in any risk groups.
  3. Type of exposure (approx. risk in 300–400 needlesticks from infected source will transmit HIV).
  4. Limited data regarding efficacy of PEP (PEP with ZDV alone reduced transmission by >80% in 1 retrospective case-controlled study—*NEJM* 337:1485, 1997).
  5. Significant adverse effects of PEP drugs.
  - Substances considered potentially infectious include: blood, tissues, semen, vaginal secretions, CSF, synovial, pleural, peritoneal, pericardial and amniotic fluids, and other visibly bloody fluids.
  - Fluids normally considered low risk for transmission, unless visibly bloody, include: urine, stool, sweat, saliva, nasal secretions, tears and sputum (*MMWR* 54(RR-9), 2005).
- If source person is **known positive for HIV** or **likely to be infected** and **status of exposure is suspected of having acute HIV infection**, antiretroviral drugs should be started **immediately** (ASAP or within hours). If source person is HIV antibody negative, drugs can be stopped **unless source is suspected of having acute HIV infection.** The HCW should not be used for dx of HIV infection because of false-positives (esp. at low titers) & these tests are only approved for established HIV infection (a possible exception is if develops signs of acute HIV (mononucleosis-like) syndrome within the 1st 4–6 wks of exposure when antibody tests might still be negative.)
- **PEP** for HIV is usually given for **4wks** and monitoring of adverse effects recommended: baseline **complete blood count, renal and hepatic panel to be repeated at 2 weeks.** 50–75% of HCW on PEP demonstrate mild side-effects (nausea, diarrhea, myalgias, headache, etc.) but in up to ½ severe enough to discontinue PEP (*Antivir Ther* 3:195, 2000). Consultation with infectious diseases/HIV specialist valuable when questions regarding PEP arise. **Seek expert help in special situations, such as pregnancy, renal impairment, treatment-experienced source.**

3 Steps to HIV Post-Exposure Prophylaxis (PEP) After Occupational Exposure: *[For latest CDC recommendations, see MMWR 54(RR-9), 2005]*

Step 1: Determine the exposure code (EC)

Is source material blood, bloody fluid, semen/vaginal fluid or other normally sterile fluid or tissue?

- Yes → What type of exposure occurred?
  - Mucous membrane or skin integrity compromised (e.g., dermatitis, open wound) → Volume
    - Small: Few drops → **EC1**
    - Large: Major splash and/or long duration → **EC2**
  - Intact skin → No PEP[1]
  - Percutaneous exposure → Severity
    - Less severe: Solid needle, scratch → **EC2**
    - More severe: Large-bore hollow needle, deep puncture, visible blood, needle used in blood vessel of source (risk 1:300/400) → **EC3**
- No → No PEP

Step 2: Determine the HIV Status Code (HIV SC)

What is the HIV status of the exposure source?

- HIV negative → No PEP[1]
- HIV positive
  - Low titer exposure: asymptomatic & high CD4 count, low VL (<1500 copies per mL) → **HIV SC 1**
  - High titer exposure: advanced AIDS, primary HIV, high viral load or low CD4 count → **HIV SC 2**
- Status unknown → Source unknown
  - HIV SC unknown
  - HIV SC unknown

[1] Exceptions can be considered when there has been prolonged, high-volume contact.

* See page 2 for abbreviations

TABLE 15D (2)

Step 3: Determine Post-Exposure Prophylaxis (PEP) Recommendation	
EC	HIV SC	PEP
1	1	Consider basic regimen[1] [a]
1	2	Recommend basic regimen[1] [a,b]
2	1	Recommend basic regimen[1] [b]
2	2	Recommend expanded regimen[1]
3	1 or 2	Recommend expanded regimen[1]
1, 2, 3	Unknown	If exposure setting suggests risks of HIV exposure, consider basic regimen[1] [c]

[a] Based on estimates of ↓ risk of infection after mucous membrane exposure in occupational setting compared with needlestick.

Modification of CDC recommendations:

[b] Or: consider expanded regimen[1].

[c] In high risk circumstances, consider expanded regimen[1] on case-by-case basis.

Around the clock, urgent expert consultation available from:
National Clinicians' Post-Exposure Prophylaxis Hotline
(PEPline) at 1-888-448-4911 (1-888-HIV-4911)

[1] **Regimens:** (Treat for 4 weeks; monitor for drug side-effects every 2 weeks)

Basic regimen: ZDV + 3TC, or FTC or + TDF, or as an alternative d4T + 3TC.

Expanded regimen: Basic regimen + one of the following: lopinavir/ritonavir *(preferred)*, or *(as alternatives)* atazanavir/ritonavir or fosamprenavir/ritonavir. Efavirenz can be considered *(except in pregnancy or potential for pregnancy—**Pregnancy Category D**), but CNS symptoms might be problematic. [**Do not use nevirapine:** serious adverse reactions including hepatic necrosis reported in healthcare workers (*MMWR 49:1153, 2001*).]

Other regimens can be designed. If possible, use antiretroviral drugs for which resistance is unlikely based on susceptibility data or treatment history of source pt (if known). Seek expert consultation if ARV-experienced source or in pregnancy or potential for pregnancy.

NOTE: Some authorities feel that an expanded regimen should be employed whenever PEP is indicated (*NEJM 349:1091, 2003; Eur J Epidemiol 19:577 2004*). Expanded regimens are likely to be advantageous with ↑ numbers of ART-experienced source pts or when there is doubt about exact extent of exposures in decision algorithm. Mathematical model suggests that under some conditions, completion of full course basic regimen (*CID 39:395, 2004*). However, while expanded PEP regimens discontinued expanded regimen (*CID 39:395, 2004*) ↑ discontinuation (*CID 40:205, 2005*). Overt or recent traumatic have ↑ adverse effects, there is not necessarily ↑ discontinuation (*CID 40:205, 2005*).

POST-EXPOSURE PROPHYLAXIS FOR NON-OCCUPATIONAL EXPOSURES TO HIV
From MMWR 54(RR-2):1, 2005—DHHS recommendations

Because the risk of transmission of HIV via sexual contact or sharing needles by injection drug users may reach or exceed that of occupational needlestick exposure, it is reasonable to consider PEP in pts who have had a non-occupational exposure to blood or other potentially infected fluids (e.g., genital/rectal secretions, breast milk) from an HIV+ source. Risk of HIV acquisition per exposure varies with the act (for needle sharing and receptive and insertive vaginal or anal intercourse, ≥0.5%, approximately 10-fold lower with insertive vaginal or anal intercourse, 0.05–0.07%). Overt or recent traumatic lesions may ↑ risk in survivors of sexual assault.

For pts at risk of HIV acquisition through non-occupational exposure to HIV+ source material having occurred ≤72 hours before evaluation, DHHS recommendation is to treat for 28 days with an anti-retroviral **expanded regimen**, using preferred regimens [efavirenz *(not in pregnancy or pregnancy risk—**Pregnancy Category D**)* + (3TC or FTC) + (ZDV or TDF)] or [lopinavir/ritonavir + (3TC or FTC) + (ZDV or TDF)] or [lopinavir/ritonavir + (3TC or ZDV)] or one of several alternative regimens [see Table 14D section B & MMWR 54(RR-2):1, 2005]. Failures of prophylaxis have been reported, and may be associated with longer interval from exposure to start of PEP (*CID 41:1507, 2005*), this suggests prompt initiation of PEP if it is to be used.

Areas of uncertainty: (1) expanded regimens are not proven to be superior to 2-drug regimens, (2) while PEP not recommended for exposures >72 hours before evaluation, it may possibly be effective in some cases, (3) when HIV status of source patient is unknown, decision to treat and regimen selection must be individualized based on assessment of specific circumstances.

Evaluate for exposures to Hep B, Hep C (see *Occupational PEP above*), and bacterial sexually-transmitted diseases (see *Table 15A*) and treat as indicated. DHHS recommendations for sexual exposures to HepB and bacterial pathogens are available in *MMWR 55(RR-11), 2006*. Persons who are unvaccinated or who have not responded to full HepB vaccine series should receive hepB immune globulin preferably within 24-hours of percutaneous or mucosal exposure or body fluids of an HbsAg-positive person, along with hepB vaccine, with follow-up to complete vaccine series. Unvaccinated or not-fully-vaccinated persons exposed to a source with unknown HepBsAg-status should receive vaccine and complete vaccine series. See *MMWR 55(RR-11), 2006* for details and recommendations in other circumstances.

TABLE 15E – PREVENTION OF OPPORTUNISTIC INFECTION IN HUMAN STEM CELL TRANSPLANTATION (HSCT) OR SOLID ORGAN TRANSPLANTATION (SOT) FOR ADULTS WITH NORMAL RENAL FUNCTION*

General comments: Medical centers performing transplants will have detailed protocols for the prevention of opportunistic infections which are appropriate to the resources and patients represented at those sites. Regimens continue to evolve and protocols adopted by an institution may differ from those of other centers. Care of transplant patients should be guided by physicians with expertise in this area. See Table 15F, page 167 for listing of timing of infections post-transplant. References: *MMWR 49(RR-10):1, 2000; CID 33:S26, 2001; CID 17:353, 2004*

OPPORTUNISTIC INFECTION (at risk)	TYPE OF TRANSPLANT	PROPHYLACTIC REGIMENS	COMMENTS/REFERENCES
Herpes simplex (seropositive)	HSCT / SOT	Acyclovir 250mg per meter-squared IV q12h or 200mg po 3x/day from engraftment to resolution of mucositis. Acyclovir 200mg po 3x/day to 400mg bid—start early post-transplant [*ClinInfectRev 10:86, 1997*]	Do not delay acyclovir if receiving CMV prophylaxis
CMV (Recipient + OR Donor +,Recipient –)	HSCT	**Preemptive therapy:** Monitor ≥ 1x/wk (days 10-100) for CMV-antigenemia or viremia by PCR test (Note: culture alone not sufficiently sensitive), start rx when + (Ganciclovir 5mg/kg IV q12h 7-14 days, then 5mg/kg IV q24h 5 days/wk to day 100 or ≥ 3wks (whichever longer) [*MMWR 49(RR-10):1, 2000*] Some use oral ganciclovir 1gm q8h after 7-14 day IV induction phase. Some use shorter courses; however, monitoring tests should be neg before stopping rx [*CID 35:999, 2002*]. Recent papers showed that 2wks valganciclovir 900mg po bid comp to ganciclovir 5mg/kg IV bid as preemptive therapy in allo-HSCT [*BMT 37:693, 2006*] & that valganciclovir 900mg bid for 2wks then 900mg po q24h for 7 days after neg. assay was effective [*BMT 37:851, 2006*]. **OR Prophylaxis:** (for high-risk pts, see *CID 35:999, 2002*, or where CMV detection tests not available) From engraftment to day 100, rx with ganciclovir IV 5 mg per kg q12h for 7 days, then 5 mg per kg q24h 5-6 days per week. **General Comments:** Review in *CMR 16:647, 2003*. Role of valganciclovir in CMV prevention is under investigation.	
	SOT	**Kidney, kidney/pancreas, heart:** Valganciclovir 900 mg po q24h for 6 months (or at least 3 mos.).[1] Some centers add CMV immune globulin. **Liver:** Ganciclovir 1 gm po q8h, start by day 10 & continue through day 100.[1] **Lung:** Ganciclovir 5 mg per kg q12h IV for 5-7 days, then valganciclovir 900 mg po q24h for 6 months (or at least 3 mos.). Some centers add CMV immune globulin 150 mg per kg within the first month [at days 2, 4, 6 & 8], then q2wks [at days 12, 16, 24] to day 120. Per Solid Organ transplantation societies, see *Am J Transpl 4(Suppl.10):51, 2004 & 5:218, 2005.* For lung, see *Transpl 80:157, 2005.* Universal prophylaxis approach (above) favored by most; there are proponents of preemptive therapy in liver transplant [*CID 40:704 & 709, 2005; Transpl 79:85 & 1428, 2005*]. Some add CMV Ig for other high-risk SOTs also. **Note:** Valganciclovir not approved by FDA for liver or lung transplantation, but some use it.	
Hepatitis B-induced cirrhosis	Liver	See Table 14A, page 136	
Candida sp. (*CID 38:161, 2004*)	Liver	Fluconazole 200-400 mg IV/po 1 time per day starting before transplant & continuing up to 3 mos. Optimal duration unknown. Concerns for ↑ non-albicans candida with fluconazole prophylaxis [*Transpl 75:2023, 2003*]	
	HSCT	Fluconazole 400 mg po 1 time per day from day 0 to engraftment or ANC > 1000. Micafungin has also been approved for prophylaxis of Candida infections in HSCT (at recommended dose of 50 mg po q24h, *CID 39:1407, 2004*).	
Aspergillus sp.	Lung/ Heart-lung	No controlled trials to determine optimal management, but regimens of an aerosolized ampho B preparation & an oral anti-aspergillus agent have been used [*Am J Transpl 4(Suppl.10):110, 2004*]. Randomized trial suggested nebulized liposomal ABLC better tolerated than nebul. ampho B deoxycholate [*Transpl 77:232, 2004*].	
	HSCT	Itraconazole iv/po solution led to significant ↓ invasive aspergillus compared with fluconazole [*AnIM 138:705, 2003*] or significant ↓ infection with ↓ toxicity/tolerance [*Blood 103:1527, 2004*]. Study of voriconazole vs fluconazole to prevent invasive fungal infections in progress (*CID 39:S170, 2004*). Von assoc. with ↑ risk of zygomycosis [*JID 191:1350, 2005*]. Posaconazole approved for prophylaxis of invasive Aspergillus and candida in high-risk, severely immunocompromised pts (eg, HSCT w/GVHD).	
Coccidioides immitis	All	Fluconazole 400 mg po q24h [*Transpl Inf Dis 5:3, 2003*] or 200-400 mg po q24h [*Am J Transpl 6:340, 2006*]. Used in liver and renal transplant patients, respectively, with prior coccidioidomycosis	
Pneumocystis carinii (P. jiroveci) & Toxoplasma gondii	All	TMP-SMX: 1 SS tab po q24h or 1 DS tab po 1x/day to 3–7days/wk. Dur: 6 mo–1yr renal; ≥6mo for allogeneic HSCT; ≥1yr to life for heart, lung, liver [*Am J Transpl 4(Suppl.10):135, 2004*]. Breakthrough pneumocystis infections reported with atovaquone doses <1500mg/day [*CID 38:e76, 2004*]. For heart transplants, 3 mos pyrimethamine/sulfa prior to lifetime TMP-SMX prophylaxis has been suggested [*see Am J Transpl 4(Suppl.10):142, 2004*] For intensive pts regimen & alternatives	
Trypanosoma cruzi	Heart	May be transmitted from organs or transfusions. Inspect peripheral blood smear of suspected cases for parasites [*MMWR 55:798, 2006*] If known Chagas' disease in donor or recipient, contact CDC for nifurtimox (phone 404-639-3670).	

* See page 2 for abbreviations

TABLE 15F – TEMPORAL APPROACH TO DIFFERENTIAL DIAGNOSIS OF INFECTION AFTER ORGAN TRANSPLANTATION*

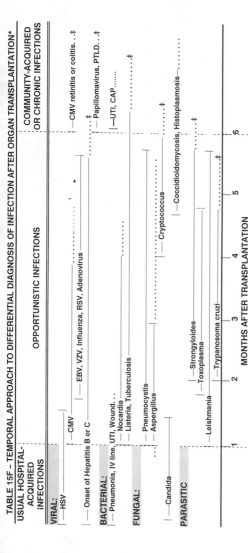

* Adapted from Fishman and Rubin, *NEJM 338:1741, 1998.* For hematopoietic stem cell transplant recipients, *see MMWR 49:RR-10, 2000.*
‡ Solid lines indicate usual time period for onset of infection; dotted lines indicate risk at reduced level. However, infection onset may be earlier or later.

[1] Symptomatic CMV antigenemia may be delayed in patients receiving 3-mo. ganciclovir prophylaxis *(Transpl Inf Dis 6:3, 2004).*

TABLE 16 – PEDIATRIC DOSAGES OF SELECTED ANTIBACTERIAL AGENTS*

*[Adapted from: (1) Nelson's Pocket Book of Pediatric Antimicrobial Therapy, 2006-2007, 16th Ed.,
J. Bradley & J. Nelson, eds., Alliance for World Wide Editing, Buenos Aires, Argentina, and
(2) 2006 Red Book, 27th Ed., American Academy of Pediatrics, pages 700–718)]*

DRUG	DOSES IN MG PER KG PER DAY OR MG PER KG AT FREQUENCY INDICATED[1]				
	BODY WEIGHT <2000 gm		BODY WEIGHT >2000 gm		>28 DAYS OLD
	0–7 days	8–28 days	0–7 days	8–28 days	
Aminoglycosides, IV or IM (check levels; some dose by gestational age + wks of life; see Nelson's Pocket Book, p. 25)					
Amikacin	7.5 q18–24h	7.5 q12h	10 q12h	10 q12h	10 q8h
Gent/tobra	2.5 q18–24h	2.5 q12h	2.5 q12h	2.5 q12h	2.5 q8h
Aztreonam, IV	30 q12h	30 q8h	30 q8h	30 q6h	30 q6h
Cephalosporins					
Cefaclor					20–40 div tid
Cefadroxil					30 div bid (max 2gm per day)
Cefazolin	25 q12h	25 q12h	25 q12h	25 q8h	25 q8h
Cefdinir					7 q12h or 14 q24h
Cefepime	30 q12h	30 q12h	30 q12h	30 q12h	150 div q8h
Cefixime					8 as q24h or div bid
Cefotaxime	50 q12h	50 q8h	50 q12h	50 q8h	50 q8h (75 q6h for meningitis)
Cefoxitin			20 q12h		80–160 div q6h
Cefpodoxime					10 div bid (max 400mg per day)
Cefprozil					15–30 div bid (max 1gm per day)
Ceftazidime	50 q12h	50 q8h	50 q12h	50 q8h	50 q8h
Ceftibuten					4.5 bid
Ceftizoxime					33–66 q8h
Ceftriaxone	25 q24h	50 q24h	25 q24h	50 q24h	50 q24h (meningitis 100)
Cefuroxime IV	50 q12h	50 q8h	50 q8h	50 q8h	50 q8h (80 q8h for meningitis)
po					10–15 div bid (max 1gm per day)
Cephalexin					25–50 div q6h (max 4gm per day)
Loracarbef					15–30 div bid (max 0.8gm per day)
Chloramphenicol IV	25 q24h	25 q12h	25 q24h	15 q12h	12.5–25 q6h (max 2–4gm per day)
Clindamycin IV	5 q12h	5 q8h	5 q8h	5 q6h	7.5 q6h
po					
Ciprofloxacin po[2]					20–30 div bid (max 1.5gm per day)
Ertapenem IV	No data	No data	No data	No data	15 q12h (max. 1g/day)
Imipenem[3] IV			25 q12h	25 q8h	15–25 q6h (max 2–4gm per day)
Linezolid	10 q12h	10 q8h	10 q8h	10 q8h	10 q8h to age 12
Macrolides					
Erythro IV & po	10 q12h	10 q8h	10 q12h	13 q8h	10 q6h
Azithro po/IV	5 q24h	10 q24h	5 q24h	10 q24h	10 q24h
Clarithro po					7.5 q12h (max. 1gm per day)
Meropenem IV	20 q12h	20 q8h	20 q12h	20 q8h	60–120 div q8h (120 for meningitis)
Metro IV & po	7.5 q24h	7.5 q12h	7.5 q12h	15 q12h	7.5 q6h
Penicillins					
Ampicillin	50 q12h	50 q8h	50 q8h	50 q6h	50 q6h
AMP-sulbactam					100–300 div q6h
Amoxicillin po				30 div bid	25–50 div tid
Amox-Clav po			30 div bid	30 div bid	45 or 90 (AM/CL-HD) div bid if over 12wks
Dicloxacillin					12–25 div q6h
Mezlocillin	75 q12h	75 q8h	75 q12h	75 q8h	75 q6h
Nafcillin, oxacillin IV	25 q12h	25 q8h	25 q8h	37 q6h	37 q6h (to max. 8–12 gm per day)
Piperacillin, PIP-tazo IV	50 q12h	100 q12h	100 q12h	100 q8h	100 q6h
Ticarcillin, T.clav IV	75 q12h	75 q8h	75 q8h	75 q6h	75 q6h
Tinidazole					> Age 3: 50mg/kg for 1 dose
Penicillin G, IV/kg IV	50,000 q12h	75,000 q8h	50,000 q8h	50,000 q6h	50,000 units/kg per day
Penicillin V					25–50mg per kg per day div q6–8h
Rifampin IV, po	10 q24h	10 q24h	10 q24h	10 q24h	10–20mg/kg per day div q4–6h
Sulfisoxazole po				120–150	120–150mg/kg per day div q4–6h
TMP-SMX po, IV; UTI: 8–12 TMP component div bid; Pneumocystis: 20 TMP component div q6h					
Tetracycline po (age 8 or older)					25–50 div q6h (>7yr old)
Doxycycline po, IV (age 8 or older)					2–4 div bid to max of 200 (>7yr old)
Vancomycin IV	12.5 q12h	15 q12h	18 q12h	22 q12h	40 div q6–8h; 60 for meningitis

[1] May need higher doses in patients with meningitis: see CID 39:1267, 2004
[2] With exception of cystic fibrosis, anthrax, and complicated UTI, not approved for use under age 18.
[3] Not recommended in children with CNS infections due to risk of seizures.
* See page 2 for abbreviations

TABLE 17A – DOSAGE OF ANTIMICROBIAL DRUGS IN ADULT PATIENTS WITH RENAL IMPAIRMENT

Adapted from DRUG PRESCRIBING IN RENAL FAILURE, 4th Ed., Aronoff et al (Eds.), American College of Physicians, 1999 and Berns et al, Renal Aspects of Antimicrobial Therapy for HIV Infection. In: P. Kimmel & J. Berns, Eds., HIV INFECTION AND THE KIDNEY, Churchill-Livingstone, 1995, pp 195–236. For review of Continuous Renal Replacement Therapy: CID 41:1159, 2005.

Drug adjustments are based on the patient's estimated endogenous creatinine clearance, which can be calculated as:

UNLESS STATED, ADJUSTED DOSES ARE AS % OF DOSE FOR NORMAL RENAL FUNCTION.

$$\frac{(140-age)(ideal\ body\ weight\ in\ kg)}{(72)(serum\ creatinine,\ mg\ per\ dL)} \quad for\ men\ (x\ 0.85\ for\ women)$$

Ideal body weight for men: 50.0 kg + 2.3 kg per inch over 5 feet
Ideal body weight for women: 45.5 kg + 2.3 kg per inch over 5 feet

For alternative methods to calculate estimated CrCl, see NEJM 354:2473, 2006.

NOTE: For summary of drugs requiring NO dosage adjustment with renal insufficiency, see Table 17B, page 176.

ANTIMICROBIAL	HALF-LIFE (NORMAL/ESRD) hr	DOSE FOR NORMAL RENAL FUNCTION§	METHOD * (see footnote§)	ADJUSTMENT FOR RENAL FAILURE Estimated creatinine clearance (CrCl), mL/min			SUPPLEMENT FOR HEMODIALYSIS, CAPD* (see footnote)	COMMENTS & DOSAGE FOR CAVH/CVVH*
				>50-90	10-50	<10		
ANTIBACTERIAL ANTIBIOTICS								
Aminoglycoside Antibiotics:			Traditional multiple daily doses—adjustment for renal disease					
Amikacin	1.4–2.3/17-150	7.5 mg per kg q12h	D&I	60-90% q12h	30-70% q12-18h **Same dose for CAVH & CVVH‡**	20-30% q24-48h	HEMO: Extra ½ of normal renal function dose AD* CAPD: 15-20 mg lost per L dialysate per day (see Comment)	High flux hemodialysis membranes lead to unpredictable aminoglycoside clearance; measure post-dialysis drug levels for efficacy and toxicity. With CAPD, pharmacokinetics highly variable—**check serum levels.** Usual method for CAPD: 2 liters of dialysis fluid placed qid or 8 liters per day (give 8Lx20 mg lost per L = 160 mg of amikacin supplement IV per day)
Gentamicin, Tobramycin	2-3/20-60	1.7 mg per kg q8h	D&I	60-90% q8-12h	30-70% q12h **Same dose for CAVH & CVVH‡**	20-30% q24-48h	HEMO: Extra ⅔ of normal renal function dose AD* CAPD: 3-4 mg lost per L dialysate per day	
Netilmicin^NUS	2-3/35-72	2.0 mg per kg q8h	D&I	50-90% q8-12h	20-60% q12h **Same dose for CAVH & CVVH‡**	10-20% q24-48h	HEMO: Extra ⅔ of normal renal function dose AD* CAPD: 3-4 mg lost per L dialysate per day	Adjust dosing weight for obesity; [ideal body weight + 0.4(actual body weight – ideal body weight)] (CID 25:112, 1997).
Streptomycin	2-3/30-80	15 mg per kg (max. of 1.0 gm) q24h	I	50% q24h	q24-72h **Same dose for CAVH & CVVH‡**	q72-96h	HEMO: Extra ½ of normal renal function dose AD* CAPD: 20-40 mg lost per L dialysate per day	

ONCE-DAILY AMINOGLYCOSIDE THERAPY: ADJUSTMENT IN RENAL INSUFFICIENCY (see Table 10D for OD dosing/normal renal function)

Creatinine Clearance (mL per min)							
Drug	>80	60-80	40-60	30-40	20-30	10-20	<10
		Dose q24h (mg per kg)				Dose q48h (mg per kg)	Dose q72h and AD*
Gentamicin/Tobramycin	5	4	3.5	2.5	4	3	2
Amikacin/kanamycin/streptomycin	15	12	7.5	4	7.5	8 q72h	3
Isepamicin^NUS	8	8	8	8 q48h	8	8 q72h	8 q96h
Netilmicin^NUS	6.5	5	4	2	3	2.5	2

‡ **CAVH** = continuous arteriovenous hemofiltration (NEJM 336:1303, 1997), usually results in CrCl of approx. 30 mL per min.; CVVH = continuous venovenous hemofiltration (CID 41:1159, 2005 & 42:436, 2006). Clearance dependent on ultrafiltration rate (21h). Dose adjustments for CAVH & CVVH are the same. * AD = after dialysis. **"Dose AD" refers to timing of dose.** §**Supplement is to replace drug lost via dialysis; extra drug beyond continuation of regimen used for CrCl <10 mL per min.**

See page 169 for other footnotes and page 2 for abbreviations.

TABLE 17A (2)

ANTIMICROBIAL	HALF-LIFE (NORMAL/ESRD) hr	DOSE FOR NORMAL RENAL FUNCTIONS	METHOD* (see footnote)	ADJUSTMENT FOR RENAL FAILURE Estimated creatinine clearance (CrCl), mL/min			SUPPLEMENT FOR HEMODIALYSIS, CAPD* (see footnote)	COMMENTS & DOSAGE FOR CAVH/CVVH*
				>50-90	10-50	<10		
Carbapenem Antibiotics								
Ertapenem	4/>4	1.0 gm q24h	D	1.0 gm q24h	0.5 gm q24h (CrCl <30)	0.5 gm q24h	HEMO: Dose as for CrCl <10; if dosed <6 hrs prior to HD, give 150 mg	↑ potential for seizures if recommended doses exceeded in pts with CrCl <20 mL per min. See pkg insert, esp. for pts <70 kg
Imipenem (see Comment)	1/4	0.5 gm q6h	D&I	250-500 mg q6-8h	250 mg q6-12h; Dose for CAVH/CVVH: 0.5-1 gm q12h (AAC 49:2421, 2005)	125-250 mg q12h	HEMO: Dose AD* CAPD: Dose for CrCl <10	
Meropenem	1/6-8	1.0 gm q8h	D&I	1.0 gm q8h	1.0 gm q12h; Same dose for CAVH/CVVH	0.5 gm q24h	HEMO: Dose AD* CAPD: Dose for CrCl <10	
Cephalosporin Antibiotics: DATA ON SELECTED PARENTERAL CEPHALOSPORINS	1.9/40-70	1.0-2.0 gm q8h						
Cefazolin	1.9/40-70	1.0-2.0 gm q8h	I	q8h	q12h; Same dose for CAVH/CVVH	q24-48h	HEMO: Extra 0.5-1 gm AD* CAPD: 0.5 gm q12h	
Cefepime	2.2/18	2.0 gm q8h (max. dose)	D&I	2 gm q8h	2 gm q12-24h; Same dose for CAVH/CVVH	1 gm q24h	HEMO: Extra 1 gm AD* CAPD: 1-2 gm q48h	CAVH/CVVH dose: As for CrCl 10-50
Cefotaxime, Ceftizoxime	1.7/15-35	2.0 gm q8h	I	q8-12h	q12-24h; Same dose for CAVH/CVVH	q12-24h	HEMO: Extra 1 gm AD* CAPD: 0.5-1 gm q24h	Active metabolite of cefotaxime in ESRD dose further for hepatic & renal failure.
Cefotetan	3.5/13-25	1-2 gm q12h	I	100%	50%	25%	HEMO: Extra 1 gm AD* CAPD: 1 gm q24h	CAVH/CVVH dose: 750 mg q12h
Cefoxitin	0.8/13-23	2.0 gm q8h	I	q8h	q8-12h; Same dose for CAVH/CVVH	q24-48h	HEMO: Extra 1 gm AD* CAPD: 1 gm q24h	May falsely increase serum creatinine by interference with assay.
Ceftazidime	1.2/13-25	2 gm q8h	I	q8-12h	q12-24h; Same dose for CAVH/CVVH	q48h	HEMO: Extra 1 gm AD* CAPD: 0.5 gm q24h	Volume of distribution increases with infection.
Cefuroxime sodium	1.2/17	0.75-1.5 gm q8h	I	q8h	q8-12h; Same dose for CAVH/CVVH	q24h	HEMO: Dose AD* CAPD: Dose for CrCl <10	CAVH/CVVH* dose: 1.5 gm, then 750 mg IV q24h
Fluoroquinolone Antibiotics								
Ciprofloxacin[NUS]	4/6-9	500-750 mg po (or 400 mg IV) q12h	D	100%	50-75%	50%	HEMO: 250 mg po or 200 mg IV q12h CAPD: 250 mg po or 200 mg IV q8h	CAVH/CVVH* dose: 200 mg IV q12h
Gatifloxacin[NUS]	7-14/36	400 mg po/IV q24h	D	400 mg q24h	400 mg, then 200 mg q24h; Same dose for CAVH/CVVH	400 mg, then 200 mg q24h	HEMO: 200 mg AD* CAPD: 200 mg q24h	CAVH/CVVH* dose: As for CrCl 10-50
Gemifloxacin	7/>7	320 mg po q24h	D	320 mg q24h	160 mg q24h	160 mg q24h	HEMO: 160 mg q24h AD*	

* **CAVH** = continuous arteriovenous hemofiltration (NEJM 336:1303, 1997) usually results in CrCl of approx. 30 mL per min; **CVVH** = continuous venovenous hemofiltration (CID 41:1159, 2005 & 42:436, 2006). Clearance dependent on ultrafiltration rate (21h). **Dose adjustments for CAVH & CVVH are the same. AD** after dialysis. **Dose at end/during of dialysis.** **Supplement is to replace drug lost via dialysis; extra drug beyond continuation of regimen used for CrCl <10 mL per min.**
See page 170 for other footnotes and page 2 for abbreviations.

TABLE 17A (3)

ANTIMICROBIAL	HALF-LIFE (NORMAL/ ESRD) hr	DOSE FOR NORMAL RENAL FUNCTIONS	METHOD (see footnote)	ADJUSTMENT FOR RENAL FAILURE Estimated creatinine clearance (CrCl), mL/min			SUPPLEMENT FOR HEMODIALYSIS/CAPD* (see footnote)	COMMENTS & DOSAGE FOR CAVH/CVVH*
				>50-90	10-50	<10		
Levofloxacin	6-51/76	750 mg q24h IV, PO	D&I	750 mg q24h	750 mg once, then 750 q48h	750 mg once, then 500 q48h	CAPD: 160 mg q24h	CAVH/CVVH* dose: As for CrCl 10-50
Macrolide Antibiotics								
Clarithromycin	5-7/22	0.5-1.0 gm q12h	D	100%	75%	50-75%	HEMO/CAPD: Dose for CrCl <10	ESRD dosing recommendations based on extrapolation
Erythromycin	1.4/5-6	250-500 mg q6h	D	100%	100%	50-75%	HEMO: Dose AD* CAPD: None	Ototoxicity with high doses in ESRD
Miscellaneous Antibacterial Antibiotics								
Colistin base	<6/≥48	80-160 mg q8h	D	160 mg q12h	160 mg q24h CrCl <30	160 mg q36h	HEMO/CAPD/CAVH: None	
Daptomycin	9.4/30	4-6 mg per kg per day	D	4-6 mg per day	4-6 mg per kg q48h	4-6 mg per kg q48h	HEMO 80 mg AD* HEMO & CAPD: 4-6 mg per kg q48h (after dialysis if possible)	LnID 6:589, 2006; CVVH: 2.5mg/kg q48h
Linezolid	6.47.1	600 mg po/IV q12h	None	600 mg q12h	600 mg q12h	600 mg q12h AD*	HEMO As for CrCl <10 CAPD: No data	CAVH/CVVH*: Accumulation of 2 metabolites—risk unknown (AAC 56:172, 2005)
Metronidazole	6-14/7-21	7.5 mg per kg q6h	D	100%	100%	50%	HEMO: Dose AD* CAPD: Dose for CrCl <10	Hemo clears metronidazole and its metabolites (AAC 29:235, 1986)
Nitrofurantoin	0.5/1	50-100 mg	D	50-100 mg	Avoid	Avoid	Not applicable	
Sulfamethoxazole	10/20-50	1.0 gm q8h	I	q12h	q18h	q24h	HEMO Extra 1 gm AD* CAPD: 1 gm q24h	
Teicoplanin^NUS	45/62-230	6 mg per kg per day	I	q24h	q48h Same dose for CAVH/CVVH‡	q72h	HEMO/CAPD: Dose for CrCl <10 CAPD: Dose for CrCl <10	
Telithromycin	10/15	800 mg q24h	D	800 mg q24h	600 mg q24h (<30 mL per min)	600 mg q24h	HEMO 600 mg AD* CAPD: No data	
Trimethoprim	11/20-49	100-200 mg q12h	D	q12h	q18h Same dose for CAVH/CVVH‡	q18h	HEMO: Dose AD* CAPD: q18h	CAVH/CVVH* dose: q18h
Trimethoprim-sulfamethoxazole-DS								
Treatment	As above	5 mg per kg IV q8h	D	100%	50%	Not recommended	HEMO/CAPD: Dose for CrCl <10	
Prophylaxis	As above	1 tab po q24h or 3 times per week	No change	100%	100%	100%		
Vancomycin	6/200-250	1 gm q12h	D&I	1 gm q12h	1 gm q24-96h	1 gm q4-7 days	HEMO/CAPD: Dose for CrCl <10	CAVH/CVVH* 500 mg q24-48h. New hemodialysis membranes ↑ clear. of vanco; **check levels**

* CAVH = continuous arteriovenous hemofiltration (NEJM 336:1303, 1997) usually results in CrCl of approx. 30 mL per min.; CVVH= continuous venovenous hemofiltration (CID 41:1159, 2005 & 42:436, 2006). Clearance dependent on ultrafiltration rate (21h). Dose adjustments for CAVH & CVVH are the same. * AD = after dialysis. **"Dose AD"** refers to timing of dose. See page 171 for other footnotes and page 2 for abbreviations. **Supplement is to replace drug lost via dialysis; extra drug beyond continuation of regimen used for CrCl <10 mL per min.**

TABLE 17A (4)

ANTIMICROBIAL	HALF-LIFE (NORMAL/ ESRD) hr	DOSE FOR NORMAL RENAL FUNCTION§	METHOD* (see footnote)	ADJUSTMENT FOR RENAL FAILURE Estimated creatinine clearance (CrCl), mL/min >50-90	10-50	<10	SUPPLEMENT FOR HEMODIALYSIS, CAPD* (see footnote)	COMMENTS & DOSAGE FOR CAVH/CVVH†
Penicillins								
Amoxicillin	1.0/5-20	250-500 mg q8h	—	q8h	q8-12h	q24h	HEMO: Dose AD* CAPD: 250 mg q12h	IV amoxicillin not available in the U.S.
Ampicillin	1.0/7-20	250 mg-2 gm q6h	—	q6h	q6-12h	q12-24h		
Amoxicillin/ Clavulanate†	1.3/4.0	500/125 mg q8h (see Comments)	D&I	500/125 mg q8h	250-500 mg AM component q12h	250-500 mg AM component q24h	HEMO: 250 mg for CrCl <10, extra dose after dialysis	If CrCl <30 per mL, **do not use 875/125 or 1000/62.5 AM/CL**
Ampicillin (AM/ Sulbactam(SB)	5-20/4.0	2 gm AM + 1.0 gm SB q6h	I	q6h	q8-12h	q24h	HEMO: Dose AD* CAPD: 2 gm AM/1 gm SB q24h	CAVH/CVVH dose: 1.5 AM/0.75 SB q12h
Aztreonam	2.0/6-8	2 gm q8h	D	100%	50-75% **Same dose for CAVH/CVVH**	25%	HEMO: Dose 0.5 gm AD* CAPD: Dose for CrCl <10	Technically is a β-lactam antibiotic.
Penicillin G	0.5/6-20	0.5-4 million U q4h	D	100%	75% **Same dose for CAVH/CVVH**	20-50%	HEMO: Dose AD* CAPD: Dose for CrCl <10	1.7 mEq potassium per million units. Potential of seizure. 6 million units per day max. dose in ESRD
Piperacillin	1.0/3-5.1	3-4 gm q4-6h	I	q4-6h	q6-8h **Same dose for CAVH/CVVH**	q8h	HEMO: Dose AD* CAPD: Dose for CrCl <10	1.9 mEq sodium per gm
Pip (P)/Tazo(T)	1.0 P/1.0 T; 3.0 P/4.0 T	3.375 gm q6h	D&I	3.375 gm q6h	2.25 gm q6h **Same dose for CAVH/CVVH**	2.25 gm q8h	HEMO: Dose for CrCl <10 + 0.75 gm AD* CAPD: Dose for CrCl <10	5.2 mEq sodium per gm
Ticarcillin	1.2/13	3 gm q4h	D&I	3 gm q4h	1-2 gm q8h **Same dose for CAVH/CVVH**	1-2 gm q12h	HEMO: Extra 3.0 gm AD* CAPD: Dose for CrCl <10	See footnote 2
Ticarcillin/ Clavulanate²	1.0 (TC)/1.0 (CL); 13 (TC)/4.0 (CL)	3.1 gm q4h	D&I	3.1 gm q4h	2.0 gm q6-8h **Same dose for CAVH/CVVH**	2.0 gm q12h	HEMO: Extra 3.1 gm AD* CAPD: 3.1 gm q12h	See footnote 2
Tetracycline Antibiotics								
Tetracycline	6-10/57-108	250-500 mg qid	I	q8-12h	q12-24h **Same dose for CAVH/CVVH**	q24h	HEMO/CAPD/CAVH: None	Avoid in ESRD
ANTIFUNGAL ANTIBIOTICS								
Amphotericin B & ampho B lipid complex	24/unchanged	Non-lipid: 0.4-1.0 mg/kg/day; ABCC: 3-6 mg/kg/day; ABLC: 5mg/kg/day; LAB: 3-5 mg/kg/day	I	q24h	q24h **Same dose for CAVH/CVVH**	q24-48h	HEMO: None CAPD: Dose for CrCl <10	For ampho B, toxicity lessened by saline loading; risk amplified by concomitant cyclosporine A, aminoglycosides, or pentamidine

1 Clavulanate cleared by liver, not kidney. Hence as dose of combination decreased, a deficiency of clavulanate may occur (JAMA 285:386, 2001).

2 Clavulanate cleared by liver, not kidney. Hence as dose of combination decreased, a deficiency of clavulanate may occur (JAMA 285:386, 2001).

* D= adjustment by Dose reduction. I= adjustment by Interval extension. CAVH= continuous arteriovenous hemofiltration (NEJM 336:1303, 1997), usually results in CrCl of approx. 30 mL per min. CVVH= continuous venovenous hemofiltration (CID 41:1159, 2005 & 42-436, 2006). Clearance dependent on ultrafiltration rate (21/l). Dose adjustment for CAVH & CVVH are based on those after dialysis + timing of dose. AD= dose after dialysis. **See page 172 for other footnotes and page 2 for abbreviations. Supplement is to replace drug lost via dialysis; extra drug beyond continuation of regimen used for CrCl <10 mL. per min.**

TABLE 17A (5)

ANTIMICROBIAL	HALF-LIFE (NORMAL/ ESRD) hr	DOSE FOR NORMAL RENAL FUNCTIONS	METHOD* (see footnote)	ADJUSTMENT FOR RENAL FAILURE Estimated creatinine clearance (CrCl) mL/min			SUPPLEMENT FOR HEMODIALYSIS, CAPD* (see footnote)	COMMENTS & DOSAGE FOR CAVH/CVVH†
				>50-90	10-50	<10		
ANTIFUNGAL ANTIBIOTICS *(continued)*								
Fluconazole	37/100	200-400 mg q24h	D	200-400 mg q24h	100-200 mg q24h Same dose for CAVH/CVVH†	100-200 mg q24h	HEMO: 100% of recommended dose AD*. CAPD: Dose for CrCl <10	
Flucytosine	3-6/75-200	37.5 mg per kg q6h	I	q12h	q12-24h Same dose for CAVH/CVVH†	q24h	HEMO: Dose AD*. CAPD: 0.5-1.0 gm q24h	Goal is peak serum level >25 mcg per mL and <100 mcg per mL
Itraconazole, po soln.	35/–	100-200 mg q12h	–	100%	100%	100%	HEMO/CAPD/CAVH/CVVH†: No adjustment with oral solution	
Itraconazole, IV	35/–	200 mg IV q12h	–	200 mg IV bid	200 mg IV bid			Do not use IV itra if CrCl <30 due to accumulation of carrier: cyclodextrin
Terbinafine	36-200/?	250 mg po per day	–	q24h				Use has not been studied. Recommend avoidance of drug.
Voriconazole, IV	Non-linear kinetics	6 mg per kg IV q12h times 2, then 4 mg per kg q12h	–	No change				If CrCl <50 mL per min, accum. of IV vehicle (cyclodextrin). Switch to po q12h. For CAVH/CVVH†: 4mg/kg po q12h
ANTIPARASITIC ANTIBIOTICS								
Pentamidine	29/118	4 mg per kg per day	I	q24h	q24h	q24-36h	HEMO/CAPD/CAVH/CVVH†: None	
Quinine	5-16/5-16	650 mg q8h	I	650 mg q8h	q8-12h Same dose for CAVH/CVVH†	650 mg q24h	HEMO: Dose AD*. CAPD: Dose for CrCl <10	Marked tissue accumulation
ANTITUBERCULOUS ANTIBIOTICS *(Excellent review: Nephron 64:169, 1993)*								
Ethambutol	4/7-15	15-25 mg per kg q24h	I	q24h	q24-36h Same dose for CAVH/CVVH†	q48h	HEMO/CAPD/CAVH/CVVH†: None	25 mg per kg q 4-6 hr prior to 3 times per wk dialysis. Streptomycin instead of ethambutol in renal failure.
Ethionamide	2.1/?	250-500 mg q12h	D	100%	100%	50%	HEMO/CAPD/CAVH/CVVH†: Dose for CrCl <10	
Isoniazid	0.7-4/8-17	5 mg per kg per day (max. 300 mg)	D	100%	100%	100%	HEMO: Dose AD*. CAPD/CAVH/CVVH†: Dose for CrCl <10	
Pyrazinamide	9/26	25 mg per kg q24h (max. dose 2.5 gm q24h)	D	25 mg per kg q24h	25 mg per kg q24h	12-25 mg per kg q24h	HEMO: 25-35 mg per kg after each dialysis. CAPD: No reduction; CAVH/CVVH†: No data	
Rifampin	1.5-5/1.8-11	600 mg per day	D	600 mg q24h	300-600 mg q24h	300-600 mg q24h	HEMO None CAPD/CAVH/CVVH†: Dose for CrCl <10	Biologically active metabolite
ANTIVIRAL AGENTS For ANTIRETROVIRALS SEE cid 40:1559, 2005.								
Acyclovir, IV	2.5/20	5-12.4 mg per kg q8h	D&I	5-12.4 mg per kg q8h	5-12.4 mg per kg q12-24h	2.5 mg per kg q24h	HEMO: Dose AD*. CAPD: Dose for CrCl <10	Rapid IV infusion can cause ↑ Cr. CAVH† dose: 3.5 mg per kg per day
Adefovir	7.5/–	10 mg po q24h	I	10 mg q24h	10 mg q48-72h	No data	HEMO: q7d AD*	
Amantadine	12/500	100 mg po bid	I	q24-48h	q48-72h	q7/days	HEMO/CAPD/CAVH/CVVH†: None	

* **CAVH** = continuous arteriovenous hemofiltration (*NEJM 336:1303, 1997*) usually results in CrCl of approx. 30 mL per min.; CVVH = continuous venovenous hemofiltration (*CID 41:1159, 2005 & 42:436, 2006*). Clearance dependent on ultrafiltration rate (21h). Dose adjustments for CAVH & CVVH are the same. **"AD"** refers to timing of dose. **"Dose AD"** refers to drug given after dialysis; extra drug lost via dialysis; **Supplement is to replace drug lost via dialysis.** See page 17:3 for other footnotes and page 2 for abbreviations.

TABLE 17A (6)

ANTIMICROBIAL	HALF-LIFE (NORMAL/ESRD) hr	DOSE FOR NORMAL RENAL FUNCTIONS	METHOD* (see footnote)	ADJUSTMENT FOR RENAL FAILURE — Estimated creatinine clearance (CrCl) mL/min >50-90	10-50	<10	SUPPLEMENT FOR HEMODIALYSIS, CAPD* (see footnote)	COMMENTS & DOSAGE FOR CAVH/CVVH*
ANTIVIRAL AGENTS For ANTIRETROVIRALS SEE *cid* 40:1559, 2005. *(continued)*								
Cidofovir Complicated dosing—see package insert								
Induction	2.5/unknown	5 mg per kg once per wk for 2 wks	–	5 mg per kg once per wk	0.5-2 mg per kg once per wk.	0.5 mg per kg once per wk.	No data	Major toxicity is renal. No efficacy, safety, or pharmacokinetic data in pts with moderate/severe renal disease.
Maintenance	2.5/unknown	5 mg per kg q2wks	–	5 mg per kg q2wks	0.5-2 mg per kg q2wks	0.5 mg per kg q2wks	No data	
Didanosine tablets¹	0.6-1.6/4.5	125-200 mg q12h buffered tabs	D	200 mg q12h	200 mg q24h	<60 kg: 150 mg q24h; >60 kg: 100 mg q24h	HEMO: Dose AD*; CAPD/CAVH/CVVH*: Dose for CrCl <10	Based on incomplete data. Data are estimates.
		400 mg q24h enteric-coated tabs	D	400 mg q24h	125-200 mg q24h	Do not use EC tabs	HEMO/CAPD: Dose for CrCl <10	If <60 kg & CrCl <10 mL per min, do not use EC tabs
Emtricitabine	10/>10	200 mg q24h	I	200 mg q24h	200 mg q48-72h	200 mg q96h	HEMO: Dose for CrCl <10	
Emtricitabine + Tenofovir	See each div q?	200-300 mg q24h	I	No change	1 tab q48h	Do not use	Do not use	Give after dialysis on dialysis days
Entecavir	128-149/?	0.5 mg q24h	D	0.5 mg q24h	0.15-0.25 mg q24h	0.05 mg q24h	HEMO/CAPD: 0.05 mg q24h	CAVH/CVVH dose: As for CrCl 10-50
Famciclovir	2.3-3.0/10-22	500 mg q8h	D&I	500 mg q8h	500 mg q12-24h; Same dose for CAVH/CVVH*	250 mg q24h	HEMO: Dose AD*; CAPD: No data	See package insert for further details

CrCl as mL per min per kg body weight—ONLY FOR FOSCARNET

			>1.4	>1.0-1.4	>0.8-1.0	>0.6-0.8	>0.5-0.6	<0.4
Foscarnet (CMV dosage) Dosage adjustment based on est. CrCl (mL per min) div. by pt's kg	Normal half-life (T½) 3 hrs with terminal T½ of 18-88 hrs. Very long with ESRD	Induction: 60mg/kg q8h;v2-3 wks IV	60 q8h	45 q8h	50 q12h	40 q12h	60 q24h	Do not use.
		Maintenance: 90-120 mg per kg per day IV	120 q24h	90 q24h	65 q24h	105 q48h	80 q48h	65 q48h Do not use

ANTIMICROBIAL	HALF-LIFE (NORMAL/ESRD) hr	DOSE FOR NORMAL RENAL FUNCTIONS	METHOD*	>50-90	10-50	<10	SUPPLEMENT FOR HEMODIALYSIS, CAPD*	COMMENTS & DOSAGE FOR CAVH/CVVH*
Ganciclovir	2.9/30	IV: Induction 5 mg per kg q12h IV	D&I	5 mg per kg q12h	2.5-5.0 mg per kg q12h	1.25-2.5 mg per kg q24h	1.25 mg per kg 3 times per wk; HEMO: Dose AD*; CAPD: Dose for CrCl <10	
		Maintenance 5 mg per kg q24h IV	D&I	2.5-5.0 mg per kg q24h	0.6-1.25 mg per kg q24h	0.625 mg per kg 3 times per wk	HEMO: 0.6 mg per kg AD*; CAPD: Dose for CrCl <10	
		po: 1.0 gm tid po.	D&I	0.5-1.0 gm q24h	0.5-1.0 gm tid	0.5 gm 3 times per week	HEMO: 0.5 gm AD*	

¹ Ref. for NRTIs and NNRTIs: *Kidney International* 60:821, 2001

* **CAVH** = continuous arteriovenous hemofiltration (*NEJM* 336:1303, 1997) usually results in CrCl of approx. 30 mL per min.; **CVVH** = continuous venovenous hemofiltration (*CID* 41:1159, 2005 & 42-436, 2006). Clearance dependent on ultrafiltration rate (21h). Dose adjustments for CAVH & CVVH are the same. **AD** = after dialysis. **Dose AD*** refers to timing of dose.
See page 174 for other footnotes and page 2 for abbreviations. **Supplement is to replace drug lost via dialysis; extra drug beyond continuation of regimen used for CrCl <10 mL per min.**

TABLE 17A (7)

ANTIMICROBIAL	HALF-LIFE (NORMAL/ ESRD) hr	DOSE FOR NORMAL RENAL FUNCTIONS	METHOD * (see footnote)	ADJUSTMENT FOR RENAL FAILURE Estimated creatinine clearance (CrCl), mL/min			SUPPLEMENT FOR HEMODIALYSIS, CAPD* (see footnote)	COMMENTS & DOSAGE FOR CAVH/CVVH†
				>50-90	10-50	<10		
ANTIVIRAL AGENTS (continued)								
Lamivudine†	5-7/15-35	300 mg po q24h	D&I	300 mg po q24h	50-150 mg q24h	25-50 mg q24h	HEMO: Dose AD*; CAPD/CAVH/CVVH†: No data	
Oseltamivir	1-3/no data	75 mg po bid	I	75 mg q12h	75 mg q24h	No data	No data	
Ribavirin	Use with caution in patients with creatinine clearance <10 mL per min.							Use with caution, little data
Rimantadine	13-65/Prolonged	100 mg bid po		100 mg q24h-bid	100 mg q24h-bid	100 mg q24h	HEMO/CAPD: No data	CAVH/CVVH† dose: As for CrCl 10-50
Stavudine, po†	1-1.4/5.5-8	30-40 mg q12h	D&I	100%	50% q12-24h **Same dose for CAVH/CVVH†**	≥60 kg: 20 mg per day <60 kg:15 mg per day	HEMO: Dose as for CrCl <10 AD* CAPD: No data	
Tenofovir, po		300 mg q24h		300 mg q24h	300 mg q48h (CrCl 30-50), 2 times per wk (CrCl 10-30)	No data	HEMO: Every 7 days or after total of 12 hr of dialysis (assumes 3 dialysis sessions of 4 hrs each).	
Valacyclovir	2.5-3.3/14	1.0 gm q8h	D&I	1.0 gm q8h	1.0 gm q12-24h **Same dose for CAVH/CVVH†**	0.5 gm q24h	HEMO: Dose AD* CAPD: Dose for CrCl <10	CAVH† dose: As for CrCl 10-50
Valganciclovir	4/67	900 mg po bid	D&I	900 mg po bid	450 mg q24h to 450 mg every other day	DO NOT USE		
Zalcitabine2	2.0/>8	0.75 mg q8h	D&I	0.75 mg q8h	0.75 mg q12h **Same dose for CAVH/CVVH†**	0.75 mg q24h	HEMO: Dose AD* CAPD: No data	CAVH/CVVH† dose: As for CrCl 10-50
Zidovudine†	1.1-1.4/1.4-3	300 mg q12h	D&I	300 mg q12h	300 mg q12h	100 mg q6-8h; if hemo, AD*	HEMO: Dose for CrCl <10 CAPD: Dose for CrCl <10	CAVH/CVVH† dose: 100 mg q8h

† **CAVH** = continuous arteriovenous hemofiltration (NEJM 336:1303, 1997); **CVVH** = continuous venovenous hemofiltration (CID 41:1159, 2005 & 42:436, 2006); ... usually results in CrCl of approx. 30 mL per min. **CVVH** = continuous venovenous hemofiltration (CID 41:1159, 2005 & 42:436, 2006) Clearance dependent on ultrafiltration rate (21h). Dose adjustments for CAVH & CVVH are the same. **AD** = after dialysis. "**Dose AD**" refers to timing of dose.
Supplement is to replace drug lost via dialysis; extra drug beyond continuation of regimen used for CrCl <10 mL per min. "**Dose AD**" refers to timing of dose.
§ Dosages are for life-threatening infections; * **D** = Dosage reduction, **I** = Interval extension; ** Per cent refers to % change from dose for normal renal function.

1 Ref. for NRTIs and NNRTIs: *Kidney International 60:821, 2001*

2 Ref. for NRTIs and NNRTIs: *Kidney International 60:821, 2001*
¶ **CVVH** = continuous arteriovenous hemofiltration (*NEJM 336:1303, 1997*) usually results in CrCl of approx. 30 mL per min., **CVVH** = continuous venovenous hemofiltration (*CID 41:1159, 2005 & 42:436, 2006*). Clearance dependent on ultrafiltration rate (21h). Dose adjustments for CAVH & CVVH are the same. **AD** = after dialysis. "**Dose AD**" refers to timing of dose. **Supplement is to replace drug lost via dialysis; extra drug beyond continuation of regimen used for CrCl <10 mL per min.**
See page 175 for other footnotes and page 2 for abbreviations.

TABLE 17B – NO DOSAGE ADJUSTMENT WITH RENAL INSUFFICIENCY BY CATEGORY*

Antibacterials		Antifungals	Anti-TBc	Antivirals	
Azithromycin	Linezolid	Andilulafngin	Rifabutin	Abacavir	Lopinavir
Ceftriaxone	Minocycline	Caspofungin	Rifapentine	Atazanavir	Nelfinavir
Chloramphenicol	Moxifloxacin	Itraconazole oral solution		Darunavir	Nevirapine
Ciprofloxacin XL	Nafcillin	Micafungin		Delavirdine	Ribavirin
Clindamycin	Pyrimethamine	Voriconazole, **po only**		Efavirenz	Saquinavir
Dirithromycin	Rifaximin			Enfuvirtide[1]	Tipranavir
Doxycycline	Tigecycline			Fosamprenavir	
				Indinavir	

[1] Enfuvirtide: Not studied in patients with CrCl <35 ml/min. DO NOT USE

TABLE 18 – ANTIMICROBIALS AND HEPATIC DISEASE DOSAGE ADJUSTMENT*

The following alphabetical list indicates antibacterials excreted/metabolized by the liver **wherein a dosage adjustment may be indicated** in the presence of hepatic disease. Space precludes details; consult the PDR or package inserts for details. List is **not** all-inclusive:

Antibacterials		Antifungals	Antivirals§	
Ceftriaxone	Nafcillin	Caspofungin	Abacavir	Indinavir
Chloramphenicol	Rifabutin	Itraconazole	Atazanavir	Lopinavir/ritonavir
Clindamycin	Rifampin	Voriconazole	Darunavir	Nelfinavir
Fusidic acid	Synercid**		Delavirdine	Nevirapine
Isoniazid	Tigecycline		Efavirenz	Rimantadine
Metronidazole	Tinidazole		Enfuvirtide	Ritonavir
			Fosamprenavir	

§ Ref. on antiretrovirals: *CID* 40:174, 2005   ** Quinupristin/dalfopristin

TABLE 19 – TREATMENT OF CAPD PERITONITIS IN ADULTS*
(Periton Dial Intl 20:396, 2000)[1]

EMPIRIC Intraperitoneal Therapy:[2] Culture Results Pending

Drug		Residual Urine Output	
		<100 mL per day	>100 mL per day
Cefazolin +	Can mix in same bag	1 gm per bag, q24h	20 mg per kg BW per bag, q24h
Ceftazidime		1 gm per bag, q24h	20 mg per kg BW per bag, q24h

Drug Doses for SPECIFIC Intraperitoneal Therapy—Culture Results Known. NOTE: Few po drugs indicated

Drug	Intermittent Dosing (once per day)		Continuous Dosing (per liter exchange)	
	Anuric	Non-Anuric	Anuric	Non-Anuric
Gentamicin	0.6mg per kg	↑ dose 25%	MD 8mg	↑ MD by 25%
Cefazolin	15mg per kg	20mg per kg	LD 500mg, MD 125mg	LD 500mg, ↑ MD 25%
Ceftazidime	1000–1500mg	ND	LD 250mg, MD 125mg	ND
Ampicillin	250–500mg po bid	ND	250–500mg po bid	ND
Ciprofloxacin	500mg po bid	ND	LD 50mg, MD 25mg	ND
Vancomycin	15–30mg per kg q5–7 days	↑ dose 25%	MD 30–50mg per L	↑ MD 25%
Metronidazole	250mg po bid	ND	250mg po bid	ND
Amphotericin B	NA	NA	MD 1.5mg	NA
Fluconazole	200mg q24h	ND	200mg q24h	ND
Itraconazole	100mg q12h	100mg q12h	100mg q12h	100mg q12h
Amp-sulbactam	2gm q12h	ND	LD 1.0gm, MD 100mg	ND
TMP-SMX	320/1600mg po q1–2 days	ND	LD 320/1600mg po, MD 80/400mg po q24h	ND

[1] All doses IP unless indicated otherwise.
   LD = loading dose, **MD** = maintenance dose, **ND** = no data; **NA** = not applicable—dose as normal renal function. **Anuric** = <100 mL per day, **non-anuric** = >100 mL per day
[2] **Does not provide treatment for MRSA.** If Gram-positive cocci on Gram stain, include vancomycin.
* See page 2 for other abbreviations

TABLE 20A – RECOMMENDED CHILDHOOD & ADOLESCENT IMMUNIZATION SCHEDULE[1]: UNITED STATES, 2006 (MMWR 54 Nos 51&52:Q1–Q4, 2006) (For overall recommendations, see MMWR 51:RR-2, 2002)

		Range of Recommended Ages			Catch-up Immunization				Assessment at Age 11–12 Years					
VACCINE	Birth	1 mo	2 mo	4 mo	6 mo	12 mo	15 mo	18 mo	24 mo	4–6 yr	11–12yr	13–14yr	15 yr	16–18yr
Hepatitis B[1]	HepB	Hep B		Hep B[1]	Hep B						HepB Series			
Diphtheria, Tetanus, Pertussis[2]			DTaP	DTaP	DTaP		DTaP			DTaP	Tdap	Tdap		
Haemophilus influenzae Type b[3]			Hib	Hib	Hib[3]	Hib								
Inactivated Poliovirus			IPV	IPV	IPV					IPV				
Measles, Mumps, Rubella[4]						MMR				MMR	MMR			
Varicella[5]						Varicella					Varicella			
Meningococcal[6]											MCV4	MCV4		
										MPSV4		MCV4		
Pneumococcal[7]			PCV	PCV	PCV	PCV				PCV	PPV			
Influenza[8]					Influenza (yearly)				Influenza (yearly)					
Hepatitis A[9]					HepA Series				HepA series					

Vaccines within broken lines are for selected populations

This schedule indicates recommended ages for routine administration of currently licensed childhood vaccines, as of 12/1/05, for children through age 18yr. Any dose not administered at recommended age should be administered at any subsequent visit, when indicated & feasible. ▨▨▨ Indicates age groups that warrant special effort to administer vaccines not previously administered. Add'l vaccines might be licensed & recommended during the year. Licensed combination vaccines may be used whenever any components of combination are indicated & other components of vaccine are not contraindicated & if approved by FDA for that dose of the series. Providers should consult respective Advisory Committee on Immunization Practices (ACIP) statements for detailed recommendations. Clinically significant adverse events that follow vaccination should be reported through the Vaccine Adverse Event Reporting System (VAERS). Guidance about how to obtain & complete a VAERS form is available at http://www.vaers.hhs.gov or by telephone, 800-822-7967.

[1] **Hepatitis B vaccine (HepB). At birth:** All newborns should receive monovalent HepB soon after birth & before hospital discharge. **Infants born to mothers who are Hep B surface antigen (HBsAg)-+** should receive HepB & 0.5 mL of Hep B immune globulin (HBIG) within 12hr of birth. **Infants born to mothers whose HBsAg status is unknown** should receive HepB within 12hr of birth. The mother should have blood drawn as soon as possible to determine HBsAg status; if HBsAg-+, infant should receive HBIG as soon as possible (no later than age 1wk). **For infants born to HBsAg-neg mothers,** birth dose can be delayed in rare circumstances but only if physician's order to withhold vaccine & a copy of mother's original HBsAg neg lab report are documented in infant's medical record. **Following birth dose:** HepB series should be completed with either monovalent HepB or combo vaccine containing HepB. Second dose should be administered at age 1–2mo. Final dose should be administered at age ≥24 wk. Administering 4 doses of HepB is permissible (e.g., when combo vaccines are administered after birth dose); however, if monovalent HepB is used, dose at age 4mo not needed. **Infants born to HBsAg-+ mothers** should be tested for HBsAg & antibody to HBsAg after completion of series at age 9–18mo(generally at next well visit after completion of series).

[2] **Diphtheria & tetanus toxoids & acellular pertussis vaccine (DTaP).** Fourth dose of DTaP may be administered as early as age 12mo, provided 6mo have elapsed since third dose & child is unlikely to return at age 15–18mo. Final dose in series should be administered at age ≥4yr. **Tetanus toxoid, reduced diphtheria toxoid, & acellular pertussis vaccine (Tdap adolescent preparation)** recommended at age 11–12yr for those who have completed recommended childhood DTP/DTaP series & have not received tetanus & diphtheria toxoids (Td) booster. Adolescents aged 13–18yr who missed age 11–12yr Td/Tdap booster should also receive single dose of Tdap if they've completed recommended childhood DTP/DTaP vaccination series. **Subsequent Td** boosters are recommended every 10yr.

[3] **Haemophilus influenzae type b conjugate vaccine (Hib).** Three Hib conjugate vaccines are licensed for infant use. If PRP-OMP (PedvaxHIB® or ComVax® [Merck]) is administered at ages 2 & 4mo, a dose at age 6mo is not required. DTaP/Hib combination products should not be used for primary immunization in infants at ages 2, 4, or 6mo but may be used as boosters after any Hib vaccine. The final dose in the series should be administered at age ≥12mo.

[4] **Measles, mumps, & rubella vaccine (MMR).** Second dose of MMR is recommended routinely at age 4–6yr but may be administered during any other visit, provided at least 4wk have elapsed since first dose & both doses are administered at or after age 12mo. Children who have not previously received second dose should complete schedule by age 11–12yr.

[5] **Varicella vaccine.** Vaccine is recommended at any visit at or after age 12mo for susceptible children (i.e., those who lack reliable history of varicella). Susceptible persons aged ≥13yr should receive 2 doses admin at least 4wk apart.

TABLE 20A (2)

6 **Meningococcal vaccine (MCV4).** Meningococcal conjugate vaccine (MCV4) should be administered to all children at age 11–12yr as well as to unvaccinated adolescents at high school entry (age 15yr). Other adolescents who wish to decrease risk may also be vaccinated. All college freshmen living in dorms should be vaccinated, pref with MCV4, although **meningococcal polysaccharide vaccine (MPSV4)** is an acceptable alternative. Vaccination against invasive meningococcal disease is recommended for children & adolescents aged ≥2yr with terminal complement deficiencies or anatomic or functional asplenia & for certain other high risk groups (see *MMWR 2005;54[No. RR-7]);* use MPSV4 for children 2–10yrs & MCV4 for older children, although MPSV4 is an acceptable alternative.

7 **Pneumococcal vaccine. The heptavalent pneumococcal conjugate vaccine (PCV)** is recommended for all children aged 2–23mo & for certain children aged 24–59mo. Final dose in series should be administered at age ≥12mo. **Pneumococcal polysaccharide vaccine (PPV)** is recommended in addition to PCV for certain high-risk groups. *See MMWR 2000;49 (No. RR-9).*

8 **Influenza vaccine.** Recommended annually for children aged ≥6mo with certain risk factors (including, but not limited to, asthma, cardiac disease, sickle cell disease, human immunodeficiency virus infection, diabetes, & conditions that can compromise respiratory function or handling of respiratory secretions or that can increase the risk for aspiration), health-care workers, & other persons (including household members) in close contact with persons in groups at high risk (see *MMWR 2005;54[No. RR-8]).* In addition, healthy children aged 6–23mo & close contacts of healthy children aged 0–5mo are recommended to receive vaccine because children in this age group are at substantially increased risk for influenza-related hospitalizations. For healthy, nonpregnant persons aged 5–49yr, the intranasally administered, live, attenuated influenza vaccine (LAIV) is an acceptable alternative to the intramuscular trivalent inactivated influenza vaccine (TIV). See *MMWR 2005;54(No. RR-8).* Children receiving TIV should be administered an age-appropriate dosage (0.25mL for children aged 6–35mo or 0.5 mL for children aged ≥3yr). Children aged ≤8yr who are receiving influenza vaccine for the first time should receive 2 doses (separated by at least 4wk for TIV & at least 6wk for LAIV).

9 **Hepatitis A vaccine (HepA).** HepA is recommended for all children at age 1yr (i.e., 12–23mo). The 2 doses in series should be administered at least 6mo apart. States, counties, & communities with existing HepA vaccination programs for children aged 2–18yr are encouraged to maintain these programs. In these areas, new efforts focused on routine vaccination of children aged 1yr should enhance, not replace, ongoing programs directed at a broader population of children. HepA is also recommended for certain high risk groups (see *MMWR 1999;48[No. RR-12]).*

Approved by the **Advisory Committee on Immunization Practices** (www.cdc.gov/nip/acip), **American Academy of Pediatrics** (www.aap.org), & the **American Academy of Family Physicians** (www.aafp.org). Add'l info about vaccines, incl precautions & contraindications for vaccination & vaccine shortages, is available at www.cdc.gov/nip or from the National Immunization Information Hotline, 800-232-2522 (English) or 800-232-0233 (Spanish).

TABLE 20B – CATCH-UP SCHEDULE (BOTH 4 MOS – 6 YRS AND 7-18 YRS)

Catch-Up Schedule For Children Aged 4 Months–6 Years

Vaccine	Min age for dose 1	Minimum interval between doses			
		Dose 1 to dose 2	Dose 2 to dose 3	Dose 3 to dose 4	Dose 4 to dose 5
DTaP[1]	6wk	4wk	4wk	6mo.	6mo.[1]
IPV[2]	6wk	4wk	4wk	4wk[2]	
HepB[3]	Birth	4wk	8wk (& 16wk after 1st dose)		
MMR[4]	12mo	4wk[4]			
Varicella	12mo				
Hib[5]	6wk	**4wk**: if 1st dose given age <12mo **8wk** (as final dose): if 1st dose given at age 12–24mo No further doses needed if 1st dose given at age ≥15mo.	**4wk**[6]: if current age <12mo **8wk** (as final dose)[6]: if current age ≥12mo & 2nd dose given at age <15mo No further doses needed if previous dose given at age ≥15mo	**8wk** (as final dose): this dose only necessary for children aged 12mo–5 yrs who received 3 doses before age 12mo	
PCV[7]	6wk	**4wk**: if 1st dose given at age <12mo & current age <24mo **8wk** (as final dose): if 1st dose given at age ≥12mo or current age 24–59mo No further doses needed for healthy children if 1st dose given at age ≥24mo	**4wk**: if current age <12mo **8wk** (as final dose): if current age ≥12mo No further doses needed for healthy children if previous dose given at age ≥24mo.	**8wk** (as final dose): this dose only necessary for children aged 12mo–5yr who received 3 doses before age 12mo	

Catch-Up Schedule for Children Aged 7–18 Years

Vaccine	Minimum interval between doses		
	Dose 1 to dose 2	Dose 2 to dose 3	Dose 3 to booster dose
Td[8]	4wk	6mo	6mo: if 1st dose given at age <12mo & current age <11 yrs, otherwise 5yr
IPV[9]	4wk	4wk	IPV[2,9]
HepB	4wk	8wk (& 16wk after 1st dose)	
MMR	4wk		
Varicella[10]	4wk		

TABLE 20B (2)

Note: A vaccine series does not require restarting, regardless of the time that has elapsed between doses.

[1] **Diphtheria & tetanus toxoids & acellular pertussis (DTaP) vaccine:** 5th dose not necessary if 4th dose given after 4th birthday.

[2] **Inactivated poliovirus (IPV) vaccine:** For children who received an all-IPV or all-oral poliovirus (OPV) series, 4th dose is not necessary if 3rd dose was given at age ≥4 yrs. If both OPV & IPV were given as part of a series, a total of 4 doses should be given, regardless of the child's current age.

[3] **Hepatitis B (HepB) vaccine:** Administer 3-dose series to all persons aged <19 yrs, if not previously vaccinated.

[4] **Measles, mumps, & rubella (MMR) vaccine:** 2nd dose of MMR is recommended routinely at age 4–6 yrs, but may be given earlier if desired.

[5] **Haemophilus influenzae type b (Hib) vaccine:** Vaccine is not generally recommended for children aged ≥5 years.

[6] **Hib vaccine:** If current age is <12 months & the first 2 doses were PRP-OMP [PedVaxHIB® or ComVax™ (Merck)], the 3rd (& final) dose should be given at age 12–15 months & at least 8wk after the 2nd dose.

[7] **Pneumococcal conjugate (PCV) vaccine:** Vaccine is not generally recommended for children aged ≥5 years.

[8] **Tetanus & diphtheria toxoids (Td):** Tdap adolescent preparation may be substituted for any dose in a primary catch-up series or as a booster if age appropriate for Tdap. A 5yr interval from the last Td dose is encouraged when Tdap is used as a booster dose. See ACIP recommendations for additional information.

[9] **IPV:** Vaccine is not generally recommended for persons aged ≥18yr.

[10] **Varicella vaccine:** Administer 2-dose series to all susceptible adolescents aged ≥13yr.

Table 20C ADULT IMMUNIZATION IN THE UNITED STATES
(MMWR 54:Q1-Q4, 2005, see also MedLett 4:47, 2006) (Travelers: see Med Lett 38:17, 1996)

Recommended Adult Immunization Schedule—United States, October 2005–September 2006

Vaccine	Age group (years)		
	19–49	50–64	≥65
Tetanus, diphtheria (Td)[1*]	1 dose booster every 10 years		
Measles, mumps, rubella (MMR)[2*]	1 or 2 doses	1 dose	
Varicella[3*]	2 doses (0, 4–8 weeks)	2 doses (0, 4–8 weeks)	
Influenza[4*]	1 dose annually	1 dose annually	
Pneumococcal (polysaccharide)[5,6]	1–2 doses		1 dose
Hepatitis A[7*]	2 doses (0, 6–12mo, or 0, 6–18mo)		
Hepatitis B[8*]	3 doses (0, 1–2, 4–6mo)		
Meningococcal[9]	1 or more doses		

☐ For all persons in this category who meet age requirements & lack evidence of immunity (eg, lack documentation of vaccination or have no evidence of prior infection)

▨ Recommended if some other risk factor is present (eg, on the basis of medical, occupational, lifestyle, or other indications)

* Covered by the Vaccine Injury Compensation Program.

NOTE: These recommendations must be read along with the footnotes.

[1] **Tetanus and diphtheria (Td) vaccination.** Adults with uncertain histories of a complete primary vaccination series with diphtheria and tetanus toxoid-containing vaccines should receive primary series using combined Td toxoid. Primary series for adults is 3 doses; administer 1st 2 doses at least 4wk apart and third dose 6–12mo after 2nd. Administer 1 dose if person received primary series and if last vaccination was received ≥10yr previously. Consult ACIP statement for recommendations for administering Td as prophylaxis in wound management (www.cdc.gov/mmwr/preview/mmwrhtml/ 00041645.htm). The American College of Physicians Task Force on Adult Immunization supports a 2nd option for Td use in adults: a single Td booster at age 50yr for persons who have completed their full pediatric series, including teenage/young adult booster. A newly licensed tetanus-diphtheria-acellular–pertussis vaccine is available for adults. ACIP recommendations for its use will be published.

[2] **Measles, mumps, rubella (MMR) vaccination.** *Measles component:* adults born before 1957 can be considered immune. Adults born during or after 1957 should receive ≥1 dose of MMR unless they have a medical contraindication, documentation of ≥1 dose, history of measles based on healthcare provider diagnosis, or lab evidence of immunity. 2nd dose of MMR is recommended for adults who 1) were recently exposed to measles or in an outbreak setting; 2) were previously vaccinated with killed measles vaccine; 3) were vaccinated with an unknown type of measles vaccine during 1963–1967; 4) are students in postsecondary educational institutions; 5) work in a health-care facility; or 6) plan to travel internationally. Withhold MMR or other measles-containing vaccines from HIV-infected persons with severe immunosuppression. *Mumps component:* 1 dose of MMR vaccine should be adequate for protection for those born during or after 1957 who lack a history of mumps based on health-care provider diagnosis or who lack laboratory evidence of immunity. *Rubella component:* administer 1 dose of MMR vaccine to women whose rubella vaccination history is unreliable or who lack laboratory evidence of immunity. For women of childbearing age, regardless of birth year, routinely determine rubella immunity and counsel women regarding congenital rubella syndrome. Do not vaccinate women who are pregnant or who might become pregnant within 4wk of receiving vaccine. Women who do not have evidence of immunity should receive MMR vaccine upon completion or termination of pregnancy and before discharge from the health-care facility.

[3] **Varicella vaccination.** Varicella vaccination is recommended for all adults without evidence of immunity to varicella. Special consideration should be given to those who 1) have close contact with persons at high risk for severe disease (health-care workers and family contacts of immunocompromised persons) or 2) are at high risk for exposure or transmission (e.g., teachers of young children; child care employees; residents and staff members of institutional settings, including correctional institutions; college students; military personnel; adolescents and adults living in households with children; nonpregnant women of childbearing age; and international travelers). Evidence of immunity to varicella in adults includes any of the following: 1) documented age-appropriate varicella vaccination (i.e., receipt of 1 dose before age 13yr or receipt of 2 doses [administered at least 4wk apart] after age 13yr); 2) US-born before 1966 or history of varicella disease before 1966 for non-US–born persons; 3) history of varicella based on health-care

TABLE 20C (2)

provider diagnosis or parental or self-report of typical varicella disease for persons born during 1966–1997 (for a patient reporting a history of an atypical, mild case, health-care providers should seek either an epidemiologic link with a typical varicella case or evidence of laboratory confirmation, if it was performed at the time of acute disease); 4) history of herpes zoster based on health-care provider diagnosis; or 5) laboratory evidence of immunity. Do not vaccinate women who are pregnant or who might become pregnant within 4wk of receiving the vaccine. Assess pregnant women for evidence of varicella immunity. Women who do not have evidence of immunity should receive dose 1 of varicella vaccine upon completion or termination of pregnancy and before discharge from the health-care facility. Dose 2 should be administered 4–8wk after dose 1.

⁴ **Influenza vaccination.** *Medical indications:* chronic disorders of cardiovascular or pulmonary systems, incl asthma; chronic metabolic diseases, incl diabetes mellitus, renal dysfunction, hemoglobinopathies, or immunosuppression (including immunosuppression caused by medications or HIV); any condition (e.g., cognitive dysfunction, spinal cord injury, seizure disorder, or other neuromuscular disorder) that compromises respiratory function or the handling of respiratory secretions or that can increase the risk for aspiration; and pregnancy during the influenza season. No data exist on the risk for severe or complicated influenza disease among persons with asplenia; however, influenza is a risk factor for secondary bacterial infections that can cause severe disease among persons with asplenia. *Occupational indications:* health-care workers and employees of long-term–care and assisted living facilities. *Other indications:* residents of nursing homes and other long-term–care and assisted living facilities; persons likely to transmit influenza to persons at high risk (i.e., in-home household contacts and caregivers of children aged 0–23mo; or persons of all ages with high-risk conditions), and anyone who wishes to be vaccinated. For healthy, nonpregnant persons aged 5–49yr without high-risk conditions who are not contacts of severely immunocompromised persons in special care units, intranasally administered influenza vaccine (FluMist®) may be administered in lieu of inactivated vaccine.

⁵ **Pneumococcal polysaccharide vaccination.** *Medical indications:* chronic disorders of the pulmonary system (excluding asthma); cardiovascular diseases; diabetes mellitus; chronic liver diseases, including liver disease as a result of alcohol abuse (e.g., cirrhosis); chronic renal failure or nephrotic syndrome; functional or anatomic asplenia (e.g., sickle cell disease or splenectomy [if elective splenectomy is planned, vaccinate at least 2wk before surgery]); immunosuppressive conditions (e.g., congenital immunodeficiency, HIV infection [vaccinate as close to diagnosis as possible when CD4 cell counts are highest]; leukemia, lymphoma, multiple myeloma, Hodgkin disease, generalized malignancy, or organ or bone marrow transplantation]; chemotherapy with alkylating agents, antimetabolites, or long-term systemic corticosteroids; and cochlear implants. *Other indications:* Alaska Natives and certain American Indian populations; residents of nursing homes and other long-term–care facilities.

⁶ **Revaccination with pneumococcal polysaccharide vaccine.** One-time revaccination after 5yr for persons with chronic renal failure or nephrotic syndrome; functional or anatomic asplenia (e.g., sickle cell disease or splenectomy); immunosuppressive conditions (e.g., congenital immunodeficiency, HIV infection, leukemia, lymphoma, multiple myeloma, Hodgkin disease, generalized malignancy, or organ or bone marrow transplantation]; or chemotherapy with alkylating agents, antimetabolites, or long-term systemic corticosteroids. For persons aged ≥65yr, one-time revaccination if they were vaccinated ≥5yr previously and were aged <65yr at the time of primary vaccination.

⁷ **Hepatitis A vaccination.** *Medical indications:* persons with clotting-factor disorders or chronic liver disease. *Behavioral indications:* men who have sex with men or users of illegal drugs. *Occupational indications:* Persons working with hepatitis A virus (HAV)–infected primates or with HAV in a research laboratory setting. *Other indications:* persons traveling to or working in countries that have high or intermediate endemicity of hepatitis A (for list of countries, see http://www.cdc.gov/travel/ diseases.htm#hepa) as well as any person wishing to obtain immunity. Current vaccines should be administered in a 2-dose series at either 0 and 6–12mo, or 0 and 6–18mo. If the combined hepatitis A and hepatitis B vaccine is used, administer 3 doses at 0, 1, and 6mo.

⁸ **Hepatitis B vaccination.** *Medical indications:* hemodialysis patients (use special formulation [40 µg/mL] or two 20-µg/mL doses) or patients who receive clotting-factor concentrates. *Occupational indications:* health-care workers and public-safety workers who have exposure to blood in the workplace and persons in training in schools of medicine, dentistry, nursing, laboratory technology, and other allied health professions. *Behavioral indications:* injection drug users; persons with more than one sex partner during the previous 6mo; persons with a recently acquired sexually transmitted disease (STD); and men who have sex with men. *Other indications:* household contacts and sex partners of persons with chronic hepatitis B virus (HBV) infection; clients and staff members of institutions for developmentally disabled persons; all clients of STD clinics; inmates of correctional facilities; and international travelers who will be in countries with high or intermediate prevalence of chronic HBV infection for more than 6mo (for list of countries, see http://www.cdc.gov/travel/diseases.htm#hepa).

⁹ **Meningococcal vaccination.** *Medical indications:* adults with anatomic or functional asplenia or terminal complement component deficiencies. *Other indications:* first-year college students living in dormitories; microbiologists who are routinely exposed to isolates of *Neisseria meningitidis;* military recruits; and persons who travel to or reside in countries in which meningococcal disease is hyperendemic or epidemic (e.g., the "meningitis belt" of sub- Saharan Africa during the dry season [December–June]), particularly if contact with local populations will be prolonged. Vaccination is required by the government of Saudi Arabia for all travelers to Mecca during the annual Hajj. Meningococcal conjugate vaccine is preferred for adults meeting any of the above indications who are aged ≤55yr, although meningococcal polysaccharide vaccine (MPSV4) is an acceptable alternative. Revaccination after 5yr might be indicated for adults previously vaccinated with MPSV4 who remain at high risk for infection (e.g., persons residing in areas in which disease is epidemic).

¹⁰ **Selected conditions for which *Haemophilus influenzae* type b (Hib) vaccine may be used.** Hib conjugate vaccines are licensed for children aged 6–71mo. No efficacy data are available on which to base a recommendation concerning use of Hib vaccine for older children and adults with the chronic conditions associated with an increased risk for Hib disease. However, studies suggest good immunogenicity in patients who have sickle cell disease, leukemia, or HIV infection or who have had splenectomies; administering vaccine to these patients is not contraindicated.

181

TABLE 20C (3)

This schedule indicates the recommended age groups for routine administration of currently licensed vaccines for persons aged ≥19yr. Licensed combination vaccines may be used whenever any components of the combination are indicated & when vaccine's other components are not contraindicated. For detailed recommendations, consult manufacturers' package inserts and the complete statements from ACIP (www.cdc.gov/nip/publications/acip-list.htm).

Report all clinically significant post vaccination reactions to the Vaccine Adverse Event Reporting System (VAERS). Reporting forms & instructions on filing a VAERS report are available by telephone, 800-822-7967, or from the VAERS website at www.vaers.hhs.gov.

Information on how to file a Vaccine Injury Compensation Program claim is available at www.hrsa.gov/osp/vicp or by telephone, 800-338-2382. To file a claim for vaccine injury, contact the US Court of Federal Claims, 717 Madison Place, NW, Washington, DC 20005, telephone 202-357-6400.

Additional info about the vaccines listed above & contraindications for vaccination are available at www.cdc.gov/nip or from the CDC-INFO Contact Center at 800-CDC-INFO (232-4636) in English and Spanish, 24hr/day, 7days/wk.

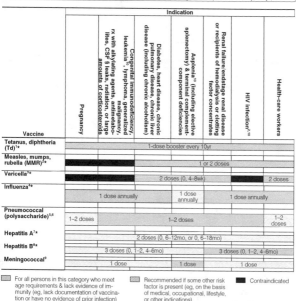

Vaccine	Pregnancy	Congenital immunodeficiency, leukemia[10], lymphoma, generalized malignancy, rx with alkylating agents, antimetabolites, CSF § leaks, radiation, or large amounts of corticosteroids	Diabetes, heart disease, chronic pulmonary disease, chronic liver disease (including chronic alcoholism)	Asplenia[10] (including elective splenectomy) & terminal complement-component deficiencies	Renal failure/endstage renal disease or recipients of hemodialysis or clotting factor concentrates	HIV infection[2,10]	Health-care workers
Tetanus, diphtheria (Td)¹*	1-dose booster every 10yr						
Measles, mumps, rubella (MMR)²*	■	■	1 or 2 doses				
Varicella³*	■	■	2 doses (0, 4–8wk)				2 doses
Influenza⁴*	1 dose annually			1 dose annually	1 dose annually		
Pneumococcal (polysaccharide)⁵,⁶	1–2 doses		1–2 doses				1–2 doses
Hepatitis A⁷*	2 doses (0, 6–12mo, or 0, 6–18mo)						
Hepatitis B⁸*	3 doses (0, 1–2, 4–6mo)				3 doses (0, 1–2, 4–6mo)		
Meningococcal⁹	1 dose			1 dose		1 dose	

░ For all persons in this category who meet age requirements & lack evidence of immunity (eg, lack documentation of vaccination or have no evidence of prior infection)   ▨ Recommended if some other risk factor is present (eg, on the basis of medical, occupational, lifestyle, or other indications)   ■ Contraindicated

* Covered by the Vaccine Injury Compensation Program
§ Cerebrospinal fluid

TABLE 20D –VACCINES LICENSED BY FDA IN US IN 2006 AND RECOMMENDED BY ACIP (NOT YET INCORPORATED INTO CDC/MMWR RECOMMENDATIONS IN TABLE 20A)

Vaccine	Comments
Human-Bovine reassortant rotavirus vaccine (RotaTeq)	Rotavirus vaccine for routine administration to infants in 3 doses at ages 2, 4, & 6mo
Live-attenuated varicella-Zoster virus vaccine (Zostavax)	Single-dose vaccine for prevention of herpes zoster in persons ≥60yr. Approved by USFDA 5/25/06. (Recommendations from ACIP expected in Q4 2006.)
Quadravalent Human Papillomavirus (Types 6, 11, 16, 18) Recombinant Vaccine (Gardasil, Cervarix)	Indicated in girls 9–26yr old to prevent cervical cancer, precancerous lesions, & genital warts caused by HPV 6, 11, 16, & 18. Administered in 3 separate IM injections in upper arm over 6mo period (months 0, 2, & 6). (Provisional recommendation by ACIP 8/14/06)

TABLE 20E –ANTI-TETANUS PROPHYLAXIS, WOUND CLASSIFICATION, IMMUNIZATION

WOUND CLASSIFICATION			IMMUNIZATION SCHEDULE				
Clinical Features	Tetanus Prone	Non-Tetanus Prone	History of Tetanus Immunization	Dirty, Tetanus-Prone Wound		Clean, Non-Tetanus Prone Wound	
				Td[1,2]	TIG	Td	TIG
Age of wound	> 6 hours	≤ 6 hours	Unknown or < 3 doses	Yes	Yes	Yes	No
Configuration	Stellate, avulsion	Linear					
Depth	> 1 cm	≤ 1 cm	3 or more doses	No[3]	No	No[4]	No
Mechanism of injury	Missile, crush, burn, frostbite	Sharp surface (glass, knife)					
Devitalized tissue	Present	Absent					
Contaminants (dirt, saliva, etc.)	Present	Absent					

[1] Td = Tetanus & diphtheria toxoids adsorbed (adult)
TIG = Tetanus immune globulin (human)
[2] Yes if wound >24hr old.
For children <7yr, DPT, DT if pertussis vaccine contraindicated);
For persons ≥7yr, Td preferred to tetanus toxoid alone.
[3] Yes if >5 years since last booster
[4] Yes if >10 years since last booster

(From ACS Bull. 69:22,23, 1984, No. 10) *(From MMWR 39:37, 1990; MMWR 46(SS-2):15, 1997)*

TABLE 20F –RABIES POST-EXPOSURE PROPHYLAXIS
All wounds should be cleaned immediately & thoroughly with soap & water. This has been shown to protect 90% of experimental animals![1]

Post-Exposure Prophylaxis Guide, United States, 2000 *(CID 30:4, 2000; NEJM 351:2626, 2004)*

Animal Type	Evaluation & Disposition of Animal	Recommendations for Prophylaxis
Dogs, cats, ferrets	Healthy & available for 10-day observation	Don't start unless animal develops sx, then immediately begin HRIG + HDCV or RVA
	Rabid or suspected rabid	Immediate vaccination
	Unknown (escaped)	Consult public health officials
Skunks, raccoons, bats,* foxes, coyotes, most carnivores	Regard as rabid	Immediate vaccination
Livestock, rodents, rabbits; includes hares, squirrels, hamsters, guinea pigs, gerbils, chipmunks, rats, mice, woodchucks		Almost never require anti-rabies rx. Consult public health officials.

* Most recent cases of human rabies in U.S. due to contact (not bites) with silver-haired bats or rarely big brown bats *(MMWR 46:770, 1997; AnIM 128:922, 1998). For more detail, see CID 30:4, 2000; JAVMA 219:1687, 2001; CID 37:96, 2003 (travel medicine advisory); Ln 363:959, 2004; EID 11:1921, 2005; MMWR 55 (RR-5), 2006.*

Post-Exposure Rabies Immunization Schedule
IF NOT PREVIOUSLY VACCINATED

Treatment	Regimen[2]
Local wound cleaning	**All post-exposure treatment should begin with immediate, thorough cleaning of all wounds with soap & water.**
Human rabies immune globulin (HRIG)	20 units per kg body given once on day 0. If anatomically feasible, the full dose should be infiltrated around the wound(s), the rest should be administered IM in the gluteal area. HRIG should **not** be administered in the **same syringe**, **or** into the **same anatomical site** as vaccine, or more than 7 days after the initiation of vaccine. Because HRIG may partially suppress active production of antibody, no more than the recommended dose should be given.[3]
Vaccine	Human diploid cell vaccine (HDCV), rabies vaccine adsorbed (RVA), or purified chick embryo cell vaccine (PCEC) 1.0 mL **IM (deltoid area[4])**, one each days 0, 3, 7, 14, & 28.

IF PREVIOUSLY VACCINATED[5]

Treatment	Regimen[2]
Local wound cleaning	All post-exposure treatment should begin with immediate, thorough cleaning of all wounds with soap & water.
HRIG	HRIG should **not** be administered
Vaccine	HDCV, RVA or PCEC, 1.0 mL **IM (deltoid area[4])**, one each on days 0 & 3

CORRECT VACCINE ADMINISTRATION SITES

Age Group	Administration Site
Children & adults	**DELTOID[4]** only (**NEVER** in gluteus)
Infants & young children	Outer aspect of thigh (anterolateral thigh) may be used (**NEVER** in gluteus)

[1] From *MMWR 48:RR-1, 1999; CID 30:4, 2000;* B.T. Matyas, Mass. Dept. of Public Health
[2] These regimens are applicable for all age groups, including children.
[3] In most reported post-exposure treatment failures, only identified deficiency was failure to infiltrate wound(s) with HRIG *(CID 22:228, 1996)*. However, several failures reported from SE Asia in patients in whom WHO protocol followed *(CID 28:143, 1999)*.
[4] The **deltoid** area is the **only** acceptable site of vaccination for adults & older children. For infants & young children, outer aspect of the thigh (anterolateral thigh) may be used. Vaccine should **NEVER** be administered in gluteal area.
[5] Any person with a history of pre-exposure vaccination with HDCV, RVA, PCEC; prior post-exposure prophylaxis with HDCV, RVA, PCEC; or previous vaccination with any other type of rabies vaccine & a documented history of antibody response to the prior vaccination

TABLE 21 SELECTED DIRECTORY OF RESOURCES

ORGANIZATION	PHONE/FAX	WEBSITE(S)
ANTIPARASITIC DRUGS & PARASITOLOGY INFORMATION *(CID 37:694, 2003)*		
CDC	Weekdays: 404-639-3670	www.cdc.gov/ncidod/srp/drugs/drug-service.html
	Evenings, weekends, holidays: 404-639-2888	
DPDx: Lab ID of parasites		www.dpd.cdc.gov/dpdx/default.htm
Gorgas Course Tropical Medicine		http://info.dom.uab.edu/gorgas
Panorama Compound. Pharm.	800-247-9767/818-787-7256	www.uniquerx.com
Parasites & Health		www.dpd.cdc.gov/dpdx/HTML/Para_Health.htm
BIOTERRORISM		
Centers for Disease Control & Prevention	770-488-7100	www.bt.cdc.gov
Infectious Diseases Society of America	703-299-0200/	www.idsociety.org
Johns Hopkins Center Civilian Biodefense		www.jhsph.edu
Center for Biosecurity of the Univ. of Pittsburgh Med. Center		www.upmc-biosecurity.org
US Army Medical Research Institute of Inf. Dis.		www.usamriid.army.mil
HEPATITIS C *(CID 35:754, 2002)*		
CDC		www.cdc.gov/ncidod/diseases/hepatitis/C
Individual		http://hepatitis-central.com
Medscape		www.medscape.com
HIV		
General		
HIV InSite		http://hivinsite.ucsf.edu
Johns Hopkins AIDS Service		www.hopkins-aids.edu
Drug Interactions		
Johns Hopkins AIDS Service		www.hopkins-aids.edu
Liverpool HIV Pharm. Group		www.hiv-druginteractions.org
Other		http://AIDS.medscape.com
Prophylaxis/Treatment of Opportunistic Infections; HIV Treatment		www.aidsinfo.nih.gov
IMMUNIZATIONS *(CID 36:355, 2003)*		
CDC, Natl. Immunization Program	404-639-8200	www.cdc.gov/nip
FDA, Vaccine Adverse Events	800-822-7967	www.fda.gov/cber/vaers/vaers.htm
National Network Immunization Info.	877-341-6644	www.immunizationinfo.org
Influenza vaccine, CDC	404-639-8200	www.cdc.gov/nip/flu
Institute for Vaccine Safety		www.vaccinesafety.edu
OCCUPATIONAL EXPOSURE, BLOOD-BORNE PATHOGENS (HIV, HEPATITIS B & C)		
National Clinicians' Post-Exposure Hotline	888-448-4911	www.ucsf.edu/hivcntr
Q-T$_c$ INTERVAL PROLONGATION BY DRUGS		www.qtdrugs.org
SEXUALLY TRANSMITTED DISEASES		www.cdc.gov/std/treatment/TOC2002TG.htm
	Slides:	http://www.phac-aspc.gc.ca/slm-maa/slides/index.html
TRAVELERS' INFO: Immunizations, Malaria Prophylaxis, More		
Amer. Soc. Trop. Med. & Hyg.		www.astmh.org
CDC, general	877-394-8747/888-232-3299	www.cdc.gov/travel/index.htm
CDC, Malaria:		www.cdc.gov/malaria
Prophylaxis		www.cdc.gov/travel
Treatment	770-488-7788	www.who.int/health_topics/malaria
MD Travel Health		www.mdtravelhealth.com
Pan American Health Organization		www.paho.org
World Health Organization (WHO)		www.who.int/home-page
VACCINE & IMMUNIZATION RESOURCES *(CID 36:355, 2003)*		
American Academy of Pediatrics		www.cispimmunize.org
CDC, National Immunization Program		www.cdc.gov/nip
National Network for Immunization Information		www.immunizationinfo.org

TABLE 22A – ANTI-INFECTIVE DRUG-DRUG INTERACTIONS

Importance: ± = theory/anecdotal; + = of probable importance; ++ = of definite importance

ANTI-INFECTIVE AGENT (A)	OTHER DRUG (B)	EFFECT	IMPORT
Amantadine (Symmetrel)	Alcohol	↑ CNS effects	+
	Anticholinergic and anti-Parkinson agents (ex. Artane, scopolamine)	↑ effect of B: dry mouth, ataxia, blurred vision, slurred speech, toxic psychosis	+
	Trimethoprim	↑ levels of A & B	+
	Digoxin	↑ levels of B	±
Aminoglycosides—parenteral (amikacin, gentamicin, kanamycin, netilmicin, sisomicin, streptomycin, tobramycin) *NOTE: Capreomycin is an aminoglycoside, used as alternative drug to treat mycobacterial infections.*	Amphotericin B	↑ nephrotoxicity	++
	Cis platinum (Platinol)	↑ nephro & ototoxicity	+
	Cyclosporine	↑ nephrotoxicity	+
	Neuromuscular blocking agents	↑ apnea or respiratory paralysis	+
	Loop diuretics (e.g., furosemide)	↑ ototoxicity	++
	NSAIDs	↑ nephrotoxicity	+
	Non-polarizing muscle relaxants	↑ apnea	+
	Radiographic contrast	↑ nephrotoxicity	+
	Vancomycin	↑ nephrotoxicity	+
Aminoglycosides— oral (kanamycin, neomycin)	**Oral anticoagulants (dicumarol, phenindione, warfarin)**	↑ prothrombin time	+
Amphotericin B and ampho B lipid formulations	Antineoplastic drugs	↑ nephrotoxicity risk	+
	Digitalis	↑ toxicity of B if K⁺ ↓	+
	Nephrotoxic drugs: aminoglycosides, cidofovir, cyclosporine, foscarnet, pentamidine	↑ nephrotoxicity of A	++
Ampicillin, amoxicillin	Allopurinol	↑ frequency of rash	++
Amprenavir and fosamprenavir	Antiretrovirals—see Table 22B & Table 22C		
	Contraceptives, oral	↓ levels of A; use other contraception	++
	Lovastatin/simvastatin	↑ **levels of B—avoid**	++
	Methadone	↓ levels of A & B	++
	Rifabutin	↑ levels of B (↓ dose by 50–75%)	++
	Rifampin	↓ **levels of A—avoid**	++
Atazanavir	See protease inhibitors and Table 22B & Table 22C		
Atovaquone	Rifampin (perhaps rifabutin)	↓ serum levels of A; ↑ levels of B	+
	Metoclopramide	↓ levels of A	+
	Tetracycline	↓ levels of A	++

Azole Antifungal Agents¹ [**Flu** = fluconazole, **Itr** = itraconazole, **Ket** = ketoconazole, **Posa** = posaconazole **Vor** = voriconazole, + = occurs, *blank space* = either studied & no interaction OR no data found (may be in pharm. co. databases)]

Flu	Itr	Ket	Posa	Vor	OTHER DRUG (B)	EFFECT	IMPORT
+	+				Amitriptyline	↑ levels of B	+
+	+	+	+	+	Calcium channel blockers	↑ levels of B	++
		+		+	Carbamazepine (vori contraind)	↓ levels of B, ↑ risk of nephrotoxicity	++
+	+	+	+	+	Cyclosporine	↑ levels of B, ↑ risk of nephrotoxicity	+
	+	+			Didanosine	↓ absorption of A	+
+	+			+	Efavirenz	↓ levels of A, ↑ levels of B	++ (avoid)
	+	+		+	H₂ blockers, antacids, sucralfate	↓ absorption of A	+
+	+	+	+	+	Hydantoins (phenytoin, Dilantin)	↑ levels of B, ↓ levels of A	++
	+	+			Isoniazid	↓ levels of A	+
		+	+	+	Lovastatin/simvastatin	Rhabdomyolysis reported; ↑ levels of B	++
+	+	+	+	+	Midazolam/triazolam, po	↑ levels of B	++
+	+	+		+	Oral anticoagulants	↑ effect of B	++
+	+	+			Oral hypoglycemics	↑ levels of B	++
		+	+	+	Pimozide	↑ levels of B—**avoid**	++
	+	+		+	Protease inhibitors	↑ levels of B	++
	+	+		+	Proton pump inhibitors	↓ absorption of A, ↑ levels of B	++
+	+	+	+	+	Rifampin/rifabutin (vori contraindicated)	↑ levels of B, ↓ serum levels of A	++
			+	+	Sirolimus (vori contraindicated)	↑ levels of B	++
+	+	+	+		Tacrolimus	↑ levels of B with toxicity	++
+	+				Theophyllines	↑ levels of B	+
	+	+			Trazodone	↑ levels of B	++
+					Zidovudine	↑ levels of B	+
Caspofungin					Cyclosporine	↑ levels of A	++
					Tacrolimus	↓ levels of B	++
					Carbamazepine, dexamethasone, efavirenz, nevirapine, phenytoin, rifamycin	↓ levels of A; ↑ dose of caspofungin to 70 mg/d	++

¹ Major interactions given; unusual or minor interactions manifest as toxicity of non-azole drug due to ↑ serum levels: Caffeine (Flu), digoxin (Itr), felodipine (Itr), fluoxetine (Itr), indinavir (Ket), lovastatin/simvastatin, quinidine (Ket), tricyclics (Flu), vincristine (Itr), and ↓ effectiveness of oral contraceptives.

TABLE 22A (2)

ANTI-INFECTIVE AGENT (A)	OTHER DRUG (B)	EFFECT	IMPORT
Cephalosporins with methyl-tetrathiozolethiol side-chain	Oral anticoagulants (dicumarol, warfarin), heparin, thrombolytic agents, platelet aggregation inhibitors	↑ effects of B, bleeding	+
Chloramphenicol	Hydantoins	↑ toxicity of B, nystagmus, ataxia	++
	Iron salts, Vitamin B12	↓ response to B	++
	Protease inhibitors---HIV	↑ levels of A & B	++
Clindamycin (Cleocin)	Kaolin	↓ absorption of A	+
	Muscle relaxants, e.g., atracurium, baclofen, diazepam	↑ frequency/duration of respiratory paralysis	+
Cycloserine	Ethanol	↑ frequency of seizures	+
	INH, ethionamide	↑ frequency of drowsiness/dizziness	+
Dapsone	Didanosine	↓ absorption of A	+
	Oral contraceptives	↓ effectiveness of B	+
	Pyrimethamine	↑ in marrow toxicity	+
	Rifampin/Rifabutin	↓ serum levels of A	+
	Trimethoprim	↑ levels of A & B (methemoglobinemia)	+
	Zidovudine	May ↑ marrow toxicity	+
Daptomycin	HMG-CoA inhibitors (statins)	DC statin while on dapto	++
Delavirdine (Rescriptor)	See non-nucleoside reverse transcriptase inhibitors (NNRTIs) and Table 22C		
Didanosine (ddl) (Videx)	Cisplatin, dapsone, INH, metronidazole, nitrofurantoin, stavudine, vincristine, zalcitabine	↑ risk of peripheral neuropathy	+
	Ethanol, lamivudine, pentamidine	↑ risk of pancreatitis	+
	Fluoroquinolones	↓ absorption 2° to chelation	+
	Drugs that need low pH for absorption: dapsone, indinavir, itra/ketoconazole, pyrimethamine, rifampin, trimethoprim	↓ absorption	+
	Methadone	↓ levels of A	++
	Ribavirin	↑ levels ddl metabolite—**avoid**	++
	Tenofovir	↑ levels of A **(reduce dose of A)**	++
Doxycycline	Aluminum, bismuth, iron, Mg++	↓ absorption of A	+
	Barbiturates, hydantoins	↓ serum t/2 of A	+
	Carbamazepine (Tegretol)	↓ serum t/2 of A	+
	Digoxin	↑ serum levels of B	+
	Warfarin	↑ activity of B	++
Efavirenz (Sustiva)	See non-nucleoside reverse transcriptase inhibitors (NNRTIs) and Table 22C		
Ertapenem (Invanz)	Probenecid	↑ levels of A	++
Ethambutol (Myambutol)	Aluminum salts (includes didanosine buffer)	↓ absorption of A & B	+

Fluoroquinolones (*Cipro* = ciprofloxacin; *Gati* = gatifloxacin; *Gemi* = gemifloxacin; *Levo* = levofloxacin; *Lome* = lomefloxacin; *Moxi* = moxifloxacin; *Oflox* = ofloxacin)
NOTE: Blank space = either studied and no interaction OR no data found (pharm. co. may have data)

Cipro	Gati	Gemi	Levo	Lome	Moxi	Oflox	OTHER DRUG (B)	EFFECT	IMPORT
+			+	+	+		**Antiarrhythmics (procainamide, amiodarone)**	↑ Q-T interval (torsade)	++
+	+		+	+	+	+	Insulin, oral hypoglycemics	↑ & ↓ blood sugar	++
+							Caffeine	↑ levels of B	+
+							Cimetidine	↑ levels of B	+
+			+		+		Cyclosporine	↑ levels of B	±
+	+					+	Didanosine	↓ absorption of A	++
+	+	+	+	+	+	+	**Cations: Al+++, Ca++, Fe+++, Mg++, Zn++ (antacids, vitamins, dairy products), citrate/citric acid**	↓ absorption of A (some variability between drugs)	++
+							Foscarnet	↑ risk of seizures	+
+							Methadone	↑ levels of B	++
+			+		+		NSAIDs	↑ risk CNS stimulation/seizures	++
+							Phenytoin	↑ or ↓ levels of B	+
+	+		+				Probenecid	↓ renal clearance of A	+
+	+	+	+		+		**Sucralfate**	↓ absorption of A	++
+							Theophylline	↑ levels of B	++
+							Thyroid hormone	↓ levels of B	++
+							Tizanidine	↓ levels of B	++
+			+	+	+	+	Warfarin	↑ prothrombin time	+

ANTI-INFECTIVE AGENT (A)	OTHER DRUG (B)	EFFECT	IMPORT
Foscarnet (Foscavir)	Ciprofloxacin	↑ risk of seizures	+
	Nephrotoxic drugs: aminoglycosides, ampho B, cis-platinum, cyclosporine	↑ risk of nephrotoxicity	+
	Pentamidine IV	↑ risk of severe hypocalcemia	++
Ganciclovir (Cytovene)	Imipenem	↑ risk of seizures reported	+
	Probenecid	↑ levels of A	+
	Zidovudine	↓ levels of A, ↑ levels of B	+

TABLE 22A (3)

ANTI-INFECTIVE AGENT (A)	OTHER DRUG (B)	EFFECT	IMPORT
Gentamicin	See Aminoglycosides—parenteral		
Indinavir	See protease inhibitors and Table 22B & Table 22C		
Isoniazid	**Alcohol, rifampin**	**↑ risk of hepatic injury**	++
	Aluminum salts	↓ absorption (take fasting)	++
	Carbamazepine, phenytoin	↑ levels of B with nausea, vomiting, nystagmus, ataxia	++
	Itraconazole, ketoconazole	↓ levels of B	+
	Oral hypoglycemics	↓ effects of B	+
Lamivudine	Zalcitabine	**Mutual interference—do not combine**	++
Linezolid (Zyvox)	Adrenergic agents	Risk of hypertension	++
	Aged, fermented, pickled or smoked foods —↑ tyramine	Risk of hypertension	+
	Rifampin	↓ levels of A	++
	Serotonergic drugs (SSRIs)	Risk of serotonin syndrome	++
Lopinavir	See protease inhibitors		

Macrolides [**Ery** = erythromycin, **Azi** = azithromycin, **Clr** = clarithromycin; **Dir** = dirithromycin, + = occurs, **blank space** = either studied and no interaction OR no data (pharm. co. may have data)]

Ery	Dir	Azi	Clr		EFFECT	IMPORT
+	+		+	Carbamazepine	↑ serum levels of B, nystagmus, nausea, vomiting, ataxia	++ (avoid w/ erythro)
+			+	Cimetidine, **ritonavir**	↑ levels of B	+
+			+	Clozapine	↑ serum levels of B, CNS toxicity	+
			+	**Colchicine**	↑ levels of B (potent, fatal)	++ (avoid)
+			+	Corticosteroids	↑ effects of B	+
+	+	+	+	Cyclosporine	↑ serum levels of B with toxicity	+
+	+	+	+	Digoxin, digitoxin	↑ serum levels of B (10% of cases)	+
			+	Efavirenz	↓ levels of A	++
+	+		+	Ergot alkaloids	↑ levels of B	++
+			+	Lovastatin/simvastatin	↑ levels of B; rhabdomyolysis	++
+			+	Midazolam, triazolam	↑ levels of B, ↑ sedative effects	+
+			+	Phenytoin	↑ levels of B	+
+	+		+	Pimozide	**Q-T interval**	++
+			+	Rifampin, rifabutin	↓ levels of B	+
+			+	Tacrolimus	↑ levels of B	++
+				Theophyllines	↑ serum levels of B with nausea, vomiting, seizures, apnea	++
+	+		+	Valproic acid	↑ levels of B	+
+	+		+	Warfarin	May ↑ prothrombin time	+
			+	Zidovudine	↓ levels of B	+

ANTI-INFECTIVE AGENT (A)	OTHER DRUG (B)	EFFECT	IMPORT
Mefloquine	ß-adrenergic blockers, calcium channel blockers, quinidine, quinine	↑ arrhythmias	+
	Divalproex, valproic acid	↓ level of B with seizures	++
	Halofantrine	Q-T prolongation	++ (avoid)
Methenamine mandelate or hippurate	Acetazolamide, sodium bicarbonate, thiazide diuretics	↓ antibacterial effect 2° to ↑ urine pH	++
Metronidazole	Alcohol	Disulfiram-like reaction	+
	Cyclosporin	↑ levels of B	++
	Disulfiram (Antabuse)	Acute toxic psychosis	+
	Lithium	↑ levels of B	++
	Oral anticoagulants	↑ anticoagulant effect	++
	Phenobarbital, hydantoins	↑ levels of B	++
Micafungin	Nifedipine	↑ levels of B	+
	Sirolimus	↑ levels of B	+
Nelfinavir	See protease inhibitors and Table 22B & Table 22C		
Nevirapine (Viramune)	See non-nucleoside reverse transcriptase inhibitors (NNRTIs) and Table 22C		
Nitrofurantoin	Antacids	↓ absorption of A	+

Non-nucleoside reverse transcriptase inhibitors (NNRTIs): For interactions with protease inhibitors, *see Table 22C.*
Del = delavirdine, **Efa** = efavirenz, **Nev** = nevirapine

Del	Efa	Nev		EFFECT	IMPORT
			Co-administration contraindicated:		
+			Anticonvulsants: carbamazepine, phenobarbital, phenytoin		++
+			Antimycobacterials: rifabutin, rifampin		++
+			Antipsychotics: pimozide		++
+	+		Benzodiazepines: alprazolam, midazolam, triazolam		++
+	+		Ergotamine		++
+	+		HMG-CoA inhibitors (statins): lovastatin, simvastatin, atorvastatin, pravastatin		++
+			St. John's wort		++
			Dose change needed:		
+			Amphetamines	↑ levels of B—**caution**	++
+		+	Antiarrhythmics: amiodarone, lidocaine, others	↓ or ↑ levels of B—**caution**	++

TABLE 22A (4)

ANTI-INFECTIVE AGENT (A)	OTHER DRUG (B)	EFFECT	IMPORT

Non-nucleoside reverse transcriptase inhibitors (NNRTIs): For interactions with protease inhibitors, see Table 22C.
Del = delavirdine, **Efa** = efavirenz, **Nev** = nevirapine

Del	Efa	Nev	Co-administration contraindicated:		
+	+	+	Anticonvulsants: carbamazepine, phenobarbital, phenytoin	↓ levels of A and/or B	++
+	+	+	Antifungals: itraconazole, ketoconazole, voriconazole	Potential ↓ levels of B, ↑ levels of A	++ (avoid)
+			Antipsychotics: pimozide		++
+		+	Antirejection drugs: cyclosporine, rapamycin, sirolimus, tacrolimus	↑ levels of B	++
		+	Benzodiazepines: as above	↑ levels of B	++
+		+	Calcium channel blockers	↑ levels of B	+ +
+		+	Clarithromycin	↑ levels of B metabolite	++
+		+	Cyclosporine	↑ levels of B	++
		+	Dexamethasone	↓ levels of A	++
+	+	+	Sildenafil, vardenafil, tadalafil	↑ levels of B	++
+		+	Fentanyl, methadone	↑ levels of B	++
+			Gastric acid suppression: antacids, H-2 blockers, proton pump inhibitors	↓ levels of A	++
+			HMG-CoA inhibitors (statins)		++
	+	+	Methadone, fentanyl	↓ levels of B	++
+	+	+	Oral contraceptives	↑ or ↓ levels of B	++
			Protease inhibitors—see Table 22C		
+	+	+	**Rifabutin, rifampin**	↑ or ↓ levels of rifabutin; ↓ levels of A—**caution**	++
+	+	+	St. John's wort	↓ levels of A	++
+		+	Warfarin	↑ levels of B	++
Pentamidine, IV			Amphotericin B	↑ risk of nephrotoxicity	+
			Foscarnet	↑ risk of hypocalcemia	+
			Pancreatitis-assoc drugs, eg, alcohol, valproic acid	↑ risk of pancreatitis	+
Piperacillin			Cefoxitin	Antagonism vs pseudomonas	++
Pip-tuzobactam			Methotrexate	↑ levels of B	++
Primaquine			Chloroquine, dapsone, INH, probenecid, quinine, sulfonamides, TMP/SMX, others	↑ **risk of hemolysis in G6PD-deficient patients**	++

Protease Inhibitors—Anti-HIV Drugs. (**Atazan** = atazanavir; **Darun** = darunavir; **Fosampren** = fosamprenavir; **Indin** = indinavir; **Lopin** = lopinavir; **Nelfin** = nelfinavir; **Riton** = ritonavir; **Saquin** = saquinavir; **Tipran** = tipranavir). For interactions with antiretrovirals, see Table 22B & Table 22C. **Only a partial list—check package insert.**

Also see http://aidsinfo.nih.gov

Atazan	Darun	Fosampren	Indin	Lopin	Nelfin	Riton	Saquin	Tipran			
									Analgesics:		
					+		+		1. Alfentanil, fentanyl, hydro-codone, tramadol	↑ levels of B	+
	+			+		+	+		2. Codeine, hydromorphone, morphine, methadone	↓ levels of B (JAIDS 41:563, 2006)	+
+	+	+	+	+	+	+			**Anti-arrhythmics: amiodarone, lidocaine, mexiletine, flecainide**	↑ levels of B; **do not co-administer**	++
	+		+	+	+	+	+	+	**Anticonvulsants: carbamazepine, clonazepam, phenytoin, pheno-barbital**	↓ levels of A, ↑ levels of B	++
+	+	+			+	+			Antidepressants, all tricyclic	↑ levels of B	++
					+	+		+	Antidepressants, all other	↑ levels of B; do not use pimozide	++
						+			**Antihistamine:** Loratadine	↑ levels of B	++
+					+	+			Antidepressants: SSRIs	↓ levels of B - avoid	+ +
+	+	+	+	+	+	+	+	+	**Benzodiazepines, e.g., diazepam, midazolam, triazolam**	↑ **levels of B—do not use**	++
					+				Beta blockers: Metoprolol, pindolol, propranolol, timolol	↑ levels of B	+
+	+	+	+	+	+	+	+	+	Calcium channel blockers (all)	↑ levels of B	++
+	+			+	+	+	+	+	Clarithro, erythro	↑ levels of B if renal impairment	+
+	+			+	+	+			Contraceptives, oral	↓ levels of B	++
	+			+	+	+			Corticosteroids: prednisone, dexa-methasone	↓ levels of A, ↑ levels of B	+
+	+	+	+	+	+	+	+	+	Cyclosporine	↑ levels of B, monitor levels	+
+	+	+	+	+	+	+	+	+	Ergot derivatives	↑ **levels of B—do not use**	++
		+	+	+		+	+		Erythromycin, clarithromycin	↑ levels of A & B	++
			+		+		+		Grapefruit juice (>200 ml/day)	↓ indinavir & ↑ saquinavir levels	++
+	+	+	+	+	+	+	+	+	H2 receptor antagonists	↓ levels of A	++
+	+	+	+	+	+	+	+	+	**HMG-CoA reductase inhibitors (statins): lovastatin, simvastatin**	↑ **levels of B—do not use**	++
+									Irinotecan	↑ **levels of B—do not use**	++
	+			+	+	+		+	Ketoconazole, itraconazole, ? vori	↑ levels of A, ↑ levels of B	+
		+		+		+		+	Metronidazole	Poss. disulfiram reaction, alcohol	+

TABLE 22A (5)

ANTI-INFECTIVE AGENT (A)	OTHER DRUG (B)	EFFECT	IMPORT

Protease Inhibitors (continued)

Column headers (vertical): Atazan | Darun | Fosampren | Indin | Lopin | Nelfin | Riton | Saquin | Tipran

Atazan	Darun	Fosampren	Indin	Lopin	Nelfin	Riton	Saquin	Tipran	OTHER DRUG (B)	EFFECT	IMPORT
										Also see http://aidsinfo.nih.gov	
+	+	+	+	+	+	+	+		Pimozide	↑ levels of B—do not use	++
+	+	+	+	+	+	+	+		Proton pump inhibitors	↓ levels of A	++
+	+	+	+	+	+	+	+	+	Rifampin, rifabutin	↓ levels of A, ↑ levels of B **(avoid)**	++ (avoid)
+	+	+	+	+	+	+	+	+	Sildenafil (Viagra), tadalafil, vardenafil	Varies, some ↑ & some ↓ levels of B	++
+	+	+	+	+	+	+	+	+	**St. John's wort**	↓ levels of A—do not use	++
	+								Sirolimus, tracrolimus	↑ levels of B	++
+									Tenofovir	↓ levels of B—add ritonavir	++
	+		+	+		+			Theophylline	↓ levels of B	+
	+			+		+		+	Warfarin	↑ levels of B	±
									Pyrazinamide INH, rifampin	May ↑ risk of hepatotoxicity	±
									Pyrimethamine Lorazepam	↑ risk of hepatotoxicity	+
									Sulfonamides, TMP/SMX	↑ risk of marrow suppression	+
									Zidovudine	↑ risk of marrow suppression	+
									Quinine Digoxin	↑ digoxin levels; ↑ toxicity	++
									Mefloquine	↑ arrhythmias	+
									Oral anticoagulants	↑ prothrombin time	++
									Quinupristin- dalfopristin (Synercid) Anti-HIV drugs: NNRTIs & PIs	↑ levels of B	++
									Antineoplastic: vincristine, docetaxel, paclitaxel	↑ levels of B	++
									Calcium channel blockers	↑ levels of B	++
									Carbamazepine	↑ levels of B	++
									Cyclosporine, tacrolimus	↑ levels of B	++
									Lidocaine	↑ levels of B	++
									Methylprednisolone	↑ levels of B	++
									Midazolam, diazepam	↑ levels of B	++
									Statins	↑ levels of B	++
									Ribavirin Didanosine	↑ levels of B → toxicity—avoid	++
									Stavudine	↓ levels of B	++
									Zidovudine	↓ levels of B	++
									Rifamycins (rifampin, rifabutin) *See footnote for less severe or less common interactions*[1] Ref.: ArIM 162:985, 2002 Al OH, ketoconazole, PZA	↓ levels of A	+
									Atovaquone	↓ levels of A, ↓ levels of B	+
									Beta adrenergic blockers (metoprolol, propranolol)	↓ effect of B	+
									Clarithromycin	↑ levels of A, ↓ levels of B	++
									Corticosteroids	↑ replacement requirement of B	++
									Cyclosporine	↓ effect of B	++
									Delavirdine	↑ **levels of A, ↓ levels of B—avoid**	++
									Digoxin	↓ levels of B	++
									Disopyramide	↓ levels of B	++
									Fluconazole	↑ levels of A[1]	+
									Amprenavir, indinavir, nelfinavir, ritonavir	↑ levels of A (↓ dose of A), ↓ levels of B	++
									INH	Converts INH to toxic hydrazine	++
									Itraconazole[2], ketoconazole	↓ levels of B, ↑ levels of A[1]	++
									Linezolid	↓ levels of B	++
									Methadone	↓ serum levels (withdrawal)	+
									Nevirapine	↓ **levels of B—avoid**	++
									Oral anticoagulants	Suboptimal anticoagulation	++
									Oral contraceptives	↓ effectiveness; spotting, pregnancy	+
									Phenytoin	↓ levels of B	+
									Protease inhibitors	↑ **levels of A, ↓ levels of B— CAUTION**	++
									Quinidine	↓ effect of B	+
									Sulfonylureas	↓ hypoglycemic effect	+
									Tacrolimus	↓ levels of B	++
									Theophylline	↑ levels of B	+
									TMP/SMX	↓ levels of A	+
									Tocainide	↓ effect of B	+
									Rimantadine	See Amantadine	
									Ritonavir	See protease inhibitors and Table 22B & Table 22C	
									Saquinavir	See protease inhibitors and Table 22B & Table 22C	

[1] **The following is a partial list of drugs with rifampin-induced ↑ metabolism and hence lower than anticipated serum levels:** ACE inhibitors, dapsone, diazepam, digoxin, diltiazem, doxycycline, fluconazole, fluvastatin, haloperidol, nifedipine, progestins, triazolam, tricyclics, voriconazole, zidovudine

[2] Up to 4wk may be required after RIF discontinued to achieve detectable serum itra levels; ↑ levels assoc with uveitis or polymyolysis

TABLE 22A (6)

ANTI-INFECTIVE AGENT (A)	OTHER DRUG (B)	EFFECT	IMPORT
Stavudine	Dapsone, INH	May ↑ risk of peripheral neuropathy	±
	Ribavirin	↓ levels of A—avoid	++
	Zidovudine	Mutual interference—do not combine	++
Sulfonamides	Cyclosporine	↓ cyclosporine levels	+
	Methotrexate	↑ antifolate activity	+
	Oral anticoagulants	↑ prothrombin time; bleeding	+
	Phenobarbital, rifampin	↓ levels of A	+
	Phenytoin	↑ levels of B; nystagmus, ataxia	+
	Sulfonylureas	↑ hypoglycemic effect	+
Telithromycin (Ketek)	Carbamazine	↓ levels of A	++
	Digoxin	↑ levels of B—do digoxin levels	++
	Ergot alkaloids	↑ levels of B—avoid	++
	Itraconazole; ketoconazole	↑ levels of A; no dose change	+
	Metoprolol	↑ levels of B	++
	Midazolam	↑ levels of B	++
	Oral anticoagulants	↑ prothrombin time	+
	Phenobarb, phenytoin	↓ levels of A	++
	Pimozide	↑ levels of B; QT prolongation—AVOID	++
	Rifampin	↓ levels of A—avoid	++
	Simvastatin	↑ levels of B (↑ risk of myopathy)	++
	Sotalol	↑ levels of B	++
	Theophylline	↑ levels of B	++
Tenofovir	Atazanavir	↓ levels of B—add ritonavir	++
	Didanosine (ddI)	↑ levels of B (reduce dose)	++
Terbinafine	Cimetidine	↑ levels of A	+
	Phenobarb, rifampin	↓ levels of A	+
Tetracyclines	See *Doxycycline*, plus:		
	Atovaquone	↓ levels of B	+
	Digoxin	↑ toxicity of B (may persist several months—up to 10% pts)	++
	Methoxyflurane	↑ toxicity; polyuria, renal failure	+
	Sucralfate	↓ absorption of A (separate by ≥2 hrs)	+
Thiabendazole	Theophyllines	↑ serum theophylline, nausea	+
Tigecycline	Oral contraceptives	↓ levels of B	++
Tinidazole (Tindamax)	See *Metronidazole—similar entity, expect similar interactions*		
Tobramycin	See *Aminoglycosides*		
Trimethoprim	Amantadine, dapsone, digoxin, methotrexate, procainamide, zidovudine	↑ serum levels of B	++
	Potassium-sparing diuretics	↑ serum K⁺	++
	Thiazide diuretics	↓ serum Na⁺	+
Trimethoprim-Sulfamethoxazole	Azathioprine	Reports of leukopenia	+
	Cyclosporine	↓ levels of B, ↑ serum creatinine	+
	Loperamide	↑ levels of B	+
	Methotrexate	Enhanced marrow suppression	++
	Oral contraceptives, pimozide, and 6-mercaptopurine	↓ effect of B	+
	Phenytoin	↑ levels of B	+
	Rifampin	↑ levels of B	+
	Warfarin	↑ activity of B	+
Vancomycin	Aminoglycosides	↑ frequency of nephrotoxicity	++
Zalcitabine (ddC) (HIVID)	Valproic acid, pentamidine (IV), alcohol, lamivudine	↑ pancreatic risk	+
	Cisplatin, INH, metronidazole, vincristine, nitrofurantoin, d4T, dapsone	↑ risk of peripheral neuropathy	+
Zidovudine (ZDV) (Retrovir)	Atovaquone, fluconazole, methadone	↑ levels of A	+
	Clarithromycin	↓ levels of A	±
	Indomethacin	↑ levels of ZDV toxic metabolite	+
	Nelfinavir	↓ levels of A	++
	Probenecid, TMP/SMX	↑ levels of A	+
	Ribavirin	↓ levels of A—avoid	++
	Rifampin/rifabutin	↓ levels of A	++
	Stavudine	Interference—DO NOT COMBINE!	++

TABLE 22B – DRUG-DRUG INTERACTIONS BETWEEN PROTEASE INHIBITORS

(Adapted from Guidelines for the Use of Antiretroviral Agents in HIV-Infected Adults & Adolescents; see www.aidsinfo.nih.gov)

NAME (Abbreviation, Trade Name)	Atazanavir (ATV, Reyataz)	Fosamprenavir (FOS-APV, Lexiva)	Indinavir (IDV, Crixivan)	Lopinavir/Ritonavir (LP/R, Kaletra)	Nelfinavir (NFV, Viracept)	Ritonavir (RTV, Norvir)	Saquinavir (SQV, Invirase)	Tipranavir (TPV, Aptivus)
Atazanavir (ATV, Reyataz)			Do not co-administer; risk of additive ↑ in indirect bilirubin	RTV 100 mg ↑ ATV AUC 238%		ATV/RTV 300/100 mg q24h	Combination not recommended	No data
Fosamprenavir (FOS-APV, Lexiva)						200 mg RTV q24h + FOS-APV 1400 mg q24h	Insufficient data	Do not combine
Indinavir (IDV, Crixivan)	Do not co-administer; risk of additive ↑ in bilirubin			IDV AUC ↑ IDV dose 600 mg bid	↑ IDV & NFV levels. Dose: IDV 1200 mg bid, NFV 1250 mg bid	Dose: IDV/RTV bid as 800/100 mg or 800/200 mg	SQV levels ↑ 4-7 fold. Dose: Insufficient data	Do not combine
Lopinavir/Ritonavir (LP/R, Kaletra)	RTV 100 mg ↑ ATV AUC 238%	Rx-naive: LP/R no dose change. Rx-experienced: LP/R 600/150 mg bid	IDV AUC ↑ IDV dose 600 mg bid		Rx-naive: LP/R no dose change. Rx-experienced: LP/R 600/150 mg bid	LP is co-formulated with RTV	SQV levels ↑ Dose: SQV 1000 mg bid; LP/R standard	Do not combine
Nelfinavir (NFV, Viracept)			↑ IDV & NFV levels. Dose: IDV 1200 mg bid, NFV 1250 mg bid	Rx-naive: LP/R no dose change. Rx-experienced: LP/R 600/150 mg bid		Dose: RTV 400 mg bid + NFV 500-750 mg bid	Dose: NFV standard. SQV 800 mg tid or 1200 mg bid	Do not combine
Ritonavir (RTV, Norvir)	ATV/RTV 300/100 mg q24h	200 mg RTV q24h + FOS-APV 1400 mg q24h	Dose: IDV/RTV bid as 800/100 mg or 800/200 mg	LP is co-formulated with RTV	Dose: RTV 400 mg bid + NFV 500-750 mg bid		Dose: 1000 mg, SQV/100 mg RTV bid or 400/400 mg bid	TPV 500 mg bid + RTV 200 mg bid
Saquinavir (SQV, Invirase)	Combination not recommended	Insufficient data	SQV levels ↑ 4-7 fold. Dose: Insufficient data	SQV levels ↑ Dose: SQV 1000 mg bid; LP/R standard	Dose: NFV standard. SQV 800 mg tid or 1200 mg bid	Dose: 1000 mg, SQV/100 mg RTV bid or 400/400 mg bid		Do not combine
Tipranavir (TPV, Aptivus)	No data	Do not combine	Do not combine	Do not combine	Do not combine	TPV 500 mg bid + RTV 200 mg bid	Do not combine	
Darunavir (DRV, Prezista)	ATV 300mg q24h + DRV 600mg + 100mg ATV bid)	No data	Do not combine				Do not combine	

TABLE 22C – DRUG-DRUG INTERACTIONS BETWEEN NON-NUCLEOSIDE REVERSE TRANSCRIPTASE INHIBITORS (NNRTIs) AND PROTEASE INHIBITORS
(Adapted from Guidelines for the Use of Antiretroviral Agents in HIV-Infected Adults & Adolescents; see www.aidsinfo.nih.gov)

NAME (Abbreviation, Trade Name)	Atazanavir (ATV, Reyataz)	Fosamprenavir (FOS-APV, Lexiva)	Indinavir (IDV, Crixivan)	Lopinavir/Ritonavir (LP/R, Kaletra)	Nelfinavir (NFV, Viracept)	Ritonavir (RTV, Norvir)	Saquinavir (SQV, Invirase)	Tipranavir (TPV, Aptivus)
Delavirdine (DLV, Rescriptor)	No data	Co-administration not recommended	IDV levels ↑ 40%. Dose: IDV 600 mg q8h, DLV standard	Expect LP levels to ↑. No dose data	NFV levels ↑ 2X; DLV levels ↓ 55%. Dose: No data.	Levels d of RTV ↑ 70%. Dose: DLV standard, RTV no data	SQV levels ↑ 5X. Dose: SQV 800 mg tid, DLV standard	No data
Efavirenz (EFZ, Sustiva)	ATV AUC ↓ 74%. Dose: EFZ standard; ATV/RTV 300/100 mg q24h with food	FOS-APV levels ↓. Dose: EFZ standard; FOS-APV 1400 mg + RTV 300 mg q24h or 700 mg FOS-APV + 100 mg RTV bid	Levels: IDV ↓ 31%. Dose: IDV 1000 mg q8h; EFV standard	Rx-naive: LP/R no dose change. Rx-experienced: LP/R 600/150 mg bid	Standard doses	Standard doses	Level: SQV ↓ 62%. Dose: SQV softgel 400 mg + RTV 400 mg bid	No data
Nevirapine (NVP, Viramune)	No data	No data	IDV levels ↓ 28%. Dose: IDV 1000 mg q8h or combine with RTV, NVP standard	Rx-naive: LP/R no dose change. Rx-experienced: LP/R 600/150 mg bid	Standard doses	Standard doses	Dose: SQV softgel + RTV 400/400 mg both bid	No data

TABLE 23 – LIST OF GENERIC AND COMMON TRADE NAMES

GENERIC NAME: TRADE NAMES	GENERIC NAME: TRADE NAMES	GENERIC NAME: TRADE NAMES
Abacavir: Ziagen	Efavirenz/Emtricitabine/Tenofovir: Atripla	Oseltamivir: Tamiflu
Acyclovir: Zovirax		Oxacillin: Prostaphlin
Adefovir: Hepsera	Emtricitabine: Emtriva	Palivizumab: Synagis
Albendazole: Albenza	Emtricitabine + tenofovir: Truvada	Paromomycin: Humatin
Amantadine: Symmetrel	Enfuvirtide (T-20): Fuzeon	Pentamidine: NebuPent, Pentam 300
Amikacin: Amikin	Entecavir: Baraclude	Piperacillin: Pipracil
Amoxicillin: Amoxil, Polymox	Ertapenem: Invanz	Piperacillin/tazobactam: Zosyn
Amox./clav.: Augmentin, Augmentin ES-600; Augmentin XR	Erythromycin(s): Ilotycin	Piperazine: Antepar
	Ethyl succinate: Pediamycin	Podophyllotoxin: Condylox
Amphotericin B: Fungizone	*Glucoheptonate*: Erythrocin	Posaconazole: Noxafil
Ampho B-liposomal: AmBisome	*Estolate*: Ilosone	Praziquantel: Biltricide
Ampho B-cholesteryl complex: Amphotec	Erythro/sulfisoxazole: Pediazole	Primaquine: Primachine
	Ethambutol: Myambutol	Proguanil: Paludrine
Ampho B-lipid complex: Abelcet	Ethionamide: Trecator	Pyrantel pamoate: Antiminth
Ampicillin: Omnipen, Polycillin	Famciclovir: Famvir	Pyrimethamine: Daraprim
Ampicillin/sulbactam: Unasyn	Fluconazole: Diflucan	Pyrimethamine/sulfadoxine: Fansidar
Atazanavir: Reyataz	Flucytosine: Ancobon	Quinupristin/dalfopristin: Synercid
Atovaquone: Mepron	Fosamprenavir: Lexiva	Ribavirin: Virazole, Rebetol
Atovaquone + proguanil: Malarone	Foscarnet: Foscavir	Rifabutin: Mycobutin
Azithromycin: Zithromax	Fosfomycin: Monurol	Rifampin: Rifadin, Rimactane
Azithromycin ER: Zmax	Ganciclovir: Cytovene	Rifapentine: Priftin
Aztreonam: Azactam	Gatifloxacin: Tequin	Rifaximin: Xifaxan
Caspofungin: Cancidas	Gemifloxacin: Factive	Rimantadine: Flumadine
Cefaclor: Ceclor, Ceclor CD	Gentamicin: Garamycin	Ritonavir: Norvir
Cefadroxil: Duricef	Griseofulvin: Fulvicin	Saquinavir: Invirase, Fortovase
Cefazolin: Ancef, Kefzol	Halofantrine: Halfan	Spectinomycin: Trobicin
Cefdinir: Omnicef	Idoxuridine: Dendrid, Stoxil	Stavudine: Zerit
Cefditoren pivoxil: Spectracef	INH + RIF: Rifamate	Stibogluconate: Pentostam
Cefepime: Maxipime	INH + RIF + PZA: Rifater	Silver sulfadiazine: Silvadene
Cefixime^{NUS}: Suprax	Interferon alfa: Roferon-A, Intron A	Sulfamethoxazole: Gantanol
Cefoperazone-sulbactam: Sulperazon^{NUS}	Interferon, pegylated: PEG-Intron, Pegasys	Sulfasalazine: Azulfidine
		Sulfisoxazole: Gantrisin
Cefotaxime: Claforan	Interferon + ribavirin: Rebetron	Telithromycin: Ketek
Cefotetan: Cefotan	Imipenem + cilastatin: Primaxin, Ticnam	Tenofovir: Viread
Cefoxitin: Mefoxin		Terbinafine: Lamisil
Cefpodoxime proxetil: Vantin	Imiquimod: Aldara	Thalidomide: Thalomid
Cefprozil: Cefzil	Indinavir: Crixivan	Thiabendazole: Mintezol
Ceftazidime: Fortaz, Tazicef, Tazidime	Itraconazole: Sporanox	Ticarcillin: Ticar
Ceftibuten: Cedax	Iodoquinol: Yodoxin	Tigecycline: Tygacil
Ceftizoxime: Cefizox	Ivermectin: Stromectol	Tinidazole: Tindamax
Ceftriaxone: Rocephin	Kanamycin: Kantrex	Tipranavir: Aptivus
Cefuroxime: Zinacef, Kefurox, Ceftin	Ketoconazole: Nizoral	Tobramycin: Nebcin
Cephalexin: Keflex	Lamivudine: Epivir, Epivir-HBV	Tretinoin: Retin A
Cephradine: Anspor, Velosef	Lamivudine + abacavir: Epzicom	Trifluridine: Viroptic
Chloroquine: Aralen	Levofloxacin: Levaquin	Trimethoprim: Proloprim, Trimpex
Cidofovir: Vistide	Linezolid: Zyvox	Trimethoprim/sulfamethoxazole: Bactrim, Septra
Ciprofloxacin: Cipro, Cipro XR	Lomefloxacin: Maxaquin	
Clarithromycin: Biaxin, Biaxin XL	Lopinavir/ritonavir: Kaletra	Valacyclovir: Valtrex
Clindamycin: Cleocin	Loracarbef: Lorabid	Valganciclovir: Valcyte
Clofazimine: Lamprene	Mafenide: Sulfamylon	Vancomycin: Vancocin
Clotrimazole: Lotrimin, Mycelex	Mebendazole: Vermox	Voriconazole: Vfend
Cloxacillin: Tegopen	Mefloquine: Lariam	Zalcitabine: HIVID
Colistimethate: Coly-Mycin M	Meropenem: Merrem	Zanamivir: Relenza
Cycloserine: Seromycin	Mesalamine: Asacol, Pentasa	Zidovudine (ZDV): Retrovir
Dalbavancin: Zeven	Methenamine: Hiprex, Mandelamine	Zidovudine + 3TC: Combivir
Daptomycin: Cubicin	Metronidazole: Flagyl	Zidovudine + 3TC + abacavir: Trizivir
Darunavir: Prezista	Micafungin: Mycamine	
Delavirdine: Rescriptor	Minocycline: Minocin	
Dicloxacillin: Dynapen	Moxifloxacin: Avelox	
Didanosine: Videx	Mupirocin: Bactroban	
Diethylcarbamazine: Hetrazan	Nafcillin: Unipen	
Diloxanide furoate: Furamide	Nelfinavir: Viracept	
Dirithromycin: Dynabac	Nevirapine: Viramune	
Doxycycline: Vibramycin	Nitazoxanide: Alinia	
Drotrecogin alfa: Xigris	Nitrofurantoin: Macrobid, Macrodantin	
Efavirenz: Sustiva	Nystatin: Mycostatin	
	Ofloxacin: Floxin	

TABLE 23 (2)
LIST OF COMMON TRADE AND GENERIC NAMES

TRADE NAME: GENERIC NAME	TRADE NAME: GENERIC NAME	TRADE NAME: GENERIC NAME
Abelcet: Ampho B-lipid complex	Garamycin: Gentamicin	Retin A: Tretinoin
Albenza: Albendazole	Halfan: Halofantrine	Retrovir: Zidovudine (ZDV)
Aldara: Imiquimod	Hepsera: Adefovir	Reyataz: Atazanavir
Alinia: Nitazoxanide	Herplex: Idoxuridine	Rifadin: Rifampin
AmBisome: Ampho B-liposomal	Hiprex: Methenamine hippurate	Rifamate: INH + RIF
Amikin: Amikacin	HIVID: Zalcitabine	Rifater: INH + RIF + PZA
Amoxil: Amoxicillin	Humatin: Paromomycin	Rimactane: Rifampin
Amphotec: Ampho B-cholesteryl complex	Ilosone: Erythromycin estolate	Rocephin: Ceftriaxone
Ancef: Cefazolin	Ilotycin: Erythromycin	Roferon-A: Interferon alfa
Ancobon: Flucytosine	Intron A: Interferon alfa	Septra: Trimethoprim/sulfa
Anspor: Cephradine	Invanz: Ertapenem	Seromycin: Cycloserine
Antepar: Piperazine	Invirase: Saquinavir	Silvadene: Silver sulfadiazine
Antiminth: Pyrantel pamoate	Kantrex: Kanamycin	Spectracef: Cefditoren pivoxil
Aptivus: Tipranavir	Kaletra: Lopinavir/ritonavir	Sporanox: Itraconazole
Aralen: Chloroquine	Keflex: Cephalexin	Stoxil: Idoxuridine
Asacol: Mesalamine	Kefurox: Cefuroxime	Stromectol: Ivermectin
Atripla:	Ketek: Telithromycin	Sulfamylon: Mafenide
Efavirenz/emtricitabine/tenofovir	Lamisil: Terbinafine	Sulperazon^NUS: Cefoperazone-sulbactam
Augmentin, Augmentin ES-600	Lamprene: Clofazimine	Suprax: Cefixime^NUS
Augmentin XR: Amox./clav.	Lariam: Mefloquine	Sustiva: Efavirenz
Avelox: Moxifloxacin	Levaquin: Levofloxacin	Symmetrel: Amantadine
Azactam: Aztreonam	Lexiva: Fosamprenavir	Synagis: Palivizumab
Azulfidine: Sulfasalazine	Lorabid: Loracarbef	Synercid: Quinupristin/dalfopristin
Bactroban: Mupirocin	Macrodantin, Macrobid: Nitrofurantoin	Tamiflu: Oseltamivir
Bactrim: Trimethoprim/sulfamethoxazole	Malarone: Atovaquone + proguanil	Tazicef: Ceftazidime
Baraclude: Entecavir	Mandelamine: Methenamine mandel.	Tegopen: Cloxacillin
Biaxin, Biaxin XL: Clarithromycin	Maxaquin: Lomefloxacin	Tequin: Gatifloxacin
Biltricide: Praziquantel	Maxipime: Cefepime	Thalomid: Thalidomide
Cancidas: Caspofungin	Mefoxin: Cefoxitin	Ticar: Ticarcillin
Ceclor, Ceclor CD: Cefaclor	Mepron: Atovaquone	Tienam: Imipenem
Cedax: Ceftibuten	Merrem: Meropenem	Timentin: Ticarcillin-clavulanic acid
Cefizox: Ceftizoxime	Minocin: Minocycline	Tinactin: Tolnaftate
Cefotan: Cefotetan	Mintezol: Thiabendazole	Tindamax: Tinidazole
Ceftin: Cefuroxime axetil	Monocid: Cefonicid	Trecator SC: Ethionamide
Cefzil: Cefprozil	Monurol: Fosfomycin	Trizivir: Abacavir + ZDV + 3TC
Cipro, Cipro XR: Ciprofloxacin & extended release	Myambutol: Ethambutol	Trobicin: Spectinomycin
Claforan: Cefotaxime	Mycamine: Micafungin	Truvada: Emtricitabine + tenofovir
Coly-Mycin M: Colistimethate	Mycobutin: Rifabutin	Tygacil: Tigecycline
Combivir: ZDV + 3TC	Mycostatin: Nystatin	Unasyn: Ampicillin/sulbactam
Crixivan: Indinavir	Nafcil: Nafcillin	Unipen: Nafcillin
Cubicin: Daptomycin	Nebcin: Tobramycin	Valcyte: Valganciclovir
Cytovene: Ganciclovir	NebuPent: Pentamidine	Valtrex: Valacyclovir
Daraprim: Pyrimethamine	Nizoral: Ketoconazole	Vancocin: Vancomycin
Diflucan: Fluconazole	Norvir: Ritonavir	Vantin: Cefpodoxime proxetil
Duricef: Cefadroxil	Noxafil: Posaconazole	Velosef: Cephradine
Dynapen: Dicloxacillin	Omnicef: Cefdinir	Vermox: Mebendazole
Emtriva: Emtricitabine	Omnipen: Ampicillin	Vfend: Voriconazole
Epivir, Epivir-HBV: Lamivudine	Pediamycin: Erythro. ethyl succinate	Vibramycin: Doxycycline
Epzicom: Lamivudine + abacavir	Pediazole: Erythro. ethyl succinate + sulfisoxazole	Videx: Didanosine
Factive: Gemifloxacin	Pegasys, PEG-Intron: Interferon, pegylated	Viracept: Nelfinavir
Famvir: Famciclovir	Pentam 300: Pentamidine	Viramune: Nevirapine
Fansidar: Pyrimethamine + sulfadoxine	Pentasa: Mesalamine	Virazole: Ribavirin
Flagyl: Metronidazole	Pipracil: Piperacillin	Viread: Tenofovir
Floxin: Ofloxacin	Polycillin: Ampicillin	Vistide: Cidofovir
Flumadine: Rimantadine	Polymox: Amoxicillin	Xifaxan: Rifaximin
Fortaz: Ceftazidime	Prezista: Darunavir	Xigris: Drotrecogin alfa
Fortovase: Saquinavir	Priftin: Rifapentine	Yodoxin: Iodoquinol
Fulvicin: Griseofulvin	Proloprim: Trimethoprim	Zerit: Stavudine
Fungizone: Amphotericin B	Prostaphlin: Oxacillin	Zeven: Dalbavancin
Furadantin: Nitrofurantoin	Rebetol: Ribavirin	Ziagen: Abacavir
Fuzeon: Enfuvirtide (T-20)	Rebetron: Interferon + ribavirin	Zinacef: Cefuroxime
Gantanol: Sulfamethoxazole	Relenza: Zanamivir	Zithromax: Azithromycin
Gantrisin: Sulfisoxazole	Rescriptor: Delavirdine	Zmax: Azithromycin ER
		Zovirax: Acyclovir
		Zosyn: Piperacillin/tazobactam
		Zyvox: Linezolid

INDEX OF MAJOR ENTITIES

PAGES (page numbers bold if major focus)   PAGES (page numbers bold if major focus)

Bold numbers indicate major considerations. Recommendations in Table 1 not indexed; antibiotic selection often depends on modifying circumstances and alternative agents.